Markets of Well-being

African Dynamics

VOLUME 9

Markets of Well-being

Navigating Health and Healing in Africa

Edited by

Marleen Dekker
Rijk van Dijk

BRILL

LEIDEN • BOSTON
2010

Cover: photos by Walter van Beek, Corine 't Hart, Nadine Beckmann, Dick Foeken, Rantimi Jays Julius-Adeoye and Marleen Dekker.

This book is printed on acid-free paper.

ISSN 1568-1777
ISBN 978 90 04 20110 1

FSC www.fsc.org MIX Paper from responsible sources FSC® C004472

PRINTED BY DRUKKERIJ WILCO B.V. - AMERSFOORT, THE NETHERLANDS

Contents

Maps

Tables

Figures

Photographs

Boxes

1

Introduction: Economic ethnographies of the marketization of health and healing in Africa

Rijk van Dijk & Marleen Dekker

Health and healing are distinctive domains in the pursuit of the well-being of people. Health is located in domains that primarily relate to bio-medical science, government policies and formal institutions, while healing indicates a cultural-historical domain of cosmologies and practices that are often termed 'traditional'. Both fields have become subject to monetization and commodification, in short, the 'market' (see Bloom & Standing 2001; Bloom, Standing & Lloyd 2008; Feierman 2008; Last & Chavunduka 1986; Luedke & West 2006). This has partly been the result of reforms in the health sector in many parts of Africa whereby the promotion of free markets, privatization and economic deregulation have entered public health systems (Turshen 1999). Yet other medical practices that are not directly incorporated in systems of public health appear to have become subject to diverse processes of marketization within a similar period of time (Pfeiffer & Chapman 2010). There is a commonality in the processes to which both domains are exposed. How patients and providers navigate these emerging markets for health and healing forms the focus of this volume.

Africa has a long history of confrontation and contestation between different models of health and healing. The introduction of bio-medical care through the establishment of missionary health facilities, which later became incorporated in colonial and post-colonial government public health services, set in motion a contestation of existing cultural-historical practices of health and healing that were increasingly placed under government scrutiny and control (Vaughan 1991). Post-colonial governments fostered the emergence of traditional healers' associations to formalize traditional healing, regularize membership and governing bodies, and standardize practices and the fees to be paid for treatment (Luedke & West 2006; Feierman 2008; Summerton 2006). While the literature euphemistically speaks of an emergent medical plurality, there is now a sense of demarcation and even competition between the two domains and the medical field has become an arena where different interests are being played out.

Each of these domains – public health on the one hand, and cultural-historical forms of healing on the other – has developed into an arena on their own account. Political, cultural, medical, pharmaceutical and economic interests have increasingly become attached to both these medical spheres. The public health systems in many African countries today are pluralistic systems where the boundaries between the public and private sectors have become porous. Markets for most medical goods and services have emerged in a largely unregulated way and are populated by a wide range of providers (Bloom & Standing 2001). In the domain of traditional healing, a wide range of forms of healing exist side by side, each having different historical origins and working with different substances or spiritual models of well-being, for example combining world religions (Christianity, Islam) with local healing traditions. In other words, there are arenas within a wider arena, battles within a battle.

One way in which these arenas are developing and manifesting themselves in the everyday lives of Africans is through monetization and commodification. Users pay a combination of fees and informal charges for most services, including those provided by the government (Bloom & Lucas 2000) and access to public health and other formal institutions, such as nutrition and social protection policies, may be brokered by informal networks or local agents. Cultural-historical forms of healing have witnessed a shift from kind to cash in the payment of treatment, as has occurred in Africa on a large scale (Last & Chavunduka 1986; Feierman 2008). Healing in its various forms has become an object of profit making, entrepreneurialism and market competition. The market of healing is conjoined in this sense by other new markets such as that of the pharmaceutical industry or religion. New forms of entrepreneurialism have emerged precisely in their use of healing practices, for example by powerful charismatic groups providing spirit healing to the general public on a huge scale. It is evident that transactions in markets for health and healing, like in many other markets in Africa (Fafchamps 2004), are not anonymous and the actors are not perfectly interchangeable. Transactions in markets for health and healing, and thus health-seeking behaviour, are personalized and relational, and in many cases involve trust (Tibandegabe & Mackintosh 2005).

This volume explores the various aspects related to the rise of markets for health and healing in nine different countries in Africa: Ethiopia, Botswana, Togo, Kenya, Cameroon, Ghana, Tanzania, Nigeria and South Africa. Although the marketization of health and healing was not the prime research subject of many of these studies, the processes of marketization and navigation of markets presented themselves in the course of the work and the cases address various aspects of the processes of marketization in the different countries. Moreover, the cases use different methodologies to look at processes around health and healing ranging from participant observation, in-depth interviews and focus-group discussions to survey questionnaires. The shared element is an interest in the manner in which people are dealing with the rapidly changing economies that surround health and healing and the way in which this informs the decisions that they make. We study how individuals, groups, families and institutions approach this situation of emergent marketization and commercialization through the lens of what we term an *economic ethnography*. Although this means that the book does not come up with definite answers to the questions raised, we believe the contributions point at important developments related to the marketization of health and healing that, in some cases, warrant further research.

The contributions not only explore the possibilities, contradictions and problems this marketization is producing for African communities, institutions, households and individuals but also the ways in which this is being translated culturally. One important aspect that we see in this cultural mediation is the way in which, through the processes of monetization and commoditization, health is being redefined in terms of 'risk' in African societies. A shift in notions of health and illness from the existential into an economic domain of understanding is occurring, especially in the public health domain. The conceptualization of illness as risk will be elaborated on in the next section. Then we set out the bio-medical context of the case study countries, followed by a review of 'navigation' in the next section. The subsequent section introduces the various contributions in more detail before the conclusion is presented.

Health and risk

Africa is not unique in its conceptualization of illness as risk. European societies too have moved a long way from Christain-Judeaic understandings of the existential and God-given social order of health and illness towards a more economized understanding of these circumstances. This process, of what Weber has termed 'the disenchantment of the world' making place for the (economic) rationalization of human affairs, has produced a shift towards the centrality of the concept of health and illness as risk. This calculus of health and illness, however, emerges differently in divergent cultural-historic settings, as is demonstrated in the review of malaria policies in colonial Kenya (Chapter 5) or in the contribution by van Beek on the divination and healing practices of the Kapsiki in Cameroon (Chapter 7).

How did the term 'risk' emerge in studies on health and healing in Africa? Vulnerability to risk is increasingly recognized as one of the defining characteristics of poverty (Bhattamishra & Barrett 2010; Elbers *et al.* 2007; Pan 2009;

Dercon 2004) and health risks constitute a major component of risk in the (rural) African context (Dercon *et al.* 2005; Bogale 2005; Krishna 2006).[1] When a person falls ill, s/he may not be able to work or may go for treatment. Depending on the nature of the ailment, patients look for bio-medical treatment or traditional healing, or a combination of the two. With the exception of self-medication (like collecting herbs), they will incur costs for most treatments, for example for transport, fees for treatment, tests and medication. These usually need to be paid on the spot and are paid from income, savings, the sale of assets, loans or with assistance from relatives and or friends. When resources to pay for treatment or healing are difficult to realize, treatment may be delayed or fore-gone, with potential consequences for a person's long-term health status.

Risk and uncertainty refer to possible events, the actual occurrence of which is referred to as a shock (Siegel & Alwang 1999). A shock can be both positive and negative. In the context of health, a positive shock is for example a reduction in the costs of medical treatment resulting from the opening of a rural clinic that offers cheap and accessible medical care, while a negative shock is the long-term illness of a family member that incurs substantial costs in treatment and possibly affects future production through reduced labour availability.

Since risk is pervasive and in our context ill health is omnipresent, the behaviour of individuals, households or institutions is shaped by strategies to prevent, mitigate and cope with any negative health shocks that may occur (Siegel & Alwang 1999; Holzmann & Jorgensen 2000; World Bank 2001). *Risk-prevention strategies* are aimed at reducing the occurrences of risk. In the case of health, households may put efforts into preventing illnesses by considering hygiene and nutrition. In the case studies presented in this book, we see examples of the government working on vector control in the fight against malaria (Chapter 5) and the promotion of school-feeding programmes in Kenya (Chapter 4.) and the activities of NGOs promoting abstinence in Botswana to try and prevent the spread of HIV/AIDS (Chapter 11). *Risk-mitigation strategies* aim to reduce the impact of a potential risk. This can be achieved by (i) diversifying income sources; (ii) accumulating and diversifying assets; and (iii) participating in insurance arrangements. Most illustrative here are financial assets like building up savings, increasing the number of cattle one has or storing food. But it also possible to invest in human capital, such as good health. In this sense, well-being but also protection may develop into a market, as is demonstrated by the use of *muti* that protects South African thieves against being caught (Chapter 6). *Risk-coping strategies* attempt to alleviate the impact

1 Illness also comes to the fore in social security studies ((Nooteboom 2003; von Benda-Beckmann 1994; Leutloff-Grandits *et al.* 2009).

of the shock once it has occurred.[2] In response to a negative health shock that requires money for treatment, households can use cash savings or sell assets that they have accumulated, such as food or cattle. Alternatively, they can borrow from neighbours, recall insurance debts or rely on other public or private transfers.[3] These strategies are discussed in more detail in the case studies on Ethiopia and Togo (Chapters 9 &10).

Opportunities and constraints in the institutional, social and policy environment of individuals or households shape the possibilities for engaging in prevention, mitigation and coping strategies. For example, the distribution of bed nets by an NGO may help prevent malaria. Such an intervention is, however, not necessarily successful: individuals or households have to decide whether to obtain a bed net and to use it in order to actually prevent malaria, and there may be all sorts of reasons for them not to do so. Similarly, governments may put efforts into guaranteeing the availability of common medicines in rural clinics. If this is the case, the sick may chose to go there for treatment but may not do so if they do not trust the providers of bio-medical healthcare or if high informal payments are linked to access to these medicines.

These examples suggest we should refrain from viewing health, risk and behaviour solely in terms of rational choice and a calculus towards optimal health in given circumstances (Buetow 2007). As illustrated in the case studies on South Africa and Zanzibar (Chapters 6 & 8), people do not always strive for a cure, good health or healing, even when this is morally expected of them. Such discordant behaviour manifests itself at different levels, for example with AIDS patients who do not take ARVs even though they are available to them, or health workers who do not protect themselves against the risk of being infected or of infecting somebody else even when they know how to do so. Although both processes go hand in hand (i.e. the turning of sickness and health into a commodity and the transformation of the patient/sufferer into a rational being), rationality should always be interpreted in its cultural setting.

The care that relatives and friends provide to the sufferer is also 'captured' by this economization as they are usually the ones faced with the problem of covering any expenses incurred. While we should not have too romantic an idea of family care for the sick (Radstake 2000), the process of commodification is transforming relational care. In some cases, providing care becomes too much of a burden for the family and friends, which leaves patients having to fend for

---

2 Although most of these risk-coping strategies are undertaken after the income shock has been realized, they will have been planned for before the risk occurred, as a risk-mitigation strategy.

3 A range of social relationships may provide security in different situations and the benefits received from such relationships or arrangements may not be directly related to premiums previously paid.

themselves. In other cases, new social formations emerge, such as self-help groups, support groups, buddies and advocacy groups that can draw attention to the plight of their members. Health activism, such as patient interest groups, has not, however, developed widely in Africa, which suggests that a mitigation of market forces in the domain of health is not taking place. Governments seem not to have much clout in mitigating this process and are weak when it comes to improving health systems, assuming they are interested in doing so in the first place. The sick are thus being confronted with market forces without much recourse to intermediary levels of mitigation or negotiation, such as that of the family or any other association, as is evident in the case of HIV/AIDS patients in Zanzibar (Chapter 8).

Intermediary levels are also involved in a process of marketization. Even charities can no longer place themselves outside the sphere of competition as they are operating in a market over which they have little control and for which there are few mitigating powers. This not only refers to the enormous increase in private hospitals and clinics that only provide treatment and care for the well-off, but also for the international players, such as NGOs, that need to deal with, for instance, the interests of the pharmaceutical industry. The relationship between health and risk is different at this institutional level compared to that of the sick and the issue of family care and resources. In the domain of AIDS for instance, religious organizations are playing an evermore important role in providing care, treatment and prevention (Prince *et al.* 2009). Yet their religious convictions may lead them to object to the promotion of condoms as a method of prevention, a rejection which they may run the risk of losing out on in the market of AIDS donor money where the ABC ideology (Abstinence, Being faithful and Condomizing) is promoted or even demanded to acquire funding. The perception of health and risk at the individual level can be different compared to the perception of health and risk at a higher level of social aggregation.

The bio-medical context of marketization and monetary risks

The country case studies presented in this book have different thematic foci and the countries themselves are diverse in terms of the current status of their national health systems and healthcare financing. Table 1.1 provides an overview of some of the key indicators on health service coverage and healthcare financing in 2006.[4]

[4] The indicators include the number of physicians, nursery and midwifery personnel and hospital beds, and gives insight into the countries' health workforce and infrastructure. Per capita expenditure on health gives an indication of total health expenditure (public and private), while the information on private health expenditure provides insight into the relative importance of government and non-government spend-

The WHO estimates that countries need 23 healthcare professionals (physicians, nurses and midwives) per 10,000 citizens to achieve adequate access to key primary healthcare. Table 1.1 indicates that with only 13 healthcare professionals per 10,000 people, African countries on average have a considerable shortage of qualified staff and rank the lowest in the world. The differences between the countries discussed in this book are great, with Botswana and South Africa scoring well, while Ethiopia, Tanzania and Togo are considerably below the African average. A similar picture emerges when looking at the availability of hospital beds, with Kenya joining the Southern African countries in their above-average scores and Nigeria and Ghana featuring below the average with just 12 beds per 10,000 inhabitants.

In terms of healthcare expenditures, which amount to, on average, US$ 111 per capita per year, Africa is second lowest in the world, after South East Asia. Here again the Southern African countries enjoy a relatively favourable position, with Ethiopia, Nigeria and Tanzania reporting extremely low levels of expenditures. The governments in Botswana, Ethiopia and Tanzania play an important role in healthcare financing, with public funds covering more than half of all expenditures. In the other countries, private expenditures are more important, with Kenya taking an intermediary position with the government providing almost half of all healthcare expenditures. The share of OOP expenditures in private healthcare financing is highest in Ethiopia, Ghana, Nigeria, Togo and Tanzania, indicating the importance of transactions in the health market, while only in South Africa is there a higher proportion of private expenditure by private prepaid plans.

The data presented in Table 1.1 are macro-level figures compiled for international comparison. However data have their limitations (WHO 2009: 7) and may not reflect the day-to-day realities of individuals, households and health workers in the country nor variations and inequalities in the system. For example, national health accounts and household expenditure surveys are likely to focus on modern healthcare facilities and may underestimate informal activities in the health sphere, such as praying and traditional healing practices. While in daily life, people can chose from a wide spectrum of health and healing prac-

ing on health issues. Private entities include corporations, commercial or mutual health insurance, NGOs and households. Finally, the contribution of out-of-pocket (OOP) expenditures by individuals or households and private prepaid plans to total private expenditures on health signals the financial burden for individuals and households when confronted with illness and the possibility of being insured against health expenditures respectively. The proportion of OOP expenditures relative to total private expenditure reflects the importance of transactions in the health markets (Tibandebage & Mackintosch 2005).

Table 1.1 Selected indicators on health workforce/infrastructure and health expenditures in the country case studies in 2006*

Country	Physicians (per 10,000 population)	Nursing & midwifery personnel (per 10,000 population)	Hospital beds (per 10,000 population)	Per capita total expenditure on health (PPP int. $)	Private expenditure on health as % of total expenditure on health	Out-of-pocket expenditure as % of private expenditure on health	Private prepaid plans as % of private expenditure on health
Botswana	4	27	24	635	23.3	27.5	5.2
Cameroon	2	16	15	379	78.8	94.8	-
Ethiopia	<1	2	2	22	39.6	80.7	3
Ghana	2	9	9	100	63.5	78.8	6.2
Kenya	1	12	14	105	51.8	80	6.9
Nigeria	3	17	5	50	69.9	90.4	6.7
South Africa	8	41	28	869	58.1	17.5	77.7
Togo	<1	4	9	70	72.2	84.7	4.2
United Republic of Tanzania	<1	4	11	45	40.8	83.4	4.5
Africa	2	11	12	111	52.9	49.8	39.6
Global	13	28	25	790	42.4	49.3	42

* These figures represent the WHO's best estimates and are based on information from national Ministries of Health and statistical offices including national health accounts, social security data and household expenditures surveys.

tices ranging from praying and spiritual or traditional healers to medical doctors in local or regional health centres, they have itineraries of health-seeking behaviour that are diffuse and concurrent. People in countries scoring high on health workforce numbers and infrastructure may still face considerable difficulties in accessing proper treatment, while people in countries that score low on these indicators can in fact have easy access to, for example, traditional midwives who may or may not be included in these figures. The country case studies presented in this volume provide micro-level experiences on health and healing in Africa and local variations in such experiences. For a thorough understanding of these experiences, it is important to contextualize them with reference to the differences in the macro-level context presented in Table 1.1.

We are highlighting this aspect of health and healing as it demonstrates the two processes that contribute to increased marketization, namely the shortage, lack and reduced access to public healthcare facilities, and the growing significance of monetarization, financial rationales and commodified morality. Some of the chapters in this volume demonstrate how and why such financial calculi are becoming relevant for understanding the dynamics that are playing out in non-bio-medical domains (see, for example, Chapters 6 & 8).

While this is a contextual reality for many people living in situations where they are faced with making fundamental and existential choices regarding expenditure on health and healing, it is epistemologically alarming. Our social-science understanding of health and healing in African situations runs the risk of becoming reductionist if we adopt such financial calculations as being self-explanatory for people's choices and behaviour. The contributions in this volume qualify and challenge such reductionism. They demonstrate the limits of such financial calculi as well as providing insight into how people in everyday situations navigate financial constraints and the overall commodification of health and healing. By introducing the term 'navigation', we acknowledge the relevance of financial aspects amidst processes of marketization and commodification and want to emphasize the way people themselves are aware of the fact that financial reasoning is one mode of thought concerning health and healing. Yet, at the same time, we argue that this mode of rationality needs to be balanced against other modalities of decision making (relational, moral or spiritual) that are relevant to this domain of social life.

Navigation

The term 'navigation' is used to analyze the ways people cope with everyday life in Africa. It was introduced in a study on how youth in Guinea-Bissau deal with war, conflict and rivalry (Vigh 2006) and was incorporated in *Navigating youth* (Christiansen *et al.* 2006). However these studies also considered how society copes with youth (particularly when youth are taking part in acts of violence, being recruited as soldiers or are involved in criminality). Navigation allows for a 'double-sidedness' to stand in between and opens up a perspective whereby analytical distinctions have to be made between the one and the other. Using this particular example, youth are developing notions, ways of conduct, lines of action that allow them to not be completely engulfed or affected by the forces and circumstances that present themselves in their lives. Hence, there is a level of reflection that appears important in understanding how youth (or any other group in society) move forward. It is not simply about coping with circumstances but includes the idea that while people are confronted with processes over which they have little control, they can still find ways of dealing creatively with them, perhaps even by taking advantage of them or by finding opportunities and challenges. In this sense, navigation is a corollary of their agency.

The way society can devise ways of dealing with a group; power, control and supervision indicates the means by which groups are navigated into a certain position. Vigh's point however is that navigation is culturally mediated. The skills, competences, experiences and emotions that come into play in how a group creates a pathway through and around various circumstances is determined by what is at hand in terms of cultural resources. The double-sidedness of navigation can well be used to understand the relationship between people and the market. Individuals, households or groups negotiate and navigate the forces of the market and the process of marketization, in this case, of practices of health and healing. Navigation allows for a perspective in which marketization is not only creating victimhood (i.e. being a victim of market forces) but is also able to grapple with these forces and take advantage of them (van Binsbergen & van Dijk 2004).

Navigating the market

To appreciate the relationship between navigation and marketization, it is important to understand the process of the increasing influence and dominance of the market in the arrangement of everyday matters. In the African setting, the process of marketization has, for example, been studied as a Marxist interpretation of the encroachment of neo-liberal capitalism (van Binsbergen & Geschiere 1985; Comaroff & Comaroff 1999) and, secondly, in studies of commodification and consumptivism (van Binsbergen & Geschiere 2003). Marxist interpretations of the expansion of the neo-liberal market on the African continent often interpreted this as being part of a victimizing process. Encroachment of the market in that sense was not neutral but perceived this process as part of the creation of deep inequalities, a subjugation of local forms of production, trade and consumption to Western-dominated forms of capitalist expansion and part of an extraction of resources in Africa for the benefit of Western wealth and prosperity. In this perspective, local forms of production, trade and consumption could not escape from this process, while the process could not benefit the local African economic spheres.

Studies of commodification and consumptivism not only explored how marketization required and was based on monetarization (i.e. turning local values into values expressed in money) but also how new appetites emerged (Miller 1987). The desire for luxury items, for instance, develops as a result of being exposed to images of the West, of its markets and consumerism. This has shaped expectations, especially among the emergent middle classes. And entrepreneurial groups have been able to engage with the expanding markets and are seeing new opportunities in this process. A literature has emerged on how marketization has been part of the creation of African forms of entrepreneurialism and mercantilism, indicating that specific forms of navigation do emerge and can be successful (Ensminger 1992). In this sense, navigation speaks critically of a former Marxist interpretation of the effects of the encroachment of neoliberalism, a process this volume seeks to understand in the context of health and healing. The contributions in this book demonstrate, for example, how AIDS patients turn to the market and begin to 'sell' their suffering to interested donors and NGOs for purposes of advocacy. And we can see how nurses become entrepreneurs within the institutional settings of public health facilities that have otherwise been marked by the effects of encroaching liberal reforms. In all these cases, despite the reforms, increasing shortages and a lack of resources, people are trying to take the market into their own hands and have become resourceful in negotiating its effects, though with varying degrees of success.

Navigating the market for health and healing

The contributions in this volume demonstrate the various dimensions of the navigation of market forces in the domain of health and healing. While assumptions can be made all too easily about the difference between the modern (i.e. modern institutions, modern state systems, bio-medicine) and the traditional (i.e. healers, traditional medicine and practice) and their engagement with the market, the question is whether or not this dichotomy is in any sense helpful in understanding the process. The same applies to assumptions about the distinction between the public and the private; what does a market of health and healing do to dichotomies of this nature? To what extent is the opposite true, namely, that it does not matter much whether or not a medical system, institution, practice or discourse is classified as modern or as traditional, or public or private? The effects of marketization and the need for a navigation of the market might be very much the same.

How far the market and related processes of commercialization blur distinctions and categorizations – making people increasingly alert to the need to be able to navigate an unclear field of medical practices and institutions – becomes clear when considering the public versus the private. In Chapter 2, Akinyoade & Bukole describe how niches are emerging in the public health systems in Nigeria where the public is turned into private gain. Medical specialists are discovering how the public domain of health provisioning can be turned into a marketable commodity by establishing private enterprises within public settings, such as government hospitals and clinics. This form of marketization of the public leads to a range of processes of navigation in which doctors and patients are jointly embedded: doctors are interested in cross-referrals between the public and the private and cleverly do so, and patients are interested in private-in-public arrangements as they hope for better care and for medical value for their money. In Chapter 3, Bohmig indicates another remarkable feature of this entrepreneurialization of public professions; the entrepreneurial nurse in Ghanaian public hospitals. Through a detailed ethnography of nursing practices, she shows how nurses commercialize elements of their nursing practice, their care for patients and the delivery of medicines and nursing materials so as to improve their performance. While much of Ghana's public health is enveloped in a cash-and-carry system whereby patients (or their families) are required to pay for care and treatment, nurses are finding ways of buying and selling on their wards so that they can continue their activities even in situations of shortage. While making modest profits, this marketization of their practice seems to comply with a wider ethic of keeping the nursing system functional in a situation where public health provisioning is marked by a serious crisis.

Entrepreneurialization in the public and the private domain that affects well-being is shown in the school feeding projects in Kenya, which are described by Foeken, Klaver, Mwangi & Owuor in Chapter 4. Schools are becoming players in local markets of food provisioning in the way they produce, sell and consume food. In situations where market prices for food have been soaring, school production may help to secure a level of food security and thus of well-being for pupils. This again causes a blurring of distinctions, as a public institution (i.e. the school) relates directly with the family system of food provisioning. In this case, schools may become the new 'shock absorbers' between the market and the family, an example of how institutions can mitigate the effect of the market. At the same time, institutions can fail in their attempts to bring health or well-being to the population, as is evident in the historical review of policies to control malaria in Kenya, which is provided by Ombongi & Rutten in Chapter 5. They argue that policy choices have clearly been affected by national and international economic, military and strategic interests. In spite of good intentions, sufficient knowledge and available funds, there is a real and significant limit to the extent to which individuals, families or institutions can navigate such a disease. To date, and despite a rapprochement between bio-medical and traditional medicine, the institutional capacity of the government has been too limited, remedies insufficient and the market too inelastic to be of any help.

In Chapter 8, Beckmann indicates another way in which the market provokes a blurring of distinctions between private lives and public presence among AIDS patients in Zanzibar who employ themselves in HIV/AIDS intervention and prevention campaigns. This shows a commercialization of private suffering and illness in the public domain where international donors are creating new markets of access to NGO-related money and wealth. While some talk of an 'NGO-ization' of the public domain, the process that Beckmann describes is one where AIDS patients are not simply victims of the disease but instead have the means to navigate the market by 'selling' their predicament. NGOs and other AIDS campaigners are particularly interested in furthering their public agendas through representation and advocacy by AIDS patients who, in exchange for money, are prepared to reveal their private status and personal suffering publicly.

The blurring of the distinction between the modern and traditional domains that emerging markets for health and healing are causing is more central in other chapters. Thornton, in Chapter 6, suggests that the market has the capacity to distort distinctions and dichotomies between a range of systems of health and healing, at least at the level of ordinary people's understanding. He demonstrates how the notion of a competing market of different medical systems makes distinctions fuzzy, and presents the making of choices for one medical system or the other as a matter of belief. In a rural town in South Africa where there is no certainty of ascertaining the effectiveness of one medical system over the other, a belief in the effectiveness of one form of health or healing becomes significant for the decisions people make. Thornton thus argues that the blurring of modern and traditional ways of healing is occurring under the impact of a rising market of beliefs. Beliefs in effectiveness compete with one another since neither the modern bio-medical system of health nor traditional systems of healing have ways of expressing their value in money. There is no particular relationship between the effectiveness of the health and healing they offer in relation to the money that is charged. Some medical remedies remain ineffective in some cases, while others are ineffective in all cases. The only certainty that exists is of entering a market of beliefs concerning the potency of certain remedies; remedies that may be applied to address illness and misfortune or that may be used to avert evil things happening.

In Chapter 7, van Beek shows how systems of divination within Kapsiki society have been translated into modern styles to deal with the unravelling of causes of disease and misfortune through the use of modern means of communication, such as the mobile telephone and marketing through advertisements. This is less of a break with the past as it is a process of constant renewal of cultural continuity that is producing even greater power with regard to healing. Engagement with these modern means of communication and of making a business out of a healing tradition that was never commercialized does not make the diviners appear weaker or less trustworthy in their practice. There is an element of skilful negotiation of the opportunities that these modern means allow, which enhances a notion of success. Divining with the mobile telephone does not replace existing forms of divination, which are elaborated and specialized in skills and competences, but adds another dimension, requiring the mastering of new skills and competences. In a sense, the commercialization of divination through the use of modern means of communication, as van Beek shows, makes the entire system more complex than it ever was before.

While these contributions discuss the potentiality of the market and processes of commercialization in blurring distinctions between the modern and the traditional, and between the public and the private, other subtle processes of navigation are taking place too. Markets of health and healing penetrate families and their resources and thus their increased monetization does not only require us to consider how individuals navigate such processes but also how collectives – such as families and households – are doing so. In Chapter 9, Dekker shows how gender-specific roles in the resource management of families and households in Ethiopia *vis-à-vis* expenses for health and healing are coming under pressure and may transform the need to be able to provide the money required to cover health-related expenses. Mothers are becoming like fathers by provisioning for care so that, internally, family structure and authority patterns may change in the process. In Chapter 10, Leliveld, t Hart, Gnimadi & Dekker similarly show that the distinctions in Togo between security and insecurity for families are changing in relation to a different market: the market of insurances. Health-seeking behaviour is determined by considerations of cost and distance, and families are having difficulty absorbing the shocks that illness and misfortune cause. While it is argued that traditional medical care is not necessarily cheaper or more readily available than modern bio-medical care, the shock remains the same on both accounts. Introducing insurance schemes could help to absorb shocks but may yet prove to be a further drain on family resources; one which families are not used to and which challenges their views and understandings of risk and insecurity.

In the context of pandemic diseases, such as HIV/AIDS and malaria, the markets of health and healing seem to provoke new and unprecedented forms of navigation by individuals, families and institutions. While the contribution by Beckmann on AIDS patients marketing their private suffering has already been mentioned, as has the wide range of forces and players in the malaria policy in Kenya, the question is how conglomerates arise interlinking private, individual, family and institutional-based forms of navigating in these markets. Both AIDS and malaria appear to produce this process and individuals, families and institutions become linked and intertwined in aligning their navigation of the ways in which these diseases produce new and specific markets and forms of commercialization. In the book's final chapter, van Dijk demonstrates how the institution of marriage in Botswana has become a target for AIDS campaigners who are pushing for the formation of stable and single-partner relationships. As the institution of marriage is perceived as a social panacea in the fight against the disease, individuals and families are negotiating increasingly costly marriage arrangements. The wedding itself has become a target for the market and in the process the extent to which the institution is a weapon in the fight against the disease is becoming more difficult to see. The market is not only blurring the distinction between traditional and modern consumerist styles in marriages, it is also confusing public display and private fortune, and affecting the level of policy making *vis-à-vis* AIDS and actual practice. For young couples, it is more difficult to navigate the demands that this consumerist style is placing on them and which is turning the institution of marriage into a problematic aspect of social life.

Conclusion

These contributions, which demonstrate how people, groups and institutions at various levels navigate the market and processes of commercialization, show how economic and anthropological studies can join together in understanding both social predicament *and* creativity. While Max Weber in his socio-economic studies has pointed at an important process of increasing rationalization and bureaucratization in analyzing modernity's progress, an economic ethnography of the kind that we have been proposing here in the field of health and healing is not satisfied with simply pointing out emerging rationalities. While these contributions demonstrate that the rise of marketization of domains of health and healing is unmistakably bringing forth a negotiation of market forces, prices, rationality and calculations of cost and investment, people do not fall victim to the logics of such emerging rationalities (Buetow 2007). Matters of belief, norms, values, hopes, expectations and desires matter a great deal in understanding how precisely such rationalities are navigated in everyday contexts.

This requires a new kind of ethnography of the prevailing economics in such situations, much akin to what Pfeiffer & Chapman (2010) called for when talking about the need to develop an ethnography of the effects of structural adjustment policies on public health systems in Africa. This economic ethnography in the realm of health and healing in Africa makes it clear that it does not help our understanding to assume that irrationalities are at play when analyzing the kind of creativity that people apply. There are serious predicaments in African systems of health and healing as these contributions demonstrate. Yet an economic ethnography of the forms of navigation that are being discussed in these contributions opens the way for setting a particular agenda for this type of research. As argued, this economic ethnography should not be limited to individual actors alone, not only to avoid methodological individualism as such but to acknowledge that everything relating to health and healing in the African context is first and foremost a communal, collective or family affair.

While marketization easily leads to individualization, an economic ethnography can demonstrate how precisely this is being negotiated. This economic ethnography also targets wider collectives (the family, the household, the institution) in the way these seem to be actors in how the market and commercialization are being navigated. While individuals are part of larger collectives, individuals and collectives may follow different paths as they negotiate the market. The economic ethnography of the state and health is all too clearly able to demonstrate how multilayered processes of navigation actually are. Public health institutions are navigating government reform policies, while within institutions individuals are negotiating the trajectories that they are developing in response to the state context.

Developing the agenda for a multilayered economic ethnography through which the present-day significance of the marketization of health and healing can be analyzed is a step this volume is aspiring to contribute to.

References

Bhattamishra, R. & C. Barrett (2010), Community-based risk management arrangements: A review. *World Development* 38(7): 923-932.

Bloom, G. & H. Lucas (2000), Health and poverty in Sub-Saharan Africa. IDS Working Paper 103. Brighton: Institute of Development Studies.

Bloom, G. & H. Standing (2001), Pluralism and marketisation in the health sector: Meeting needs in context of social change in low and middle-income countries. IDS Working Paper No. 136. Brighton: Institute of Development Studies.

Bloom, G., H. Standing & R. Lloyd (2008), Markets, information asymmetry and health care: Towards new social contracts. *Social Science and Medicine* 66: 2076-2087.

Bogale, T., D.H. Mariamand & A. Ali (2005), Cost of illness and coping strategies in a coffee-growing rural district of Ethiopia. *Journal of Health Population and Nutrition* 23(2): 192-199.

Buetow, S. (2007), Non-attendance for health care. When rational beliefs collide. *The Sociological Review* 55(3): 592-610.

Christiansen, C., M. Utas & H. Vigh, eds (2006), *Navigating youth, generating adulthood: Social becoming in an African context*. Uppsala: Nordiska Afrikainstitutet.

Comaroff, J. & J. Comaroff (1999), Alien-nation: Zombies, immigrants, and millennial capitalism. *CODESRIA Bulletin* (3/4): 17-28.

Dercon, S. (2004), Growth and shocks: Evidence from rural Ethiopia. *Journal of Development Economics* (74): 309-329.

Dercon, S., J. Hoddinnott & T. Woldehanna (2005), Shocks and consumption in 15 Ethiopian villages, 1999-2004. *Journal of African Economies* 14(4): 559-585.

Elbers, C., J.W. Gunning & B. Kinsey (2007), Growth and risk: Methodology and micro evidence. *World Bank Economic Review* 21: 1-20.

Ensminger, J. (1992), *Making a market: The institutional transformation of African society*. Cambridge: Cambridge University Press.

Fafchamps, M. (2004): *Market institutions in Sub-Saharan Africa: Theory and evidence*. Cambridge: MIT Press.

Feierman, S. (2008), Money heals: Traditional medicine and the meanings of exchange. *Palabres actuelles* 2: 5-26.

Holzmann, R. & S. Jorgensen (2000), Social risk management: A new conceptual framework for social protection and beyond. Social Protection Discussion Paper 6. Washington D.C.: World Bank.

Krishna, A.; D. Lumonya, M. Markiewicz, A. Kafuko, J. Wegoye, & F. Mugumya (2006), Escaping poverty and becoming poor in 36 villages of Central and Western Uganda. *Journal of Development Studies* 42(2): 346-370.

Last, M. & G.L. Chavunduka (1986), *The professionalisation of African medicine*. Manchester: Manchester University Press (in association with the International African Institute).

Leutloff-Grandits, C., A. Peleikis & T. Thelen, eds (2009), *Social security in religious networks. Anthropological perspectives on new risks and ambivalences*. New York: Berghahn.

Luedke, T. & H. West, eds (2006), *Borders and healers: Brokering therapeutic resources in southeast Africa*. Bloomington: Indiana University Press.

Meillasoux, C. (1971), *The development of indigenous trade and markets in West Africa*. Oxford: Oxford University Press.

Miller, D. (1987), *Material culture and mass consumption*. Oxford, Basil Blackwell.

Nooteboom, G. (2003), A matter of style. Social security and livelihood in upland East Java. PhD Thesis, Nijmegen University. Rotterdam: Optima Grafische Communicatie.

Pan, L. (2009), Risk pooling through transfers in rural Ethiopia. *Economic Development and Cultural Change* 57(4): 809-835.

Pfeiffer, J. & R. Chapman (2010), Anthropological perspectives on structural adjustment and public health. *Annual Review of Anthropology* 39: 149-165.

Prince, R., Ph. Denis & R. van Dijk (2009), Introduction: Engaging Christianities. Negotiating HIV/AIDS, health and social relations in East and Southern Africa. In: R. Prince, Ph. Denis & R. van Dijk, eds, *Christianity and HIV/AIDS in East and Southern Africa*. Special Issue of *Africa Today* 56(1): v-xviii.

Radstake, M. (2000), *Secrecy and ambiguity: Home care for people living with HIV/AIDS in Ghana*. Leiden: African Studies Centre.

Siegel, P. & J. Alwang (1999), An asset-based approach to social risk management: A conceptual framework. Social Protection Discussion Paper no. 9926. Washington D.C.: World Bank.
Summerton, J.V. (2006), The organisation and infrastructure of the African traditional healing system: Reflections from a sub-district of South Africa. *African Studies* 65(2): 297-319.
Tibandebage, P. & M. Mackintosh (2005), The market shaping of charges, trust and abuse: Health care transactions in Tanzania. *Social Science and Medicine* (61): 1385-1395.
Turshen, M. (1999), *Privatizing health services in Africa*. New Brunswick: Rutgers Publications.
van Binsbergen, W. & R. van Dijk, eds (2003), *Situating globality. African agency in the appropriation of global culture*. Leiden: Brill.
van Binsbergen, W. & P. Geschiere, eds (1985), *Old modes of production and capitalist encroachment: Anthropological explorations in Africa*. London: Kegan Paul.
van Binsbergen, W. & P. Geschiere, eds (2005), *Commodification. Things, agency, and identities*. Hamburg: LIT Verlag.
Vaughan, M. (1991), *Curing their ills. Colonial power and African illness*. Cambridge: Polity Press.
Vigh, H.E. (2006), *Navigating terrains of war: Youth and soldiering in Guinea-Bissau*. New York: Berghahn Books.
von Benda-Beckmann, F. & K. von Benda-Beckmann (1994), Coping with insecurity. *Focaal* 22/23: 7-31.
World Bank (2001), *Attacking poverty. World development report 2000/1*. New York: Oxford University Press.
WHO (2009), *World Health Statistics*. Geneva: WHO.

2

Milking the sick: Medical pluralism and the commoditization of healthcare in contemporary Nigeria

Akinyinka Akinyoade & Bukola Adeyemi Oyeniyi

This chapter examines the commoditization of healthcare and variations in the delivery of services as perceived by users of healthcare facilities in Lagos and Ibadan in southwestern Nigeria. Commoditization, access, effectiveness and forms of healthcare services were measured in five local government councils in the two cities. Healthcare seekers appear to have evolved a pragmatic accommodation between the usage of local herbal medical practitioners and the modern formalized healthcare system. The commoditization of healthcare services is gaining ground and new forms of healthcare institutions, such as private-in-public healthcare units, are being entrenched, The relatively high costs associated with healthcare procurement in these units is commensurate with the higher quality of care that patients receive. Questions arise as to who the revenue should go to when health workers deliver services using government facilities during working hours when they are already being paid. The implications of the private-in-public system on inequality and exclusion remain a conjecture for healthcare access and provisioning in contemporary Nigeria.

Introduction

This chapter examines the commoditization, entrepreneurization, access and effectiveness of Nigeria's healthcare delivery system following the introduction of privatization and liberalization policies by the Nigerian government in the early

2000s. Data sets obtained from oral interviews conducted in selected local government areas in Oyo and Lagos States between March and June 2009 and in the first quarter of 2010, combined with information from questionnaires, personal observations and the existing literature on healthcare delivery, were used in the analysis. Entrepreneurization is an environment in which public healthcare workers who have a stake in both the public and private bio-medical healthcare infrastructure set up a system whereby patients in public hospitals are referred to private clinics for medical treatment. A unique form of private service provision that is gaining ground in Nigeria is the establishment and entrenchment of privately run units in public hospitals. Commodification, as used in this chapter, describes situations where healthcare services suddenly became a commodity that is subjected to market fundamentals such as supply, demand and profitability. Central to the thesis of the study is the contention that economic liberalization, with its emphasis on profitability, is spawning new forms of delivering healthcare that take it beyond the reach of the poor in both urban and rural areas. In this context, healthcare providers, such as doctors, nurses, auxiliary workers and consultants, have commodified public health service provision and formed a new layer of entrepreneurs who are milking the sick in the name of providing healthcare. Given the prevalence of this scenario in Nigeria, the nation presents itself as a mosaic through which the place of market and economic liberalization in delivering healthcare can be examined.

Following the return to democratic rule in May 1999, the Obasanjo administration renewed attempts to implement a privatization policy, which has since had an important and unanticipated impact on healthcare. Prior to 2000 when privatization became official government policy, successive Nigerian governments verbally committed themselves to providing healthcare services. This was, however, limited to free diagnosis in the public health system, especially in southwestern Nigeria, as treatment and drug procurement had to be paid for. Since the quality of healthcare diminished in the public sector, especially following the implementation of the IMF- and World-Bank-orchestrated Structural Adjustment Programme (SAP) in the late 1980s, the liberalization of the healthcare sector has become one of the options taken to ensure access to treatment. Under this new healthcare regime, which is inadvertently underlined by profit concerns, those who can afford it choose private bio-medical care while those who cannot afford it opt for 'traditional' treatment, which is offered at lower prices compared to treatment in the public sector.

The chapter is divided into five parts. The introductory section sets out the basic arguments and direction of the entire chapter. The second offers a panoramic view of healthcare delivery in Nigeria and the place of market and economic liberalization in it, especially since 2000. The third section examines the entrepreneurization of healthcare services and its effect on healthcare in general as well as on the dynamic coping strategies Nigerian medical personnel have evolved to cope with the changes. The fourth section, which uses data sets from selected healthcare centres in Lagos and Oyo, focuses on access to healthcare services in the urban and rural areas in Nigeria. The concluding section draws together the study's major findings and suggests ways of preventing a healthcare catastrophe in Nigeria.

Healthcare and economic liberalization in Nigeria

Nigeria's healthcare system offers primary healthcare delivered by clinics and dispensaries in local areas; secondary healthcare provided by maternity homes and hospitals; and tertiary healthcare, which comprises medical centres, teaching hospitals and specialized and professional hospitals such as the Nigeria Army Hospital and the Nigeria Dental Hospital.

Prior to 1999, healthcare delivery in Nigeria was essentially a public-sector concern. This was not to say that private individuals had no stake in healthcare provisioning, but they were few and far between. It must be noted though that standardized privately run healthcare infrastructures (as well as mushroom units)[1] have been in existence for several decades. Most of today's public hospitals were set up by the military governments in the 1970s but were neglected over time and exposed to corruption, as were almost all sectors of socio-economic and political life under military autocracy.[2]

Coupled with the brain drain and the mass migration of health professionals (Eastwood *et al.* 2005; Connell *et al.* 2007) that followed the implementation of SAPs in 1986; corruption, neglect and a decaying infrastructure contributed to the parlous state of public and private healthcare infrastructure across the country (Onwudiegwu 1997). Public healthcare provisioning declined and public healthcare institutions were anecdotally referred to as mere consulting clinics. This labelling came against a backdrop of gradual paucity of government funding that eroded public hospitals' capacity to deliver a full range of services. Patients were mostly limited to prescriptions for drugs that could only be obtained in pharmacies outside hospital precincts, and in other cases patients were referred to private hospitals that could deliver a wider range of health services but at a fee.[3] In addition, doctors and nurses were emigrating, job losses and

---

1 These are healthcare units labelled clinics that are run by nurses and/or healthcare auxiliary workers in their private homes.

2 See 'Lagos Launches 34th Mini Medical Mission, Stresses Its Importance To Improved Healthcare Services' at:
http://www.lagosstate.gov.ng/index.php?page=news&nid=244.

3 Admission of patients for a long stay and the lack of drugs at pharmacies in hospitals gradually became the norm.

retrenchments as a result of SAPs compounded the situation, and people's purchasing power dropped as salaries lost value due to the devaluation of the currency and increasing debt (Onwudiegwu 1997; Evans 1995). Public funding gradually declined and the government placed a ceiling on employment and promotions.

A doctor attached to Ibarapa Local Government in Oyo State noted that this development stimulated two things in Nigeria's health sector. The first was that 'healthcare professionals who decided to remain in the country were forced to turn inward for solutions' and secondly that 'healthcare delivery lost its allure'. The solutions included obtaining licences and setting up private clinics and sometimes full-fledged hospitals while at the same time remaining in government employment. This practice was not limited to doctors alone: some pharmacists, for example at the Ladoke Akintola University Teaching Hospital in Oyo State, established their own pharmacies so that they could earn extra money by directing patients from government hospitals to these private concerns.

At its zenith, the referral system involved nurses, paramedics and ward maids who set up consultation clinics, shops and premises where all forms of medical, paramedical and even pseudo-medical services were offered. Besides referrals, private, specialized services in government clinics, maternity centres and hospitals have also been developed. Today, the practice is such that healthcare practitioners have turned parts of government healthcare centres into private wards, where those who can afford the costs associated with such services are treated at exorbitant rates. This raises the question about who accrues the revenue when health workers deliver services using government facilities during their regular working hours for which they are being paid.

Both the referral and private-within-public service delivery systems are coping strategies devised by medical practitioners to cushion the effects of government neglect, dwindling allocation, SAP conditions, the brain drain and other problems that beset the nation between 1986 and 1999 (NISER 2005: 22). These issues have contributed to a decline in the health sector.

The development inadvertently weaned two healthcare delivery systems that had been in existence prior to the troubles that beset the health sector. On the one hand, there is a traditional and informal system made up of herbalists, seers, traditional birth attendants or midwives, and faith healers (pastors and imams offering a spiritual dimension to healing),[4] and on the other hand a modern, public/semi-private modern bio-medical system run by formally trained personnel (doctors, nurses and administrators). These two systems, which are not mutually exclusive, are juxtaposed spatially and socially in a structure of medical pluralism. Generally in Nigeria, the two are either mutually supportive or

---

4 See Adib (2004); Barnes *et al.* (2000) and Vecchiato (1993).

intricately but almost imperceptibly linked. Traditional healthcare has become a dominant feature among the Nigerian poor, both rural and urban, while Western or public healthcare is dominant among the affluent (urban and rural). Caught in this quagmire, Nigerians, especially urban dwellers, have evolved a pragmatic accommodation between the traditional and informal system; and the modern, public/semi-private and formalized system (Logan & Mengisteab 1995). In many parts of Nigeria today, herbal medicine providers are locked in competition with hospitals and clinics. Bizarrely, herbal medicine shops are located next to hospitals and clinics, and both compete for patronage on radio and television.

In addition to herbal medicine, faith healing, which is a non-bio-medical but religious intervention that is gaining prominence especially in Pentecostal Christianity and radical Islam, has also presented itself as a credible alternative in the field of healthcare in Nigeria. Churches and mosques are today making claims about unprecedented healing, even of HIV/AIDS, diabetes and sickle cell anaemia (Ezeome & Anarado 2007; Adogame 2007).

In southwestern Nigeria where Lagos and Ibadan are located, public health services were delivered freely by the Unity Party of Nigeria (UPN) state governments between 1979 and 1983. Services such as consultations, laboratory tests, surgical operations and medical record-keeping were either provided free of charge or were heavily subsidized. After 1983, user fees were gradually introduced in all health facilities in Nigeria. With the return to democratic rule in May 1999 and the renewed attention by the Obasanjo-led administration to privatization, full user fees and charges were introduced in all public hospitals as the government removed subsidies. When Obasanjo's government introduced privatization, two forms of care emerged in Nigeria's healthcare sector. On the one hand, the government democratized space to establish private clinics and related health services, such as medical laboratories. These services were offered by private individuals and were located outside regular public hospitals, which were ordered to charge user fees for a range of services from medical record-keeping (called card acquisition in local parlance) to complex surgery. Healthcare services in these hospitals were charged at market rates. On the other hand, public hospitals were not turned over to private management. This new privatization initiative allowed entrepreneurs, either medical practitioners or those who could command their labour, who met the requirements for establishing and running private health institutions to obtain licences and open premises to offer healthcare services. Drug quality, under this new privatization regime, is primarily controlled by the government's National Agency for Food and Drug Administration and Control (NAFDAC).[5] In addition, standard practices and

---

[5] See http://thenationonlineng.net/web2/articles/15879/1/ for a description.

benchmarks have been set by the state for privately-owned healthcare facilities to comply with, and breaches have led to the withdrawal of licenses in some cases. And to ensure that private practitioners adhere to the ethical standards set by the state, health officers and inspectors are regularly deployed to visit health facilities to determine their effectiveness and adherence to the rules.

The government also took steps to 'unbundle' the existing public healthcare services and privatized services, either in part or as a whole. A more expansive description of the economic liberalization process is provided by Heald (1985) and Logan (1995) on how economic liberalization could be achieved through the deregulation of government controls, franchising, contracting and the sub-contracting of services.

With the development in the telecommunications sector in Nigeria serving as a beacon,[6] if not a lure; it was hoped that the privatization and marketization of healthcare would facilitate unprecedented progress in terms of access to healthcare and the quality of the care provided. It was hoped that healthcare would become affordable through competition. Profitability, it was argued, would drag entrepreneurs away from the urban centres into the rural areas. Proponents of the liberalization of healthcare argued that, beyond basic health provisioning by government, individuals should be able to choose to purchase additional protection for themselves. Diametrically opposed to this argument is the perception that healthcare is a fundamental right and not a privilege for the rich alone. The privatization of healthcare is thus believed to discriminate against the poor as entrepreneurs focus on profitability rather than social welfare provisioning. Given its importance to human development; can concern for healthcare be juxtaposed with a concern for profit?

It is not in the purview of this chapter to engage in an ideological debate on economic liberalization and the specific characteristic of healthcare delivery in Nigeria. However we will examine how it has spawned a new type of entrepreneurial and referral system among medical personnel, especially doctors in public hospitals in Ibadan and Lagos. In the first instance, we trace how patients are promised effective, efficient, affordable healthcare when referred by medical practitioners in government/public hospitals to private units within public hospitals manned by health workers in government employment. In addition, an analysis is offered of access and the efficiency of public hospitals using retrospective experiences of sampled users of units in local government areas (LGAs) of Lagos and Ibadan cities.

---

6 Privatization of the telecommunications sector has helped to revolutionize communications and has since served as benchmark to measure privatization as a panacea for development in Nigeria.

Entrepreneurization of healthcare services in Nigeria

One important dimension of Nigeria's healthcare system is its entrepreneurization, which has adopted two different forms: the referral system and the public-in-private system. The referral system describes the setting up of private healthcare centres by medical practitioners in public service to which they refer patients from public healthcare centres for better, but often costly, medical care. The private-in-public system is the practice of setting up private wards manned by government officials within public healthcare centres. It should be noted that while these two forms of entrepreneurization involve the higher echelons of the medical profession, such as doctors, nurses, pharmacists, paediatricians and radiologists, the lower echelons have also been detected profiting from either the sale of consumables such syringes, cleansing agents and cotton wool or the renting out (to patients) of amenities like sheets and pillow cases. Medical practitioners who have a stake in both public bio-medical and private bio-medical healing practices are involved here.

To obtain data on healthcare entrepreneurization, semi-structured interviews were conducted with fifteen randomly selected doctors and pharmacists in public hospitals in Lagos and Oyo States. In addition, twenty in-patients were interviewed in both states. Although two of the respondents were staff at Redeemer's University in Ogun State, the interviews were held at the Lagos Teaching Hospital. The interviews aimed to understand the prevalence of the referral system, its patterns, aims and objectives, its transformations and the consequences it has had on healthcare delivery.

All the respondents confirmed the existence and prevalence of the referral system. Chief among the reasons cited for its existence and prevalence were the paucity of funding, government neglect of the health sector, low salaries and the poor pension system that necessitated medical practitioners to insure their future by engaging in private practice alongside government employment. A retired hospital matron based in Oyo State rated poor remuneration as the chief factor driving the trend. She noted that the medical profession began to witness its development from the late 1980s and early 1990s onwards and adduced the development as, on the one hand, being the result of the devaluation of the Naira and the austerity measures that followed the implementation of SAPs, and, on the other hand, reduced government expenditure on healthcare. One pharmacist in government employment who was running a private pharmacy noted that low salaries in the face of the crushing economic downturn were the impetus for the development.

Medical doctors however, differed, citing greed and not SAPs as the reason for the development of entrepreneurization among medical personnel. Some

Map 2.1 Nigeria, showing research locations

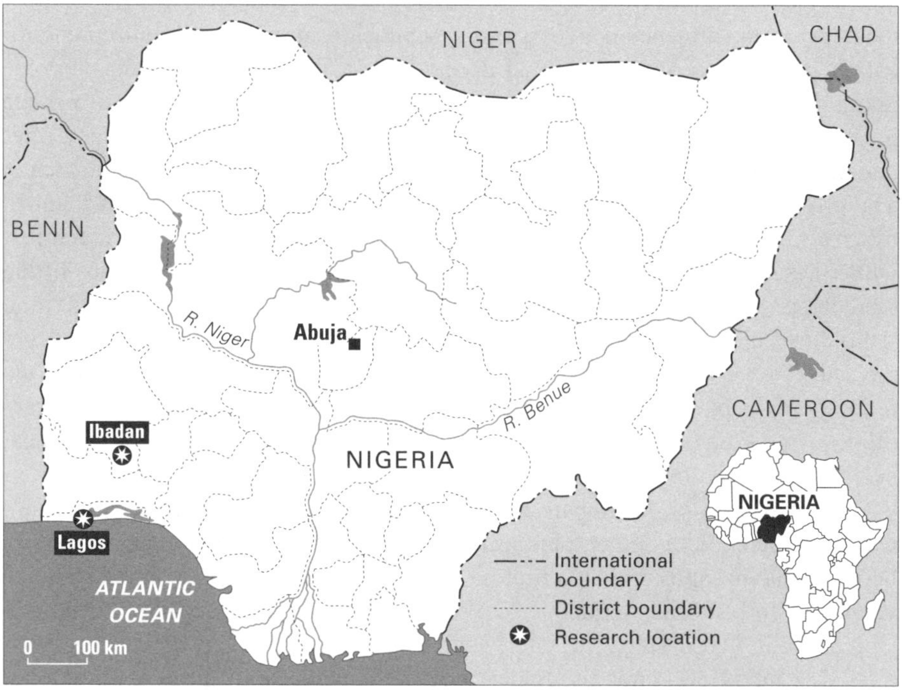

argued that cuts in budgetary expenditure did not apply to the health sector alone but ran across other sectors too. When asked why such development did not occur in other sectors, it was noted that medical practitioners first adopted the measure as a way of cushioning the effects of the SAP. A former resident doctor at Redeemer's University, who had resigned to further his studies in Poland, mentioned that the implementation of SAPs also stimulated out-migration of health professionals from Nigeria and led to situations in which medical practitioners began to set up private practices while, at the same time, holding down their positions in public healthcare centres.

Another medical doctor at the privately run Eko Hospital in Lagos noted, however, that the referral system owed its existence not only to SAPs but also to a different dynamic brought about by them. He claimed that his father, like many others, had left Nigeria in 1987 but that he had returned to Nigeria in 1994 to set up a private practice in Lagos. He remarked that the prevalence of such returnees, especially since 1999, to set up in private practice has encouraged the expansion of the referral system, as serving medical practitioners joined these returnees to either help out in setting up new healthcare centres or to generate extra income. The absence of vital equipment and drugs in most public hospitals as well as a lack of on-the-job training, which the returnees had overcome, drew many medical practitioners into the referral system. A medical doctor at the privately owned Halleluyah Hospital in Lagos added that medical practitioners, who were impressed by the feat achieved within a short time by returnees, began to import medical equipment into the country in order to set up their private premises.

One unique development has been the private-in-public system, where units are operated as a private entity within a government hospital. The afore-mentioned matron, while not denying the existence of private practices within the public healthcare system in Nigeria, noted that it developed first when public figures were admitted to private wards to reduce disturbance and interference from the public and to allow medical practitioners private access to their celebrity patients. She argued that the financial benefits that followed were usually in the form of gifts. A lecturer at Redeemer's University in Ogun State, who has been using private wards in public hospitals since 2006, mentioned that the practice had gone beyond establishing private wards to include full-scale private medical care within the public healthcare system. He confirmed that at Lagos University Teaching Hospital (LUTH) where his wife had recently been admitted with a liver-related ailment, there was efficient private-in-public medical care that was costly but effective. Narrating a recent experience, the lecturer claimed that when he took his wife in for urgent medical attention, the nurses and other assistants on duty promptly advised him to move her to the private ward given her critical condition. He confirmed that doctors and other medical personnel were quickly on hand to treat her. He initially paid N 50,000 (€250) as a deposit and admission fee, which enabled his wife to be admitted to the ward; N 10,000 (€50) in consultation fees; N 5,000 (€25) a night for a bed; and N 1,200 (€6) for food. In addition, there were the costs of drugs, lab tests and so on. The quality of care within the private-in-public system was, however, high and not in any way comparable to what his wife would have received on the general ward. For instance, he noted that patients in private wards would not be affected if medical practitioners went on strike or undertook any other form of industrial action. Despite the care received, his wife sadly passed away a few weeks after receiving medical attention in one of these units.

A female patient in the LUTH private ward noted that 'money generated from the running of this private-in-public system is used to run the ward as well as to pay its staff, as the ward derives no special funding from the government'. The lecturer, however, added that these private-in-public 'hospitals' have management styles that are different from those of the main hospitals. Unlike in the general ward where patients queue, sometimes for days, to consult doctors, on the private ward, 'you have access to your doctor on the dot of your appointment time, the nurses attend to you specifically, you get a room or a blind corner to yourself, you are served the meal of your choice, etc'.

A patient who preferred not to divulge her name claimed that the management of LUTH and other hospitals where such practices abound put measures in place to ensure that only the rich could access healthcare, as doctors in these public hospitals prefer to work on the private wards where consulting rooms have been arranged rather than in their offices where they see those who cannot afford the high cost of healthcare requested in the private wards.

One senior non-teaching staff member at Ladoke Akintola University of Technology in Oyo State said that the practice was not limited to only government hospitals. She claimed to have used private wards at the Nigerian Baptist Medical Center, a religious mission hospital in Oyo State where she had her three children. She was introduced to the private ward by staff at the hospital and said that, given the quality of care available, she elected to use a private ward for all her deliveries and did not mind paying the higher costs demanded. In contrast, another patient who delivered her first child in the regular ward at the same Baptist Medical Center noted that she could not afford the cost of a private ward but that she did know of its existence. In the regular ward, N 6,500 (€32.5) is demanded for services whereas N 40,000 (€200) is needed to gain access to the private labour ward.

Despite the fact that Nigerian Baptist Medical Center is a mission-owned healthcare centre, patients in the general wards use common facilities, which were deemed unhygienic for the most part by our respondents, and they lack amenities and essential equipment. On the other hand, private wards were compared to ensuite hotel rooms with facilities such as televisions and video games, and patients could receive visitors at any time.

The former matron noted that in a situation where all actors from nurses who sell cotton wool and cleansing agents obtained from government hospital stores to patients to doctors who use government facilities to treat patients in private hospitals and junior staff who clean wards work for a fee on top of their salaries, the profit motive cannot be ignored. A doctor at the University of Ibadan Teaching Hospital (UCH) in Ibadan remarked that any medical practitioner who engages in either the referral or private-in-public system is a medical entrepreneur and for such practitioner, she argued, profit rather than healthcare delivery is the driving force. This is a breach of the Hippocratic Oath. Whatever factors may underlie entrepreneurization, it should be noted that medical practitioners have also confirmed its prevalence. The referral system simply translates to the personalization of power (Kunz 1991): 'The king in every man' or in this case the potential authority in a medical doctor employed in a public hospital that uses his/her office to engage in private practice for private gain. One of our respondents, a pharmacist, asserted that not only was the entrepreneurization of healthcare rampant in Nigeria but that a new dimension in its development is a situation whereby doctors, pharmacists and laboratory technicians who had no private premises are now combining public service with private practice in healthcare premises set up by those who could afford to establish such premises. Some of them were not even medical practitioners.

Two arguments have been offered on entrepreneurization. On the one hand, there is the argument that entrepreneurization portends a serious danger for healthcare delivery as it allows medical practitioners to take advantage of not just the government but also patients. This, it is argued, invariably erodes the equality of healthcare. On the other hand, there is the argument that the referral system is good as a way of increasing access to healthcare. Notwithstanding these two positions, it should be noted that the system allows for double payment for healthcare, as patients pay not only at government healthcare centres but also in private healthcare centres. In all, medical practitioners involved in the referral system benefit in both cases as their remuneration for government services are assured while patients also pay for the same services. As one of our respondents argued, entrepreneurization is one reason why Nigeria has not lost all its medical practitioners to the brain drain. Besides stemming the brain drain, it can also be argued that entrepreneurization, especially the private-in-public system, has helped healthcare providers to realize additional resources in the wake of reduced government provisioning.

Access to healthcare services in Nigeria

According to the World Health Organization (2000), the goals of any health system include ensuring good health, a responsiveness to the expectations of the population and a fair financial contribution. Unarguably, none of these existential ideals can be achieved if people, the very target of healthcare system, cannot access healthcare. This section examines patients' access to healthcare in Nigeria as a function of the spatial allocation of healthcare centres and healthcare effectiveness in relation to the delivery of the WHO's ideals. These indicators of measurement have been adapted from a two-dimensional model used by Duckett (2004) to measure the healthcare delivery system in Australia. Access, as it is used in this study, encompasses both the spatial allocation of healthcare centres and the effectiveness of healthcare. Effectiveness of healthcare in Nigerian society in the context of this study describes the ability of a healthcare system to deliver the expected end, which includes patients getting well within two or three weeks of seeking medical attention. Access and effectiveness therefore form the core values when measuring Nigeria's healthcare systems in the context of this study. The chapter uses Lagos State to measure access to healthcare services in urban centres while Oyo State is used to measure healthcare access in peri-urban and rural areas.

The choice of Ibadan and Lagos was made on account of their respective strategic importance. Lagos, the former capital of Nigeria whose socio-economic and political importance lies in it still being widely perceived as the country's economic capital, is a coastal city with twenty local government areas and an estimated population of 9 million.[7] It remains a major centre of commerce and administration. Lagos State is administered by a democratically elected parliamentary government at the head of which is a governor. Despite its modest beginnings, Lagos remains one of the major cosmopolitan cities in Nigeria and this perception, coupled with it being the most populous city in Nigeria, makes it a location of choice for most public and private programmes and policies. This advantage makes Lagos a strategic location for testing the access and effectiveness of public healthcare delivery mechanisms. Ibadan (the capital of Oyo State), with a land mass five times that of Lagos; is one of the largest cities in Nigeria with a population of just under the 5 million mark. It is divided administratively into nine local government areas (5 municipal, 4 peripheral). Although Ibadan is an important centre of trade and commerce, Lagos outdistances it in terms of economic activity and its associated developments. In this study, we are measuring healthcare delivery in urban areas and have used Lagos as a case study. Our use of Ibadan is somewhat different and more complex. Ibadan is a moderately well developed urban area but is ringed by numerous village communities. Together, Ibadan and these villages were used to test the access and effectiveness of healthcare delivery in both urban and rural areas.

There are three categories of healthcare services in Nigeria in general and also in Lagos and Ibadan:[8]

Primary Healthcare: In Lagos and Ibadan, primary healthcare centres offer medical and other healthcare services such as maternity services, treatment and the diagnosis of common diseases and infections, treatment for injuries and prescriptive services. Primary healthcare centres do not usually provide surgical services or have resident doctors because of the basic nature of their services. They often employ consultants to provide medical services on their behalf.

Secondary Healthcare: Healthcare in centres in this category include the Federal Medical Center, general hospitals, specialist hospitals and other professional/specific hospitals. Secondary healthcare centres in Lagos and Ibadan are owned and operated by the state governments. In addition to the services men-

[7] See Lagos State's website: http://www.lagosstate.gov.ng/index.php?page=projectdetail&ptype=Programme&poid=108&mnu=module&mnusub=ministry&mpid=32&pocat=ministry&pocatsub=32

[8] See: http://www.lagosstate.gov.ng/index.php?page=news&nid=244

tioned above, secondary healthcare facilities provide general medical services including surgery. In Lagos State, most of the facilities in these institutions have been upgraded and better conditions of service have been instituted for healthcare personnel. Secondary healthcare institutions usually have resident doctors, pharmacists and medical representatives, laboratory technicians and specialists, nurses, midwives, matrons and other medical personnel. They also have more space to accommodate emergencies such as gunshot and accident victims or people suffering heart problems or similar conditions.

Like the publicly-owned health facilities, privately-owned facilities in Lagos and Ibadan also offer primary and secondary healthcare services. More often than not, they provide basic health services, consultancy services and treatment for common diseases and illnesses including infections of various kinds.

In general, although privately-owned healthcare service providers offer services that are the same as those on offer at the publicly-owned centres, privately-owned healthcare service providers are regarded as faster and more convenient and flexible and it is felt that they offer more satisfactory treatment. In Lagos, the privately-owned Eko hospital, St Nicholas Hospital, could rival some of the general hospitals in terms of facilities and skilled personnel although it is beyond the reach of most Nigerians in terms of distance and cost. Characteristically, privately-owned healthcare facilities are more expensive, as their private owners place a premium on profit ahead of all other considerations.

Tertiary Healthcare: The biggest providers of healthcare services in Nigeria are the tertiary healthcare centres. They, therefore, receive the government's highest priority in terms of facilities, funding, staffing and functioning. These hospitals, in addition to providing healthcare services, also train medical personnel for the country's health sector while rendering diverse medical services at the same time. Structurally, they may be larger than the general hospitals and can include world-class facilities as well as providing complex medical services, such as heart surgery, organ transplants and other complex surgical procedures. Notable examples of hospitals in this category in Lagos and Ibadan are University College Hospital, Oritamefa, Ibadan; Lagos University Teaching Hospital, Idi-Araba; National Orthopaedic Hospital, Igbobi and the Yaba Psychiatric Hospital.

It is important to note that most healthcare institutions in Lagos and Ibadan were constructed during the military administration in the 1970s and early 1990s and have suffered from chronic neglect and unprecedented inefficiency.[9] Healthcare services, whether delivering primary, secondary or tertiary level

---

[9] See 'Lagos launches 34th mini medical mission, stresses its importance to improved healthcare services' at: http://www.lagosstate.gov.ng/index.php?page=news&nid=244

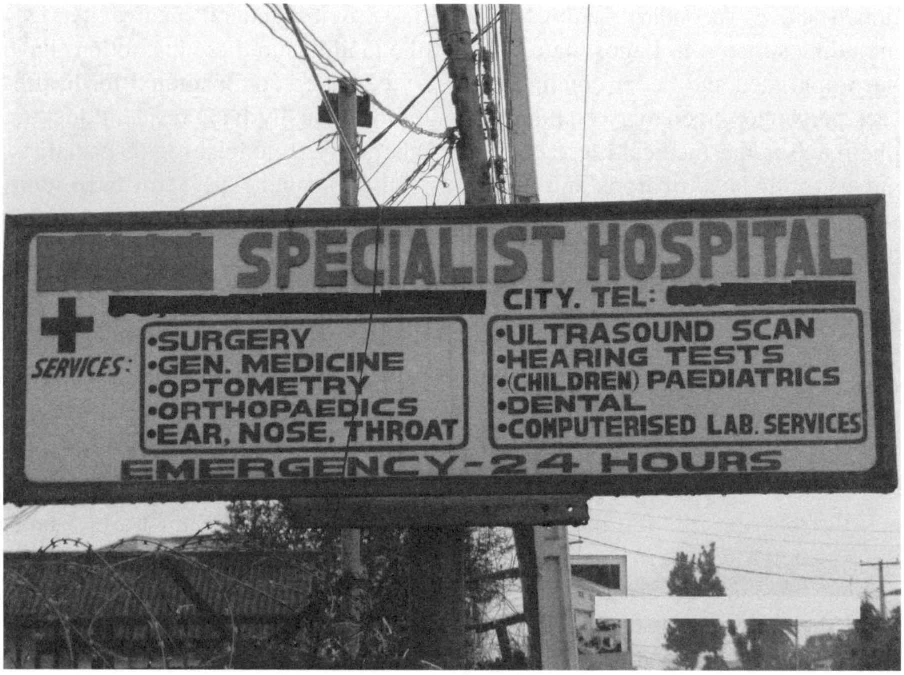

Photo 2.1 Signpost of a range of services offered by a privately-run hospital [Photo: Akinyinka Akinyoade]

care, have experienced frequent strikes, shortages of drugs and other equipment, and many other problems (Ogunbekun *et al.* 1999; Orubuloye & Oyeneye 1982). With Nigeria's return to multiparty democracy in 1999, service delivery appears to have been restored to normalcy and a sense of order has returned to these institutions.

Ironically, the government is talking about free medical care in most states in Nigeria today but in reality, all that is free in hospitals today is the diagnosis. And even this free diagnosis must be taken with caution; patients are made to pay for the retrieval of their medical records during subsequent visits for treatment of the same ailment.

In the remaining part of this section, healthcare delivery in Lagos and Ibadan is measured using two indices: (a) access: with the percentage of hospital visits as a ratio of the estimated population of an area; and (b) effectiveness:[10] measured as a function of healthcare delivering the expected results to patients within two or three weeks of seeking medical attention. Table 2.1 shows the number of

[10] See Okafor & Rizzuto (1994) and Ayeni *et al.* (1987).

healthcare institutions in Lagos and Ibadan. There has been considerable debate about the number of local government councils in Lagos State.[11] For this study, we have taken the federal government's officially recognized number of 20.[12] Ibadan's urban agglomeration, with its seven local government areas, has a total of 42 government-owned healthcare institutions delivering bio-medical/Western-style medical services. Lagos has three times more healthcare institutions than Ibadan.

Table 2.1 Government-owned healthcare institutions in Lagos State and local government areas of Ibadan in Oyo State

State	Local Government Councils	Healthcare institutions
Lagos[13]	20	155
Ibadan (Oyo State)[14]	7	42

In Lagos State, four new public healthcare facilities were built between 1999 and 2009.[15] However, Oyo State recorded none. Paradoxically, the different states in Nigeria earmarked huge financial outlays to refurbish and re-equip existing facilities, but a cursory look at the scorecards of most states shows that the nation's political class are long in rhetoric but short on delivery. The health institutions in these two states cater for a combined population of more than 13 million. Using the 2006 population census figures, this means that each public health institution serves about 60,000 people in Lagos and 95,000 people in Ibadan. From primary data obtained for this study, Ibadan appears to be relatively worse off than Lagos in terms of absolute numbers and has less than a third of the total number of government-owned health institutions; and in terms

11 See: http://www.lagosstate.gov.ng/index.php?page=news&nid=244

12 While we consider this sanguinary to ownership and control, we have considered that the refusal of the federal government to recognize a total of 57 local council development areas (LCDAs) has not in any way passed ownership and control of the healthcare institutions under these LCDAs to either the federal government or to private business. Consequently, ownership is seen as belonging to the state and it is believed that the result of the study is not in any way distorted by the development. There is no controversy In Oyo State about the number of local government councils.

13 See: http://www.lagosstate.gov.ng/index.php?page=projectdetail&ptype=Programme&poid=108&mnu=module&mnusub=ministry&mpid=32&pocat=ministry&pocatsub=32

14 See: http://oyostate.gov.ng/local-govt-areas.

15 See: http://www.lagosstate.gov.ng/index.php?page=news&nid=244

of the ratio of health institutions to the population, Ibadan is not well served either.

We also looked at the utilization of these institutions, using hospital attendance records as a standard of measurement and comparison in the period between 2005 and 2009. The data presented below on hospital attendance were collated from the hospital management boards of both Lagos and Oyo States. The figures include in-patients, referred patients as well as out-patients in the areas covered. The implications of this patient mix is that it gives no specific picture of the nature of healthcare services provided by the institutions, the kinds of ailments that were treated or the multiple nature of patients' visits. The information obtained offers a general view of healthcare access in Lagos and Ibadan. Figure 2.1 presents patient hospital attendance figures in Lagos and Ibadan for the 2005-2009 period.

Figure 2.1 Average annual hospital attendance in selected local government areas in Lagos and Ibadan (2005-2009)

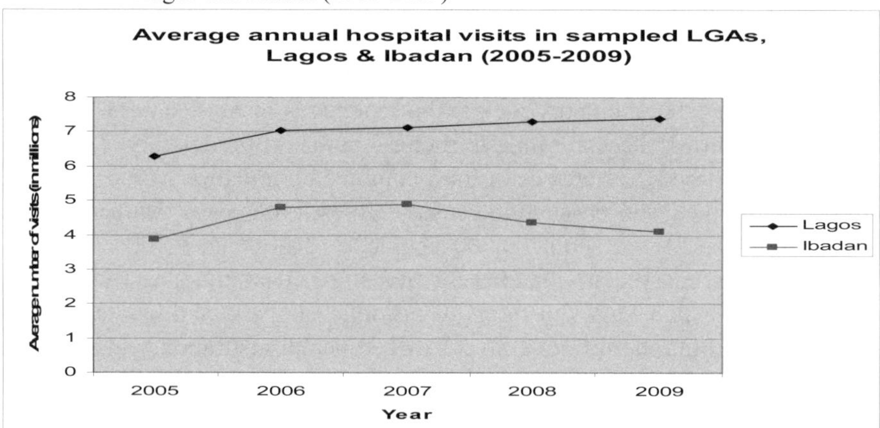

Source: Lagos Medical Records Department, Hospital Management Board, Lagos State Secretariat, Alausa, Lagos State. Ibadan Medical Record Unit, Hospital Management Board, Lagos State Secretariat, Agodi, Ibadan, Oyo State.

The data presented in Figure 2.1 on access to healthcare, using the annual number of hospital visits for the utilization of services, shows an increase in visits of about 17.5% between 2005 and 2009 in Lagos. The natural growth rate of the population was measured at about 3.1% in Nigeria in this period. In Ibadan, hospital attendance increased remarkably by 25.6% from 2005 to 2007, after which it declined by about 16% to the level recorded in 2009. A host of qualifications could be made with respect to the decline. It could be that the population's health improved, thereby reducing hospital attendance. Another possibility relates to patients' inability to afford the costs. There could also be a level of distrust or dissatisfaction regarding the services obtained in these institutions. There is the additional likelihood that the number of patients seeking or patronizing public hospitals is decreasing while those seeking alternative medical care – herbal cures or faith healing – are increasing in number. There is also the possibility that new healthcare facilities have opened in neighbouring states, for instance, in Ogun, Ondo, Ekiti and Kwara States which has changed the flow of patients.

Although the figures do not illustrate the quality of healthcare, they do show an increase in the number of hospital users. However when this is juxtaposed by the number of healthcare facilities, it can be assumed that the number of healthcare facilities in Lagos and Ibadan has not been commensurate with population growth, though there was a dearth of accurate data on the number of hospitals in both locations two decades ago. Invariably, pressure is mounting on services in government-owned hospitals. It has also been recorded that the cost of securing treatment for various health conditions is on the rise since subsidies were removed from the health sector. For instance, it was shown that the cost of x-rays increased by 250% between 1994 and 1996, and the cost of treating malaria increased by 100% in 1994, 1500% in 1995 and 2100% in 1996 (Fatiregun *et al.* 2007). Based on a trend that has been noted since the early 1990s (Orubuloye *et al.* 1991), the cost of treating malaria has risen from US$ 2.22 to a current (2010) estimate of approximately US$ 15 for bio-medical treatment. It can thus be argued that healthcare costs have risen in the past two decades. When healthcare seekers become frustrated by costly and inadequate services, they are more willing to seek alternative care that is less costly in terms of time and money. We will return to this later on.

To measure the effectiveness of healthcare services accessed by users in Lagos and Ibadan, 300 questionnaires were administered to randomly sampled patients in five local government areas in Lagos and Ibadan respectively. The questions were tailored to elicit information on past health conditions and the results of any bio-medical services received during their previous illnesses. The questions were based on doctors' requirements that effectiveness is measured by wellness and patients' responses to bio-medical services. As noted above, these respondents were issued with the questionnaires in the general waiting rooms of government-owned hospitals while they were waiting for services ranging from consultations with doctors, to treatment and/or the mundane task of applying for a sick note to present at work to justify an application for sick leave, a requirement for civil servants in government employment. As a general rule, the questionnaires were administered to those who had previous medical records. All the interviewees therefore had a positive score on bio-medical care use. The questions covered (i) the length of time of the illness;[16] (ii) healthcare use; (iii) the medication taken; and (iv) the results after medication. While many patients combine bio-medical healthcare with alternative remedies, the survey concentrated mainly on those who used only bio-medical healthcare. On the duration of the illness, we used information from patients who were sick for more than two weeks (since this has implications for job security). We also focused mainly on patients who, during their illness, visited healthcare facilities more than three times.[17] Service effectiveness was defined in this context by finding the percentage of people who were healed as a function of their number over the sample size of 300. Patients' responses to these basic questions were collated and are presented in Table 2.2.

The patient/data selection concentrated on patients who returned more than three times and those who used bio-medical services; thereby omitting those

Table 2.2 Distribution of respondents according to effectiveness of healthcare access in sampled metropolitan LGAs of Lagos and Oyo States (%)

Location	Local Government Area (LGA)	Sick for at least two weeks	Took drugs prescribed	Cured
Lagos	Agege	78.0	51.5	70.7
	Ajeromi-Ifelodun	64.0	69.0	43.0
	Alimosho	83.3	50.0	66.0
	Amuwo-Odofin	28.3	77.5	20.3
	Apapa	92.0	58.9	42.7
Ibadan	Egbeda	65.7	59.3	32.7
	Ibadan North	95.7	91.7	70.0
	Iddo	43.0	34.3	66.0
	Ibadan North-West	93.0	51.5	59.3
	Ibadan South East	70.3	82.1	59.3
Lagos	All 5 LGAs above	69.1	58.9	48.5
Ibadan	All 5 LGAs above	73.5	67.2	57.5

Source: Primary data, 300 respondents per LGA interviewed in bio-medical health institutions

[16] Doctors and pharmacists interviewed in the pilot stage recommended 'two weeks' as a benchmark to measure the length of an illness. Diseases have a period of gestation and incubation before the symptoms are visible. After drugs have been administered, visible signs of healing would show for most illnesses within the first 3 to 5 days, or at most 10 to 15 days.

[17] Doctors explained that when cases are not critical enough to warrant admission, they monitor progress in drug administration at appointments and that a patient's reaction to a drug should be determinable on the third appointment.

who came less frequently and/or those who may have decided that bio-medical care was too expensive. We concede that we do not know the proportion of 'infrequent' patients, those who were not cured and/or those who used some form of alternative care. This way of looking at the data is, no doubt, biased, and it is but one way of looking at them.

From Table 2.2, we observe that about 70% of the respondents for the two cities under review were sick for two weeks prior to seeking bio-medical intervention. The reasons for this delay range from trying alternative means of healing to just waiting to see if the person's health would change for the better. For example, those who had a high temperature thought they had an ordinary fever before seeking treatment for malaria, for which a proper diagnosis is available at hospital, We also noticed that the proportion of respondents who were sick for more than two weeks was marginally higher in Ibadan than in Lagos. Ibadan, having more rural and peri-urban LGA respondents, stated delays such as the distance to hospital and a longer waiting time for consultations as barriers to seeking immediate bio-medical care, until they realized their condition was not improving. Despite this, patients in urban parts of Ibadan (the southeast and the north) seemed to trust the care they received more (or they could afford the drugs prescribed) as it is shown that two-thirds of the respondents obtained and used prescriptions from the pharmacy that were prescribed by the doctors. However, the data obtained did not show if such patients had more money or if there was a better availability of medicines in urban areas of Ibadan than Lagos. In Lagos, a little more than half of the respondents who were sick for two weeks or more took their doctor's prescription, thereby indicating a lower level of distrust of services dispensed at government-owned Western-style medical service delivery units; or a relative lack of financial resources to procure healthcare services. While a lack of trust could be related to population pressure on facilities that caused delays, some respondents claimed that the care they received was inadequate as doctors and other medical personnel did not have enough time to give proper diagnosis and treatment to patients. When probed further on why they then repeatedly visit such institutions, it was revealed that on the one hand they might be lucky and get good treatment on one such visit if there were fewer patients there; and on the other hand, more importantly, 'excuse from work' or 'sick leave' notes from government healthcare institutions have more weight when patients want to defend or apply for sick leave. It is important to note that without 'excuse from work' notes, sick workers could be treated no better than erring ones and sick workers might be queried about their absence or could have part of their salary deducted for the days they are absent.

The percentage of the population that is healed as a ratio of the total population in the sample size of those seeking healthcare in the local government

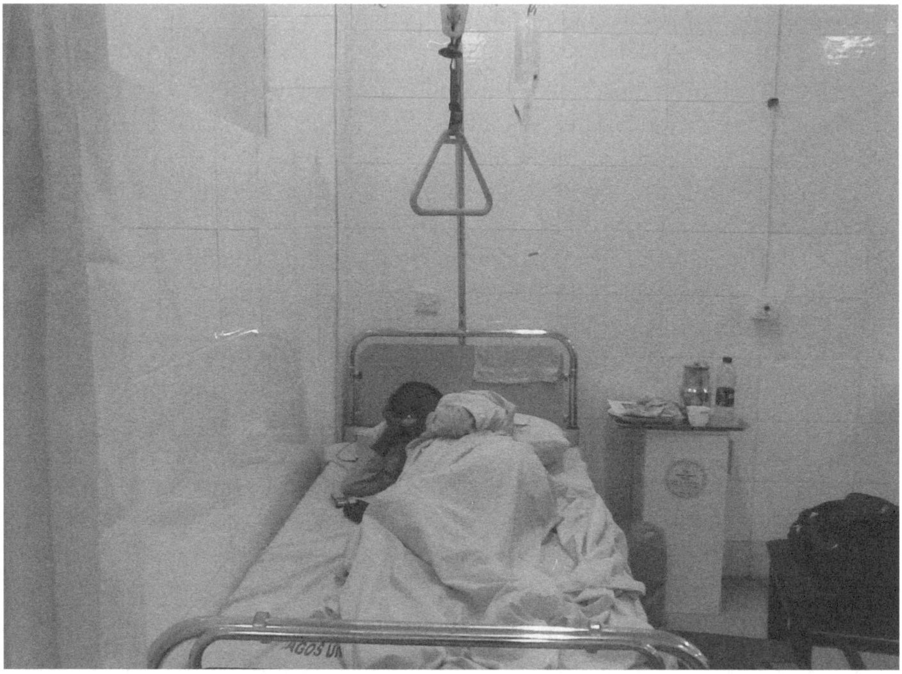

Photo 2.2 A patient in the private ward of Lagos University Teaching Hospital [Photo: Rantimi Jays Julius-Adeoye]

areas examined is not as high as in the two states. This could have arisen from the following scenarios: healthcare seekers taking their medication incorrectly; using fake drugs purchased cheaply from the ubiquitous street vendors; an outright refusal to use the medications prescribed or possible drug failure. While it must be conceded that a patient's behaviour plays an important role here, all the factors stated are capable of eroding healthcare quality in Lagos and Ibadan. When this is juxtaposed with the fact that relative to the population, the number of healthcare centres in Lagos and Ibadan is inadequate, one gets the picture that healthcare delivery in Lagos and Ibadan is grossly flawed. However, this number may have been underestimated since data on those who sought private hospitals and other non-bio-medical units were not considered.

Another important qualification that must be made concerns the differences observed in the data among the local government areas. One important factor is the distinction between rural and urban areas. The data presented on access demonstrated that it is higher in urban areas. Similarly, government interventions and control are higher in urban areas than in peri-urban areas, where their presence is felt less and in the rural areas where little or no presence can be seen to exist. In Ibadan, for instance, the study found that local government areas have no fewer than three resident doctors each, while those in peri-urban areas each have one resident doctor. Local councils in these peri-urban areas, it should be noted, do have between three and five dispensaries, maternity homes and other health facilities. This important development has serious implications for healthcare delivery not just for the study areas of Lagos and Ibadan, but for Nigeria as a whole.

Locality-specific factors are also at play. If we take Amuwo-Odofin as a guide, the local government here had the lowest number of ill people, a higher number of patients who were seeking medical care but a lower number of patients that got better. The hazy picture this presents could be seen to result from many different factors. On the one hand, there are factors associated with respondents' general living conditions or characteristics such as (i) the nature of the illness or (ii) the geographical location (especially when residents sleep in one place and work somewhere else where they seek medical care, which is known as 'sleeping locality'). Sleeping locality underscores lower hospital attendance, as noticed in Amuwo-Odofin. On the other hand, there are factors related to the sales of fake and/or sub-standard drugs there. The data show that despite high intakes of prescribed drugs, a low proportion of patients were reportedly cured. These and many other differences are noticed in the local government areas' data, but owing to space and the need for focus, these and many other issues have been excluded from the analysis in this chapter.

Some other obstacles to healthcare delivery include infrastructural requirements such as pipe-borne water, electricity, roads and recreational facilities (Bokhari 1982: 11-14). The impact of the relative absence of these infrastructures in peri-urban and rural areas negatively impacts on healthcare delivery (Okafor 1984; Stock 1983). For instance, ambulance services that require deploying medical personnel to deliver healthcare services are often unavailable although they are supposed to be provided in rural parts of Nigeria. Where these services do exist, bad roads stand as a major obstacle to the prompt movement of healthcare personnel even in emergency situations. While some of these infrastructural requirements abound in urban centres, the relative absence of such facilities in peri-urban and rural areas portends untoward danger for healthcare delivery. The situation becomes complex as 53% of Nigerians live in rural areas (Population Reference Bureau 2009). While launching the 34th initiative to revive healthcare delivery in the state in November 2009, Mr Raji Fashola, the Executive Governor of Lagos State, noted that 'the services at the Primary Healthcare Centers suffered a major setback in the country and this has brought decay and loss of confidence in the Primary Healthcare Systems. We cannot allow this to continue as the health of our people in this state is a top priority and it must be given the prime attention it deserves. It is in this spirit that the state government embarked on the journey of overhauling the decayed healthcare system.'[18]

To increase access to healthcare, the Nigerian government instituted a number of measures between 1999 and 2003, the main one being the National Health Insurance Scheme (NHIS).[19] But only a few people currently fall within the group that the NHIS covers as the scheme encompasses government employees, the organized private sector and the informal sector. Legally, the scheme also covers children under five, those who are permanently disabled and prison inmates. In 2004, the government further empowered the scheme by bringing in a couple of amendments to the original 1999 legislation. Healthcare facilities in the NHIS scheme are to provide healthcare services to registered members who, in turn, pay for these services through monthly premiums. Privately-owned healthcare facilities are expected to join publicly-owned ones for the programme to attain its aims. To fund the programme, the costs of diagnosis, surgery and medication are initially borne by the insurance scheme and are paid for by patients over a period of time. The beauty of the NHIS is that it allows access to healthcare by removing the barriers earlier posed by equity and distance. Its effectiveness is still being assessed (Oshi 2009). Under the programme, public and private institutions have been designated as NHIS centres where individuals are encouraged to register to access healthcare at fixed and affordable prices. To assure quality care, the government set minimum benchmarks for participating institutions and practitioners. It was hoped that through the NHIS, healthcare delivery would reach everyone and at an affordable cost, but this is yet to happen. Other measures taken to ameliorate these and the many other problems besetting healthcare delivery in Nigeria include the expansion of healthcare provision, which has given further credence to the use of alternative healthcare such as faith healing and herbal cures. While this development has served to validate the impact or belief in the efficacy of alternative healthcare, it also suggests that the government (for example Lagos State) has admitted its inability to provide adequate, effective and efficient healthcare for its citizens. Although no state has yet set up any alternative/herbal healthcare facilities, the states have passed bills that have given an impetus to the provision of alternative/herbal cure. Alternative/herbal cure usage is not only prominent amongst peri-urban and rural dwellers, its use even predominates in urban centres (Obi *et al.* 2006; Ajaiyeoba *et al.* 2003). This is due more to the fact that healthcare is relatively cheaper to access for herbal cures compared to the costs associated

---

[18] 'See: http://www.lagosstate.gov.ng/index.php?page=news&nid=283.

[19] See 'National Health Insurance Launched in Abuja', *The Nation*, 23 July 2000, pp. 2, 5 and 45.

Table 2.3 Comparative costs of securing treatment in hospitals and in alternative (traditional) service centres

Illness	Relative costs of securing treatment (in Naira)	
	Bio-medical/Western hospitals	Alternative healthcare
Delivery without complications	15,000.00	5,000.00
Common cold, headache and fever	3,000.00	100.00
Fever	5,000.00	200.00
Fracture (arm)	25,000.00	7,000.00
Fracture (leg)	30,000.00	7,000.00
Ulcer	30,000.00	2,000.00
Hernia	35,000.00	1,200.00
Diabetes	15,000.00	3,000.00

Source: Retired nurse and chief matron, based in Ibadan.
Note: €1 = N200 (April 2010)

with treatments in bio-medical hospital units. Table 2.3 highlights the differential rates of treatment in the two systems.

The cost of securing treatment for ailments in bio-medical hospital units is relatively higher compared to the cost of using alternative healthcare. The cost differential in absolute terms could, for example, be three times higher if women used maternity delivery services in formal bio-medical hospitals, and would be thirty times higher if they sought treatment for fever, compared to the costs of local herbal medicine. In this situation, the retired chief matron who provided data on costs said that some patients inadvertently 'use Western hospitals to get a proper diagnosis of their health condition but [then] procure drugs from local herbal sources'. While this elucidates on cost differentials, it says nothing about effectiveness. Other respondents interviewed in formal hospitals concurred that there are two healthcare systems in Nigeria: a traditional and informal system made up of herbalists, seers, midwives, pastors and imams, and a modern, public/semi-private, formalized bio-medical service delivery system. They argued that medical pluralism, whose provenance could not be ascertained, is gaining prominence in Lagos and Ibadan, and has been orchestrated by a pragmatic combination of Western/bio-medical and alternative healthcare systems, manifesting medical pluralism in a variety of forms.

Conclusion

Since the arrival of the third wave of democracy in Nigeria in 1999, two healthcare services have increasingly gained in prominence: the traditional and informal system; and the modern, public and semi-private, formalized system with its bio-medical treatments, doctors and nurses. While none of this is a recent development, the two systems, which are mutually supportive and intricately linked, are juxtaposed spatially and socially in a structure of medical pluralism. In Lagos and Ibadan, the two cases used in this chapter, problems associated with access to and the effectiveness of bio-medical healthcare services have served as the impetus for a burgeoning landscape of the traditional and informal system.

Various attempts by the government to intervene in healthcare delivery, especially in the privatization and liberalization of the health sector through the National Health Insurance Scheme and other options, have brought unanticipated developments, the main one being entrepreneurization, which is characterized by the referral and private-in-public systems. Opinions differ even among medical practitioners as to the impact and necessities of these developments on healthcare delivery. For some, the development signals eroding standards, which is impinging on healthcare delivery. For others, it enables the sector to rise above dwindling government funding and to lift healthcare delivery above the line, although at a cost. Caught in the dividing lines of both arguments is the patient who either pays more for healthcare or seeks alternative care with faith healers and herbal-medicine dealers.

This unfolding argument challenges the role of the state in healthcare provisioning in Lagos and Ibadan in particular, and in Nigeria in general. When healthcare is privatized and private entrepreneurs whose concerns are primarily a return on investment are allowed to dictate the pace, healthcare ceases to be a public good.

While this development could be blamed on many factors, the nation's economic situation is not helpful. In addition, Nigeria used to have long-term plans for the different sectors of the economy laid out in five-year development plans, but its current political leadership appears to place more emphasis on rhetoric rather than on delivering on promises. Between 1999 and 2010, the number of newly constructed healthcare facilities in Nigeria has not seen a significant increase but this is not because governments have been static. Attempts have indeed been made to right some of these wrongs and programmes have been orchestrated such as the introduction of free health (for example in Lagos and Ondo States by the current political leadership) based on the perspective that healthcare is a public and a merit good, and not a private good. But more often than not, free healthcare in public health facilities is limited to diagnosis. Another development has been the current privatization of healthcare delivery, which is premised on the concept that the market mechanism potentially posses in-built valves to ensure access and quality healthcare even for the rural poor. For now, evidence weighs on the inability of market mechanisms to deliver on promises, rather than making healthcare accessible to all. The commoditization of healthcare services and delivery is gaining ground and new forms of healthcare institutions, such as the private-in-public healthcare units, are being entrenched. But the huge costs associated with healthcare procurement in the private-in-public system are commensurate with the quality of care received by patients. The costs of service are relatively high in private-in-public healthcare units yet public patronage indicates that they perceive such units as providing better services. It is too early to conjecture the implication of private-in-public healthcare facilities on class formation but evidence from this study indicates that a large proportion of the population are excluded from accessing this service due to cost considerations.

With these and many other concerns in mind, such as inefficient public utilities and infrastructure, there are limitations on access to public healthcare by the urban and rural poor. A section of the populace is thus cut off from public service; thereby imposing greater pressure on areas where relatively affordable or accessible healthcare services abound. It will not be surprising if in the not too distant future, informal healthcare provisioning, faith healing and alternative or traditional healing practices overtake Western bio-medical healthcare provision, summing up institutional failure to revamp the PUBLIC healthcare delivery system in Nigeria.

References

Adib, S.M. (2004), From the biomedical model to the Islamic alternative: A brief overview of medical practices in the contemporary Arab world. *Social Science and Medicine* 58: 697-702.

Ajaiyeoba, E.O., O. Oladepo, O.I. Fawole, O.M. Bolaji, D.O. Akinboye, O.A.T. Ogundahunsi, C.O. Falade, G.O. Gbotosho, O.A. Itiola, T.C. Happi, O.O. Ebong, I.M. Omoniwu, O.S. Osowole, O.O. Oduola, J.S. Ashidi & A.M.J. Oduola (2003), Cultural categorization of febrile illnesses in correlation with herbal remedies used for treatment in Southwestern Nigeria. *Journal of Ethnopharmacology* 85(2-3): 179-185.

Ayeni, B., G. Rushton & M.L. McNulty (1987), Improving the geographical accessibility of health care in rural areas: A Nigerian case study. *Social Science and Medicine* 25(10): 1083-1094.

Barnes, L.L., G.A. Plotnikoff, K. Fox & S. Pendleton (2000), Spirituality, religion, and pediatrics: Intersecting worlds of healing. *Pediatrics*, Supplement 106(4).

Bokhari, R.H. (1982), *Subvention policy and practices for public enterprises*. Ljubljana: International Center for Public Enterprises in Developing Countries.

Connell, J., P. Zurn, B. Stilwell, M. Awases & J-M. BracheT (2007), Sub-Saharan Africa: Beyond the health worker migration crisis? *Social Science and Medicine* 64(9): 1876-1891.

Duckett, S.J. (2004), *The Australian health care system*. Melbourne: Oxford University Press.

Eastwood, J.B., R.E. Conroy, S. Naicker, P.A. West & J. Plange-Rhule (2005), Loss of health professionals from Sub-Saharan Africa: The pivotal role of the UK. *The Lancet* 365(9474):1893.

Evans, I. (1994), Editorial, structural adjustment too painful? *The Lancet* 344: 1377-1378.

Ezeome, E.R. & A.N. Anarado (2007), Use of complementary and alternative medicine by cancer patients at the University of Nigeria Teaching Hospital, Enugu, Nigeria, *BMC Complementary and Alternative Medicine* 7(28).

Fatiregun, A.A., I.O. Yisa & A.E. Olumide (2007), Utilization and costs of medical services at military health facilities in Ibadan, Nigeria. *Journal of Medical Systems* 31: 505-509.

Heald, D. (1985), Privatization policies, methods and procedures. Conference on privatization policies, methods and procedures. Manila, Philippines, 31 January - 1 February.

Kunz, F.A. (1991), Liberalization in Africa: Some preliminary reflections. *African Affairs* 90(359): 223-235.

Logan, B.I. (1995), Can Sub-Saharan Africa successfully privatize its health care sector?. In: K. Mengisteab & B.I. Logan, eds, *Beyond economic liberalization in Africa: Structural adjustment and the alternatives*, pp. 59-65. London: Zed Books.

Logan, B.I. & K. Mengisteab, eds (1995), *Beyond economic liberalization in Africa: Structural Adjustment and the alternatives*. London: Zed Books.

Nigerian Institute of Social and Economic Research (EC-EMCAP/NISER) (2005), *Study on effectiveness of public expenditure in Nigeria, Final report volumes 1 & 2*. Nigeria: Okley Printers.

Obi, E., D.N. Akunyili, B. Ekpo & O.E. Orisakwe (2006), Heavy metal hazards of Nigerian herbal remedies. *Science of the Total Environment* 369(1-3): 35-41.

Ogunbekun, I., A. Ogunbekun & N. Orobaton (1999), Private health care in Nigeria: Walking the tightrope. *Health Policy and Planning* 14(2): 174-181.

Okafor, C.B. & R.R. Rizzuto (1994), Women's and health-care providers' views of maternal practices and services in rural Nigeria. *Studies in Family Planning* 25(6): 353-361.

Okafor, F.C. (1984), Accessibility to general hospitals in rural Bendel State, Nigeria. *Social Science and Medicine* 18(8): 661-666.

Onwudiegwu, U. (1997), The effect of a depressed economy on the utilization of maternal health services: The Nigerian experience II. *Journal of Obstetrics and Gynaecology* 17(2): 143-148.

Orubuloye, I.O., J.C. Caldwell, P. Caldwell & C.H. Bledsoe (1991), The impact of family and budget structure on health treatment in Nigeria. *Health Transition Review* 1(2): 189-209.

Orubuloye, I.O. & O.Y. Oyeneye (1982), Primary health care in developing countries: The case of Nigeria, Sri Lanka and Tanzania. *Social Science and Medicine* 16(6): 675-686.

Oshi, D.C. (2009), *Rural women and the financing of health care in Nigeria*. Maastricht: Shaker Publishing.

Population Reference Bureau (2009), *World population data sheet*. Population Reference Bureau, Washington DC. www.prb.org

Stock, R. (1983), Distance and the utilization of health facilities in rural Nigeria. *Social Science and Medicine* 17(9): 563-570.

Vecchiato, N.L. (1993), Illness, therapy, and change in Ethiopian possession cults. *Africa, Journal of the International African Institute* 63(2): 176-196.

World Health Organization (2000), *The world health report 2000: Health systems: Improving performance*. Geneva: WHO.

3

Organizing monies: The reality and creativity of nursing on a hospital ward in Ghana

Christine Böhmig

The introduction of Western medicine in Africa changed perceptions of health and appropriate healthcare. The subsequent globalization of the health sector has presented new ways of treating patients and has opened the door to modern facilities and professions. Looking at the situation in Ghana, the concept of health and expectations about the delivery of care on hospitalization are complex. While traditionally health and illness are perceived as social conditions, modern definitions have transformed health into a traded good and assess its weight as a commodity. This chapter presents the perspective of nurses as agents in the health sector where ideas on good care collide with the reality of badly equipped hospital wards, and Christian convictions of serving the suffering with financial restraints and delayed treatments as patients face unpredictable costs. Nurses are finding themselves engaged as creative entrepreneurs who need to develop tools to navigate through uncertainties and respond to the needs put before them. It is argued that nurses are oscillating between professional standards and socioeconomic demands.

Introduction

Visiting hour starts at seven o'clock in the morning on the female medical ward in Accra's main hospital. Family members enter the building and hurry to see their wives, daughters, aunties or sisters, bringing food, assisting in washing and praying with them. They also check whether a new prescription has been written by the doctors indicating the start of a new course of medication, whether an examination is to be done or additional dressing material is needed. Hardly any patient is covered by insurance and in addition to the regular costs of hospital admission, all medications, dressing materials and examinations like blood tests, X-rays and CT scans have to be paid for by the family. A young woman moves between the beds selling toothbrushes, toilet paper and buckets, snacks and soft drinks. The nurses are keen to spot family members because as part of their work, they sell diapers for incontinent patients and blood-sugar strips to check the sugar level of newly admitted patients and those with diabetes. Outstanding costs are carefully itemized on a list next to the nurses' table and collected during visiting hour. Less than an hour later, the matron asks the visitors to leave the ward and the sick lie quietly in bed as the nurses gather for a prayer before starting their morning shift.

This scene is typical of many wards and health centres in Ghana. Patients feel overwhelmed and intimidated by the organization and requirements when admitted, nurses serve as guides, direct activities and are in control of the ward and its patients. Looking more closely, we can identify mechanisms of coping with illness and economic demands and ways of incorporating them into nursing concepts. They help us understand the organization and functioning of the current healthcare system and its place in daily life in Ghana. While traditional healing and the treatment of disease have always been connected to financial costs and various forms of reciprocity, the role of money is of high importance in a successful treatment programme in a biomedical setting. This chapter explores the impact of financial constraints on the delivery of care in hospitals in Ghana. Nursing today cannot be understood without some historical framing and conceptual considerations of the reality of modern Ghana. The hospital as a place of healthcare delivery thus needs to be positioned within the surrounding society. Cultural norms, social roles and economic mechanisms are manifest in hospital routines, challenge their organization and offer solutions. By highlighting developments and shifts in the understanding of nursing, current forms of care in modern Ghana can be examined and the commodification of care questioned. Focusing on the ideas and actions of nurses, the factors that influence their work and the framework within which care is delivered will be shown. To understand the impact and functioning of money and the processes in the marketization of healthcare delivery, the chapter describes the development and financing of biomedicine and the working reality of nurses today, analyzes the situation of patients and nurses on the ward itself and considers the forms of navigation that deliver nursing care and ensure a successful healing process for patients. The chapter is based on extensive fieldwork and anthropological research carried out on a medical female ward in Accra's teaching hospital be-

Map 3.1 Ghana

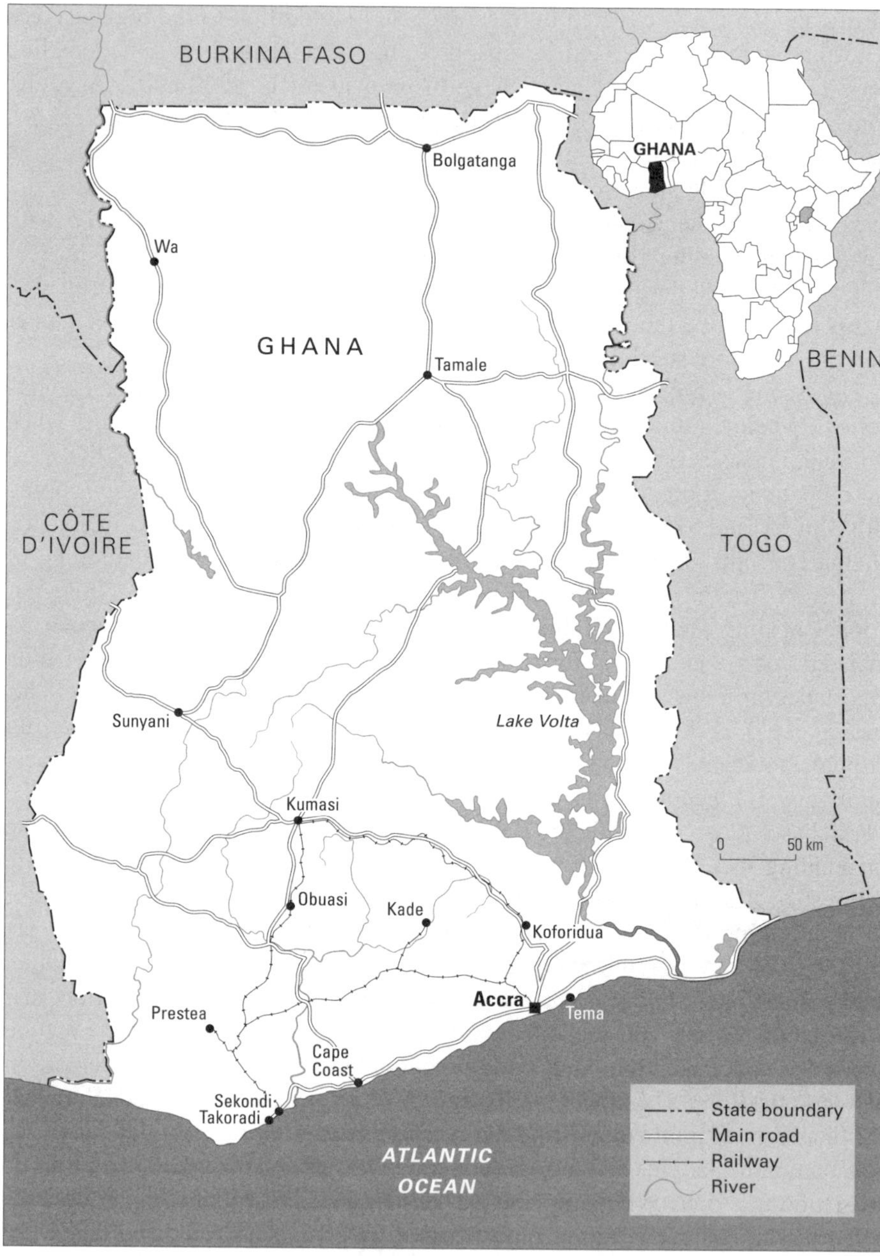

BURKINA FASO
GHANA
BENIN
TOGO
CÔTE D'IVOIRE
GHANA
Bolgatanga
Wa
Tamale
Lake Volta
Sunyani
Kumasi
Obuasi
Kade
Koforidua
Accra
Tema
Prestea
Cape Coast
Sekondi-Takoradi
ATLANTIC OCEAN
0 50 km
State boundary
Main road
Railway
River

tween 2003 and 2007 (Böhmig 2010b). It focuses on the nurses who are the main actors on the ward day and night and are in regular contact with the patients. By working alongside the nurses, sharing their daily routine and talking about their motives and challenges, their working reality and its underlying perceptions became visible.

The concept of health and healing in Ghana

Having celebrated 50 years of political independence in 2007, Ghanaian society is facing various changes. Traditional norms of rendering respect, upholding the solidarity of the family, recognizing the authority of older members and striving for a balanced reciprocity remain crucial values. Children are socialized with the notion of respect towards older family members and society as a whole. Religion offers a stabilizing factor. Ghanaians young and old confirm that Ghana is a religious country: 'If we talk about all things and don't add the religious part, it's like there's nothing inside' (nurse, aged 57). In addition to traditional beliefs, Christian denominations predominate in the south and centre of the country, while in most people in the north are Muslim. Whether a person attends a more established church or one of the countless Charismatic and Pentecostal churches is of less concern. Disputes about beliefs and dogmas play a subordinate role: what is important is that a person is a practising believer (Nukunya 2003; Senah 2004; De Witte 2008). To be 'a good Christian' one has to go to church regularly and lead a life according to the Bible. Since the liberalization of the media in 1992, television and radio stations have continuously reported religious developments and have broadcast Bible studies and church services. The Church plays an important role in regulating the daily lives of Christians in Ghana. Church welfare committees support members in times of hardship, helping to finance health expenditures and funerals; and prayer groups support church members in times of illness. Years of political unrest and economic hardship have led to migration, changes in labour practices and shifts in social cohesion (Hagopian *et al.* 2005). But Ghanaian society has also been influenced by globalization and new growing markets characterized by mass labour migration and the transfer of monies. Trends in urbanization and monetarization can be seen in the rise of mobile phones and Internet cafés in both urban and rural settings.

Ghanaians have traditionally always understood health and illness as being integrated. Illness is seen as a combination of social events and the supranatural, and health and illness are part of the whole magico-religious fabric (Twumasi 2005: 8). Disease is seen as 'a painful thing' (Ventevogel 1996: 15) that reflects a disturbance in the harmony between elements of social and physical life. In this framework, the causes of disease are sought in witchcraft, bad medicine, misfortune or spiritual forces and almost never in natural forces alone. Traditional healers explain disease on physical and social causation, and their services include consultations, treatment and prevention. Knowledge of traditional medicine has evolved over generations and skills are passed on through apprenticeship training. Traditional healers use an individualized approach to diagnose and treat patients, and the low number of patients per healer is attractive to many Ghanaians. The biomedical setting in hospitals forms a contrast to this understanding, representing hope and 'do-ability', also through images and reports transported in the modern media, the unpredictability in outcome and the economic consequences. Bierlich (2000) describes the ambivalence towards biomedicine that is seen as attractive and powerful but also feared, positioning the sick individual in a dilemma (see also Horton 2001; Vaughan 1991).

The individual is caught between tradition and change when it comes to health-seeking behaviour. When someone becomes ill, the patient and his family have to determine a plan of action and navigate their way through the various healthcare options. The choice of treatment is often based on experience. Combining traditional and Western treatments is not perceived as a contradiction but instead as a powerful and promising mixture. The complex formal and informal health facilities and the problem of accessibility given the urban-rural bias of health facilities form, together with cultural norms and post-colonial experiences, a continuum to which the individual looks for an explanation and therapeutic options (Senah 1997; Ventevogel 1996; Takyi 2003). The advantages of Western medicine are recognized, such as the impressive reduction in infant mortality rates[1] from almost 250 to 58 per 1,000, compared to 76 in low-income countries and 6 in high-income countries (Buor 2004), the eradication and/or reduction in levels of various diseases, and nationwide immunization programmes that have led to a rise in the quality of life and higher life expectancy – 57 in Ghana compared to 78 in Germany and 49 in Nigeria (WHO 2006). However when they become ill, people often hesitate to visit a health centre or hospital. Research shows that about 20% of the population need medical help but of these only about 20% can afford the costs involved (Korle Bu 2006: 8). WHO country health indicators indicate that Ghana had a per capita gross national income of US$ 320 in 2003, with almost 45% of the population living below the poverty line, and per capita health expenditure was US$ 17 (see also Appendix B & C). The monthly income of a general nurse was approximately US$ 250, placing, the profession among the range of middle-class jobs accessible to women, and comparable with school teachers and secretaries. Most of the patients in public hospitals are market

[1] According to health statistics, 60% of infant deaths are caused by malnutrition.

women, workers and farmers with much lower and less certain incomes. An unforeseen hospital admission forms a personal, social and financial threat to many.

The organization of (biomedical) healthcare in Ghana

Formal medical work officially started in Accra in 1878 when huts were erected to serve as medical posts for government forces (Twumasi 2005: 65). In 1880, the Gold Coast Medical Department was established to organize and supervise preventive services like vaccinations and sanitation. The first British nursing sisters arrived in Ghana in 1899 to start caring for the white administrators, soldiers, traders and their accompanying family members. There was little understanding of the existing traditional health system. Medicine was an instrument of power (Vaughan 1991). The parallel introduction of formal education and upcoming urbanization had an additional influence on the process of acceptance. Understanding that healthy workers increased the economic and political wealth of the colony, the indigenous population was soon forced to seek Western medicine in case of illness (Curtin 1992). At the beginning, there was much resistance within the African population to consulting Western sources, let alone assisting the doctors and nurses. The traditional system opposed the concept and practices of Western medicine that were so different to the traditional cosmological order. Patterson (1981: 15) wrote:

> The colonial physician was often a puzzling figure for Africans. He was usually a white male stranger who had to use an interpreter. He often asked impolite questions, demanded, for reasons unknown to the patient, samples of blood, urine and faeces; and sometimes cut open the bodies of the dead. On the other hand, he frequently had great power over sickness and injury.

The health problems then can be described as mainly environmental (Twumasi 2005: 66). In hospitals, the main diagnoses were pulmonary tuberculosis, lobar pneumonia, anaemia and epidemics of yellow fever, while malaria was the main cause of infant mortality (Hawe 1962: 16). Reflecting on the introduction of Western medicine in Africa, it is necessary to touch on the underlying ideology in Europe. Medicine in the nineteenth century was characterized by scientific discoveries, imperialistic politics and colonial power constellations. This led to a shift in thought towards an objectification of the human body and the de-individualization of the person in Europe and the colonies alike. Foucault (2003), analyzing the rise of hospitals in France, shows its social implications and the construction of power between actors and the formation of the body as the site of these power relations. These ideological and social changes led to the increased use of scientific medicine and the establishment of a rigid medical group. In Africa, biomedicine was presented as superior and was not questioned.

After independence in 1957, the building of more health centres became a priority in Ghana. The number of medical doctors increased from 330 to about 960 in the late 1980s while that of nurses grew from 800 to over 5,000. The start of the country's own nursing training in 1945 and the opening of the medical school in Accra in 1964 were aimed at improving the situation further. However political unrest and Ghana's economic decline led to poor health facilities and an unsatisfactory supply of drugs and materials. Patients seeking help in hospitals had to provide their own medication, bed linen and even stationery for their medical records (Senah 1997). The key health problems during this period were worsened by an absence of organization, poor procedures and an unrealistic budget. Healthcare was either not available or was of poor quality. Unequal access to facilities and the concentration on hospital-based curative care instead of on preventive and educational programmes led to continuous health problems. The political instability, socio-economic crisis and financial constraints increased self-medication and visits to traditional healers. The exodus of health workers continued and by the 1990s, about 30% of Ghana's trained health workers had left the country to work abroad.

The 2000 census counted more than 1,100 doctors and 13,000 nurses, of whom a third were working within the Greater Accra Region. These numbers indicate a shortfall of 50% to 65% in the public health sector (Nyanotor 2004). Most health workers want to live within Accra or Kumasi where there are better-equipped hospitals, better living conditions and the patient population is more educated. While only about a third of Ghana's population live in these urban centres, more than two-thirds of the health personnel work there (Twumasi 2005, Ventevogel 1996). This is in sharp contrast to the needs of the health service (see Appendix B). Although more hospitals are being built and health workers trained, the provision of healthcare facilities has not kept pace with the growing population, which has led to a population: doctor/nurse ratio of 1: 17,900 and 1:1508 respectively. In terms of access to care, about 40% of the population is estimated to live more than 15 km from a health facility, with rural areas being generally less well served (Ghana Ministry of Health 2003; Arhinful 2003).

Nursing in Ghana

In 1878 the first European nurses arrived on the Gold Coast to care for European officials. The aim was to care for the sick and maintain a healthy living environment for both Europeans and Africans (Holden 1991). These nurses were carefully selected and instructed to represent their home country and its moral norms. This order and discipline was symbolized in their working attitude and spotless white uniform. The 'right type of woman' was often compared to a soldier, as Tooley wrote: 'No place is too remote, no climate too deadly for the nurse to ply her ministrations. Like the soldier she obeys the call of duty and if need be gives her life for the cause' (in Holden 1991: 68). With the formal beginning of medicine in 1878, it became apparent that there were too few British nurses and that locals were needed to support the doctors, bathe and feed patients and dress their wounds. But nursing had a low status and working in these new institutions (hospitals) where white doctors practised an unknown healing system was unattractive. Another new element was the content of the work, namely dealing with naked bodies, blood, faeces and bad smells; it was seen as menial work and not considered 'proper'. The recruitment of candidates constituted a formidable problem (Addae 1996; Kisseih 1968). Dr Henderson, the Chief Medical Officer, reported: 'No native of intelligence would like to be a nurse because the pay is low and conditions of service are not good' (Owusu 1980: 1). It was a long time before perceptions changed and nursing became an accepted and well-rewarded profession (Böhmig 2010a, Sumani 2005). Work on these wards was from the beginning characterized by a shortage of nurses and a heavy workload, which put limitations on the work and led to frustrations (Akiwumi 1971; Opare & Mill 2000).

The start of formal nursing in Ghana brought about an interesting development. While caring in homes and compounds was the domain of women, nursing in health institutions was a new phenomenon. Cultural barriers forbade women from joining the nursing profession, and it was male school-leavers who were trained as the first nursing assistants. The European perception of the good woman caring for the sick could not immediately be translated into this context. Although working outside the house was possible for women, for example as market women or traders, dealing with sick strangers was initially regarded as inappropriate. It took time before formal school education was introduced and girls were admitted to secondary education. Secretarial work, teaching and midwifery became options for these girls, professions that were imported from Europe and labelled 'typical female activities'. Nursing was added to this group of 'female professions' slightly later. It underwent a change in perception and since it meant direct work under and with the colonial power, it was perceived as respected and venerable. The white nursing uniform reinforced this idea. Some 45 years after the arrival of the first nurses in Ghana, the nursing profession became attractive and accepted for women to choose after they had finished school. The rationale and practical work were copied from the British model without cultural adaptations. A similar approach was chosen in Uganda and Zambia (Martin 2006; Schuster 1980). Schuster (1980: 78) criticizes this as a 'cultural process of imitation … the perpetuation of colonial dependency'.

Even today, there is little place for traditional healing in hospitals, with nurses and doctors following the imported Western understanding of healing and care. Akiwumi (1995) researched nurses' ideas about their role and competencies and found that newly trained nurses experienced feelings of insecurity and a lack of practical routine when entering the work floor. The qualities required of a nurse continued to be defined as observant, responsible, punctual, accurate and patient, attributes that are generally labelled as female and Christian, confirming the existing gender perception of the 'good woman'.

Financing healthcare

Ghanaian society is based on reciprocity and solidarity within the family and kinship (van der Geest 1997). In times of need, individuals turn to their family to mobilize financial resources in exchange for past or future investment in social-capital formation. With urbanization and migration, this system of social security is under threat and is failing. The state introduced a new organizational model that was based on the market and formal sector. In 1954 the newly established Ministry of Health recommended the abolition of hospital fees and charges, but kept prices for drugs. As there was no functioning tax system, financing of the health system soon became difficult (Arhinful 2003: 47). After independence in 1957, the President of the First Republic, Dr Kwame Nkrumah, launched a ten-year plan that included the reduction and in most cases abolition of costs for users of the health service, but this led to an escalation of the financing problem. The military regime that overthrew Nkrumah re-introduced fees and enforced their collection. The Second Republic under President Busia passed the Hospital Fee Act 1971. However the economic and social crisis in Ghana between 1975 and 1985 led to the collapse of many health facilities and to problems in implementing the new primary healthcare strategy. The necessary drugs were not available and many health workers, nurses and doctors left Ghana to work abroad.

Around the millennium, the decision was taken to introduce the National Health Insurance Scheme (NHIS). As in other Sub-Saharan countries, this new insurance system met much initial resistance (Vogel 1999; Arhinful 2003). The NHIS, organized by communities and districts, was to replace the individualized out-of-pocket payment at service delivery points, the so-called 'cash and carry', which placed unpredictable financial burdens on family resources. The concept is based on the notion of the authority of the state demanding a new form of solidarity built on the vision of a nation to which all members, irrespective of lineage connection or tribal background, contribute. The government defined a minimum package of illnesses that all scheme would cover, comprising around 95% of all diseases in Ghana. It also included outpatient services like consultations, X-rays and ultrasounds, medications and physiotherapy, and inpatient services such as general care and accommodation, examinations and medication, surgical operations, cervical and breast cancer treatment and physiotherapy. Other services included were oral and eye-care services, maternity care including antenatal check ups, deliveries, caesarean sections and postnatal care, all emergencies (medical and surgical), and dialysis for acute renal failure. Fees were graded according to one's income (see Appendix A).

In addition to problems with social acceptance and trust, the registration process faced structural problems. Ghana has a system of non-existent or irregular street- and house-numbering and as all users had to register by address, this led to an additional delay. All houses needed to receive a traceable cluster of numbers for identification before registration could start. Many Ghanaians doubted whether the system would work; trusting the state's responsibility and liability in providing continuous healthcare and the notion of national solidarity remained complex concepts. At the time of this research, the scheme had not yet been implemented and was not operational, and payments still had to be made by patients themselves.[2] In a culture where illness (especially a serious condition) can be perceived as a punishment for individual misbehaviour or as being caused by magical powers, saving money for possible healthcare costs can be understood as creating an illness. For a patient, being hospitalized means

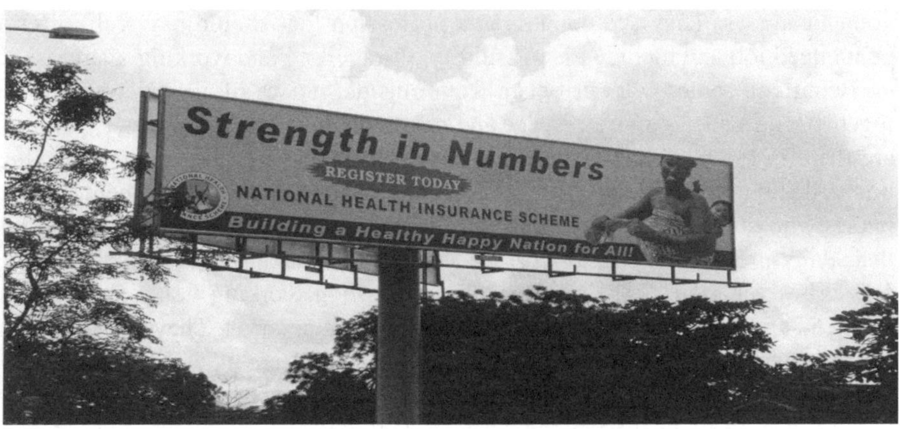
Strength in Numbers
REGISTER TODAY
NATIONAL HEALTH INSURANCE SCHEME
Building a Healthy Happy Nation for All!

Photo 3.1 Advertisement for the National Health Insurance Scheme, autumn 2005 [Photo: Christine Böhmig]

[2] In 2004, there was one Christian hospital in the Ashanti region working with the NHIS. It treated registered patients for free and claimed the costs back from the insurers. Many other hospitals were waiting to hear its experiences before implementing similar systems.

a combination of challenges and leads to physical pain, psychological uncertainties, socially embedded fears and an unpredictable financial burden. Health has become and remains a commodity; with possibilities for diagnosis and treatment depending on a person's economic means.

Motives for nursing and the concept of good care

When asked about their reasons for becoming a nurse, the current group of nurses presented various motives. There is a clear generational difference: older nurses mentioned guidance from their family and religious convictions. The decision of respected family members to enter nursing was followed up without hard feelings, although a certain romanticizing of the image and professional ignorance plays a role here. They feel like pioneers in the profession, copying and fulfilling the role of the British sisters: to be a true Christian and a well-educated woman with a spotless reputation as represented in the neatly ironed white dress, the symbol of 'the good woman'. The younger generation are also influenced by the wishes and demands of their families and exposed to existing role expectations of being a decent woman. They want to live the ideal of 'being a good woman', especially the image of an obeying, helping, trusting, humble and serving woman. Such personal beliefs strengthen the nurse and form a supportive element when carrying out their challenging work on the ward. But financial pressures and uncertainty about the future crop up in the answers of younger nurses. They see nursing as a profession that should pay well, offer a guaranteed job and include the possibility of travelling and working overseas.

Being confronted with criticism from outside, nurses of all generations join together and call for more respect and acknowledgement from society. Nurses are there in the hospitals, clinics and health posts all over the country working under difficult conditions with inadequate manpower and equipment. Those nurses who do not leave the country or the profession want to be recognized for their daily presence and hard work. Local and national strike actions take place regularly over salaries. Nurses feel that their long working hours and regular weekend and night duties should justify better remuneration. They verbalize this claim by stating that they are 'not being motivated enough'. Using the term 'motivation' is unanimously interpreted as 'sufficient money' to cover daily living costs and take part in modern markets and consumerism. This money should come in the form of enhanced salaries and additional incentives like 'extra hour allowances', preferential treatment when renting housing nearby, buying a car or purchasing land. The claim is that raising the financial reward will guarantee more satisfied workers. In this way, nurses are trying to cope with the pressure of an unsatisfying work environment and growing demands from society and the desire to (re)gain control and influence over the processes in the health service (Böhmig 2010a).

Today, there are extreme shortages of nursing personnel and a decline in the availability of working equipment. Dealing with a decrease in status and experiencing shortcomings can be difficult to handle for the older generation, which has led to a romanticizing of the pioneering period. Younger nurses find themselves caught between transmitted values, the influence of their families and modern wishes, and are struggling to find a balance. When one looks at the statements of professional bodies, it becomes clear that they define caring for the sick as the main focus of nursing. In 1997 the President of the Ghana Registered Nursing Association (GRNA) wrote:

> Colleagues of the noble nursing profession … I have confidence in you all and believe that you are all a 'CARING' dedicated people who are challenged to give best nursing care … We must be compassionate, tolerant and empathic. However, we must understand also that the best of our efforts requires a structure for skill at making decisions. (*The Ghanaian Nurse* 1997: 4)

But the GRNA's slogan does not seem powerful enough to form a stable basis within today's nursing body. Career prospects, better financial compensation and satisfying working conditions are pressing issues among today's generation and are likely to remain so. Nurses have to be creative and innovative on a daily basis to manage the challenges on the ward and to care for seriously ill patients.

Negotiating 'good care' and the role of religion

Based on Western nursing theories and rooted in Ghanaian norms of respect and authority, there are clear ideas of what constitutes a 'good nurse'. The President of GRNA stated that

> … the Ghanaian nurse has certain qualities: she is honest, punctual, qualified and intelligent, yes she must be intelligent. Nurses have to dress moderately and not overdress. A health worker has to be neat when talking about health, otherwise it is not good. We are a role model and people watch us.[3]

As mentioned above, the work of the British nurses was first seen as inappropriate and dirty but soon came to be perceived as a 'service to God and mankind'. Nurses formed a well-organized group in the face of sickness, dirt and death. Taking care of severely ill and dying patients and carrying out the Christian idea of servitude soon came to be highly valued. The nursing profession turned into the perfect activity for God-fearing and mankind-respecting women who wanted to serve society.

3 Personal communication, autumn 2005.

Building on this understanding and in combination with their religious convictions, nurses today see their attitude as empathetic. Even so, their working conditions are unforgiving and unpredictable, and their reward comes from wishing to 'touch somebody's life and be useful to the community'. But they remain psychologically distanced from their patients and control their emotions, 'crying with them does not help'. The nurses on the ward organize their work within the given framework and, unlike situations in other parts of Africa or Asia, the involvement of patients' families is restricted to short visiting hours (cf. Zaman 2005; Andersen 2004). Even so, the workload is high, basic care like washing, feeding and bed-making is carried out by nurses and their assistants; relatives are discouraged and corrected in their attempts. This can be understood as an attempt to fit the expectations of the hard-working nurse who is in charge in all situations and lives up to the prestigious image that results in high status. They are directive towards patients and try to present their profession as a necessary complement to that of the doctors. All nurses present themselves as confirmed Christians and see this as a prerequisite for being a good nurse. Praying and accepting God's ultimate plan for patients is inherent in their definition of nursing care. This way nurses fulfil the role model of a well-educated woman who is morally pure and whose behaviour is indisputable (Böhmig 2010c).

Respect for more senior nurses is another important factor that guides a nurse's actions and understanding of care. Experienced nurses are seen as role models for their younger colleagues and knowledgeable authorities in their families and neighbourhoods. They expect younger nurses to be humble and, even stronger, that 'you should be in a servant-hood attitude, you should always serve'. The younger generation perceives this demand as problematic. They learn new concepts of individualized care and specific nursing techniques and want to discuss and implement them. The intergenerational gap leads to friction and frustration within the group of nurses and open discussion is impossible. A few matrons understand the wishes of their junior colleagues and see the need to include them and their ideas in the nursing organization but traditional norms of respect and disciplining younger members remain crucial. One nurse formulates it thus: 'As a nurse, you must be humble and outspoken, that is the trick'.

Nurses encourage and support patients by referring to God as the ultimate healer. Praying in front of and with patients is a part of nursing care. 'If you are a Christian like the patient, you pray with her and assure her that God will take care of everything. It helps the patient calm down and find rest.' Nurses encourage patients to pray and promise to pray for them. The departmental director of nursing talks to the patients, stating that: 'We are doing our best. We keep on praying for you.' She encourages patients to pray: 'If you want to say something to God, you say it in the air, and He will be sure to hear.' Patients are grateful for such encouragement and agree on the importance of religion. Indeed, most patients have a Bible with them, read it and pray during the day and at night. In visiting hours, family members regularly pray with the sick, ask for blessings and sing out loud. On Sundays, the songs and prayers from the nearby chapel can be heard on the ward and patients follow religious programmes on the ward TV all day. Being religious is an important aspect of rendering good care. Through public praying and worship, nurses show their personal belief, form a group that encourages and confirms their basic convictions and calms patients who are afraid and worried by their hospitalization. It also has the function of reinforcing the image and status of a good woman and preventing criticism. Religious expression shows patients, doctors and visitors that the nurses' work is grounded not only in professional theories but also in heavenly foundations. The nurses 'do good' and 'serve God in the patient'; criticism of their work is therefore out of place. Nursing in an understaffed and poorly equipped environment means improvisation and a balancing act between the ideals and reality of nursing care. Religion is a way of dealing with that stress and the uncertainties on the ward, and is also a supportive factor for nurses and patients in dealing with illness One patient concluded: 'If you ask me about nurses, they must be called by God. If He does not call you, you cannot be a good nurse. You deal with human beings so you have to have this calling.' Ideas on caring and nursing concepts characterized by 'dedication, attachment and caring as indirect self-fulfilment', as discussed by Kleinmann & van der Geest (2009) in which the patient and his/her wishes are central to nurses' work, are theoretically shared by nurses and taught at college. In reality, contact usually remains impersonal and emotionally detached.

The reality of nursing on a medical ward

This research project is based on fieldwork undertaken over several years on a medical ward in the academic hospital in the capital. Since it was built in 1923 during the British administration, it has grown to be the leading national hospital with 1,600 beds and a staff of 3,000 working in 17 departments (Korle Bu 2003: 10). The average length of admission is 11 days, with most cases being referred for specialized treatment from regional hospitals or clinics. The main reasons for outpatient attendance are malaria, diarrhoeal diseases and hypertension. HIV/AIDS, for which there is a specialized unit, ranks almost last comprising 560 new official cases in 2005. The three medical wards with 85 beds (30 female, 55 male) reported in 2005 a total of 465 admissions, 595 discharges and 222 deaths, which amounted to 47% of admissions. Patients form a cross-section of the population regarding age, profession and disease (Appendix D). The main diseases diagnosed are hypertension, cardiovascular attacks

(CVA), nephritic problems and heart failure in addition to diabetes, pneumonia and cancer.

On the 30-bed female ward, 20 nurses work in three shifts. The beds are occupied with women of all ages who have been hospitalized for diseases like hypertension and CVA, liver or kidney diseases, lung problems, diabetes and cancer. The nursing routine is characterized by basic care delivery (making up beds, assisting in washing and feeding), the distribution of medication, the dressing of wounds and the completion of paper work in the form of documentation and notes. The hospital setting and its equipment is outdated and suboptimal, which results in insufficient sheets and dressing materials, incidental water shortages and a lack of privacy for both nurses and patients. The system forces patients to pay in cash for medical treatment and care, which presents a problem as most patients come from poor neighbourhoods and fear unmanageable costs. Given the limited financial means of the patients and their families, medications are not available, examinations are delayed and treatment may be stopped prematurely. As a result, many patients die on the ward and nurses have to cope with death on an almost daily basis. While they discuss the reasons for the high mortality rate and introduce arguments such as patients coming in too late, bringing in too little money or being just 'too ignorant', the death of a patient forms a major challenge in the nurses' work. In addition to the material limitations and medical difficulties, the constant understaffing of the ward challenges the nurses in their attempts to offer good care. The workload is high and the routine unpredictable. Working on a medical ward is considered not to be rewarding and may even be seen as a punishment (Böhmig 2010b).

Unlike the situation in other hospitals in Ghana and elsewhere in Africa, family members are not included in care giving. Visiting hours are restricted to two times 30 minutes when families bring in food, wash their relatives and pray with them while also checking for new prescriptions and medication. The nurses are in charge of keeping order on the ward, maintaining cleanliness and radiating serenity.

They view nursing as a responsible and busy profession encompassing, in addition to bedside nursing, writing and documentation, and communicating with patients and other medical groups. Nurses communicate in clearly defined styles with patients and among each other. While private conversations are conducted in Ga, Twi or Ewe, nursing issues and written forms of communication and documentation are in English. All the medical and nursing terminology is English and this allows nurses the chance to demonstrate a form of professionalism and educational level, both in speaking and writing. Patients reply to questions by calling the nurses 'Sister' or 'Auntie', a respectful and dignifying naming even when the nurse is much younger than the patient. Most descriptions, reports and briefs contain limited details but the nurses display their control over the patients and the work on the ward as a whole with their written work. While the training schools teach a more individualistic and personal approach to nursing and caring, the reality on a ward demands a functionalistic approach to nursing. The space for personal specifications on a patient's condition or her psychological state of mind remains blank in her notes. Patients are labelled as cases that are 'fairly ill', 'ill', 'ill but conscious', 'weak' or 'weak and restless', describing the condition as a whole. While the first term refers to less seriously ill patients who are mobile and improving, the latter indicates a serious health threat, possibly approaching death. This is never mentioned out loud, indeed there is no structural communication about a patient's well-being and psycho-social state either with the patient or among the nurses.

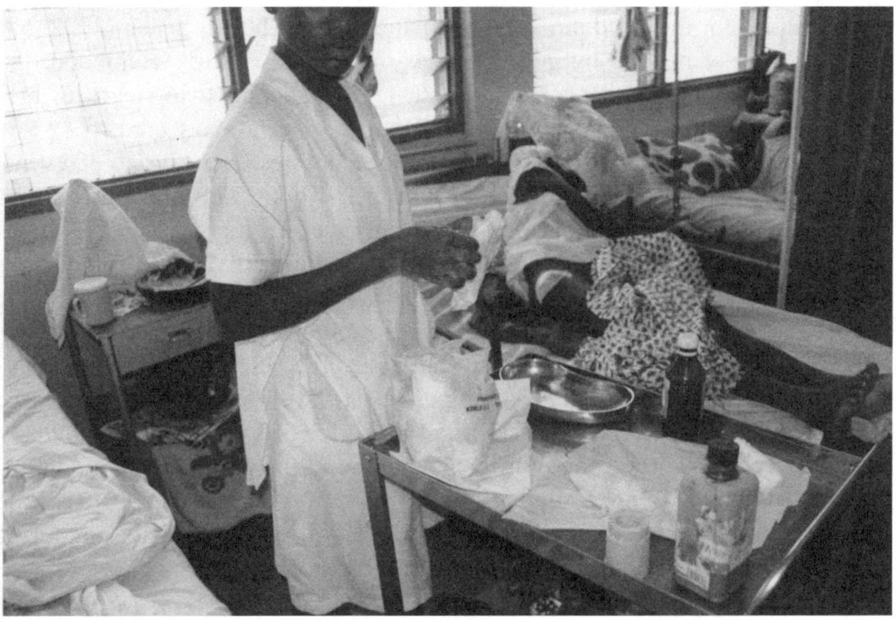

Photo 3.2 A nurse on the medical ward, dressing a patient's wound
[Photo: Christine Böhmig]

By carrying out their work well and handing over a clean and well-ordered ward to the next shift, nurses show responsibility towards their patients. The nurses are aware of their position: they define themselves as knowledgeable and educated and their role is to guide their patients through their stay on the ward in a directive way. Discussions or extensive questioning of their orders and activities through the patients is neither expected nor appreciated. The patients respect the nurses. Being authoritative is the professional role nurses are expected to adopt. Patients often call them 'Auntie Nurse', reflecting their high status. Gibson (2004) analyzed the role of nurses when trying to catch the doctor's attention for a special patient in the South African context. On the medical ward, the risk of 'falling out of the gaze' of both doctor and nurse starts during admission with the nurses. And in a hospital in the north of Ghana, Andersen (2004) found that nurses did not treat all their patients in the same way, claiming that many of them, mainly the poorer ones, were ignorant and less educated. The degree of integration and 'focus in the gaze' is determined on admission and hardly changes until the patient is discharged. The financial means of the patient play a role in this ranking. Younger or wealthier patients can influence and negotiate their position on the ward and catch the regular attention of nurses and doctors. Too knowledgeable patients are seen as difficult and unhelpful for the ward's routine and patients' well-being. Senah (2002: 58) explains this perspective by cultural background: 'From early childhood, the Ghanaian is made to understand that knowledge is acquired in stages of biological maturation and precocity is evil. Authority is said to be sacred.'

The irregular supply of equipment and the unforeseeable order of events during shifts require nurses to improvise in their work. That procedures learnt during training need to be adjusted to the reality faced is a process typical of all professions (see Melia 1987; Du Toit 1995). While this is true for nursing worldwide, the African or in this case Ghanaian situation is intensified by the financial situation of patients and the unpredictability of the working conditions of nurses. Shortcomings must be managed and solved creatively, be they managing with insufficient laundry, running understaffed shifts or caring for a large number of seriously ill patients asking for elaborate and individualized nursing care. But by being very visible in their white uniforms, nurses display and represent 'shelter' in all uncertainties and display control and order. They radiate authority and power. And looking closer, it is clear that both patients and nurses have found ways to create responses to the needs and demands on the ward.

Challenges and solutions in navigating financial risks in care

The Ghanaian health sector faces several challenges regarding its financing, which have implications for the health workers and the patients. Health delivery functions as a process of commodification. Admission, diagnosis, treatment and daily care are part of the health market and all the actors involved have to deal with this reality. Patients have to invest money and nurses have to manage financial constraints and develop strategies to successfully do their work and satisfy external and individual expectations. In this section, the patient's reality is displayed first and then the position and reaction of nurses. How both parties try to react to the needs they face and how nurses cope with the mechanisms of the modern health sector are discussed.

Patients' creativity in organizing monies

On admission, every patient is supposed to pay a deposit of ¢ 300,000 (€ 30). This is used for medications required immediately and covers the daily costs of accommodation and food. The patient's final bill is set off against it. Regular medications and costs for items like dressing materials, syringes, gloves and catheters are not included but calculated separately. On average, patients stay on the ward for 11 days and their final bill varies between ¢ 400,000 and ¢ 800,000 (€ 40-80), in addition to charges for medications and dressing materials (see Appendix E and F). As an autonomous referral and teaching hospital, the government's policy directive for free treatment to children under five and patients over seventy years of age does not apply. Patients unable to pay their bills may be referred to the Social Welfare Department. Between 2001 and 2005, the hospital paid ¢ 3.1 billion[4] in bills for 1,614 poor patients, and 1,977 patients left without paying their bill. In 2005, the Social Welfare Department decided on the cases of 1,120 patients who could not afford to pay what they owed, with the majority of cases being resolved by requesting patients pay in instalments.

While in the traditional setting family members would negotiate treatment and its costs with the healer directly, the delivery of medicines and care in this hospital has standard and non-negotiable prices. On admission, a deposit is paid and prescriptions for medication and examinations start right away. The family is expected to assist in paying these bills but this creates friction and possibly revives past conflicts. One relative visiting a sick relation on the ward said: 'She [the patient] never contributed to family issues, so now, we cannot support her either.' This shows the dependency within the larger family system. Unless somebody manages to become finically independent and rich, growing individualization carries the risk of unbearable costs in cases of serious sickness. A nurse commented that: 'some time ago, the Ghanaian had an extended family. Now, we're all going back, falling back on our nuclear family in order to help us. The extended family system is not working well because if you don't contribute to the coffers, you don't benefit.' As patients have to provide dressing materials for wounds, specific disinfectants and medications themselves, the nurse in charge makes sure that relatives buy these items in the hospital pharmacy and sterilization department. Sometimes fellow patients show solidarity and donate items to their neighbours, and in emergency cases nurses actively

4 In 2005, ¢ 10,000 were equivalent to € 1. The exchange rate changed in 2007 ¢1 = € 1, but the old amounts are reported here.

ask for an item or just take it. Discharged patients may leave supplies behind and help refill the nurses' supply. And fearing high costs, many patients delay a hospital consultation or negotiate an early discharge or a termination of their treatment to spare the limited household budget. The new health insurance scheme promises to end such hardship and facilitate medical treatment. However at the time this research was carried out, only a few patients had registered and hospitals had not yet started reimbursements. The idea of national solidarity had not yet reached an acceptable level. Almost all patients had to bear the costs of hospitalization, medical treatment and medication themselves; and only a few civil servants and employees of big companies and institutions were eligible for a refund from their employers.

Most patients come from the immediate neighbourhood and work as traders, farmers or shop keepers, and almost no one is insured or receives a regular income. A short-term admission can often be managed and organized with the help of the extended family. Chronic illness and acute health problems form a more serious threat, and families may then be forced to decide whether to continue treatment or stop it prematurely. The situation of several patients is illustrated here to show the impact of hospitalization.

Akosua is a very friendly young woman who was diagnosed with acute lymphatic leukaemia two years ago. She lives with her mother about an hour's drive from Accra. She is regularly admitted for medical check-ups and chemotherapy and reads the Bible and prays for healing. Normally her mother, a nurse herself, stays with her and brings her fresh fruit and juices. Her treatment involves regular lumbar punctures, with her medication being injected straight into the spinal chord. Akosua tries hard to put up with the pain but suffers most from being dependant on others for help. Her condition has not improved over the months of treatment and financing it has become a problem. One chemotherapy treatment costs more than US$ 100 and she will need 12 to 14. Her aunties and uncles are trying to support her financially, but money is scarce. From talking to her, it appears that some of her costs are covered by the insurance of her late father who worked for an international water company, but only as long as she is under 18. Later I learn that it was her maternal uncle's insurance and she was declared as his daughter in order to get coverage. At a certain point all efforts prove in vain, her blood count is low and she is discharged and sent home to rest and regain strength. She died later at home.

Elisabeth Kwasie is 59 years old, divorced and lives in the eastern region where she works as a cocoa farmer. She is admitted to the ward with pleural effusion on the right side and pneumonia. She has never been hospitalized before. Her brother visits her every week and takes the decisions concerning her treatment and medication. Her youngest (eighteen-year-old) daughter stays in the capital to look after her. She brings her food every day and washes her clothes and sheets. The nurses accuse the patient of having arrived too late and she is labelled as ignorant for first looking for healing through alternative medicine and prayer camps.[5] The doctors decide to insert a tube into her right lung and give her brother a prescription to buy it. Looking at this instrument, the matron explains: 'It is a single-use system that is meant to be disposable, but we are here in Ghana, we cannot afford that. We will have to empty it and use it again. We cannot just throw it away.' In the course of the weeks, there is no improvement in Elisabeth's health. A CT scan is done but reveals no new insight into her condition. Her family is angry as the test was expensive and did not provide a new diagnosis. It is decided she should be treated for tuberculosis. The doctor says: 'The treatment for TB is free. If you as a doctor do not know what the matter is and the patient is short of money, you put her on TB treatment. From then on, they do not have to pay. In many cases the real problem is a malignant tumour. We would need a biopsy, but there is no money.' After four months, she is discharged, weak and coughing. The diagnosis remains unclear. Her bill totals ¢ 1.5 million (€ 150). Her brother needs several days to organize the money. Elisabeth says when leaving: 'My family is fighting about the money. My daughter, too, left me today in anger. At home, they have to give me medicine, Blackman medicine, you know? It will help me, so I will take some, together with your medicine. If only God wakes me up.'

Another strategy for manipulating the cost of biomedical treatment is to look for medical treatment elsewhere. One option seems to be healthcare in neighbouring countries where costs are supposed to be lower, and also in private clinics where healing is promised. While there are no official statistics and medical histories available, such a strategy is high risk and the long distances involved prohibit patients from attending post-treatment check ups. For example, a young woman had undergone surgery on her hyperactive thyroid in a neighbouring country. She had been released and sent home but soon afterwards experienced severe complications. On admission to hospital in Ghana, she was diagnosed with severe hypothyroidism, a life-threatening situation. After three weeks of intensive medical treatment she was released with medication for her illness and with a big bill.

Having sufficient money changes the prerequisites for admission. Rich patients can afford first-class treatment in hospital. Several wards have small rooms for better-off patients and there is a so-called VIP ward that promises a hygienic environment, sufficient nurses and fast treatment. It is reported that there is the option to have all kinds of surgery carried out in the well-equipped

---

[5] Prayer camps are healing sessions organized by Pentecostal churches. For further details, see van Dijk (1997).

and sterile heart-surgery unit at excessive prices.[6] Such surgery is likely to run fewer risks of complications, such as wounds not healing. This option is a coping strategy for patients who face serious illness and who are looking for a way to get treatment and improve their health using the biomedical health system.

Such stories show the reality of hospital admission and the various approaches to organizing treatment from the patient's point of view. The availability of money is crucial: wealthier patients have more options while poorer ones depend on the solidarity and support of their family, the kindness of religious groups or the functioning of welfare schemes. Cultural, traditional and religious explanations for the disease are given and healing is often sought outside the biomedical health system before admission. The whole family support the sick and share the costs by organizing money 'from the coffers'. As the hospital is not an isolated space but is embedded in the surrounding society, the hopes of expected results, perceptions about the medical conclusion and threads of the unpredictable outcome are present in the individual patient and the family.

The inventiveness of nurses

Nurses on the ward know about patients' fears but also have to solve problems concerning their work. In addition to dealing with the given reality, they also develop strategies to improve the situation.

Nurses regularly put their problems in coping with the workload on the ward down to poor working conditions, especially the provision and use of equipment. To measure patients' vital signs, the ward has three digital thermometers, two working blood-pressure gauges with stethoscopes and one machine to check blood-sugar levels. All wards are regularly supplied with general equipment like gloves, normal and sterile cotton wool and gauze, syringes and plasters. The laundry service is supposed to deliver clean sheets every morning and collect the dirty ones.[7] The main laundry regularly encounters problems with water and electricity supplies, resulting in less linen or no delivery at all. In the rainy season, the drying process is slower, leading to additional shortages. Once a week, the nurse in charge files a request to the hospital's pharmacy for disinfectant spirit, parasol and plasters. In addition, there is a basic supply of drips (normal saline and glucose), sterile urinal catheters with urine bags and

[6] These stories wee revealed to the researcher in private conversations. Surgeries that were supposed to be carried out there were caesarean sections and hysterectomies. This could not be verified with hospital officials.

[7] The number of sheets collected is recorded in a booklet. Each ward marks its own sheets and makes sure it receives back all those collected.

stomach probes. The reality however is that stocks of sheets and disposable gloves are limited, which leads to delays. A nurse in charge reported:

> Supply is our problem. We make an annual budget and estimate the number of patients, gloves and everything that will be needed. You know, on other wards, they are not so ill, so you do not need so many gloves there. But here, people are sick. Normally they should supply us with equipment twice a week. We write down what we need and it is brought to us from the main supply. I think the shortage has to do with general hospital policy. There are people who say the hospital owes the main supplier money and that is why nothing is given out. Like this, all work is affected. And you know we also had a water shortage last week. There are still not enough sheets for us. On Monday they brought only a few sheets, yesterday none at all, and today five. And these are for the whole ward. And we just have two boxes of gloves for the whole day. What will happen tonight? The night nurse won't have enough gloves to protect herself if something happens.

Every morning, the nurse in charge provides her team with sheets, a box of gloves and some spirit to disinfect wounds. She keeps the stock locked up in her office: managing the supply carefully and anticipating shortages is part of her responsibility. Depending on the number of sheets, all or just some of the beds are changed. There are sheets of different sizes, and the nurses have to try their best to guarantee no patient is lying on plastic. Nurses refuse to use the patients' own colourful cloth as they aim to have a 'clean white ward'. Nurses, doctors and orderlies use disposable gloves for making beds, feeding, dressing wounds, examining a patient, cleaning the ward and so on. An opened box of gloves seems to encourage staff to take several pairs and keep them for later. In the morning, a box (100 pairs) can disappear within half an hour. When later that morning, a doctor needs gloves to set a line, nurses need to insert a urinal catheter or students have to dress wounds or change a soiled sheet, searching for gloves is part of the preparatory procedure. Nurses and doctors alike complain about the shortage, while the students are frustrated and joke about it. One morning, a nursing student feeds a patient suffering from tuberculosis through a tube without wearing gloves. She says: 'You know they have a strict glove economy here'. The matron justifies her hesitant supply: 'I give out full boxes. Where do they all go? How can we work without equipment? I am responsible and we need to have enough in store for the doctors' rounds, then we need to present our ward well.'

Facing shortage and shortcomings, nurses have invented several procedures to manage the situation. Most are combined with market activities, be they selling products or requesting supplies. This way they manage to organize the ward's finances and arrange for the necessary equipment, thus coming close to realizing their idea of good nursing.

The hospital offers one way of ensuring supplies. The official measure is to fill in cost sheets per patient. This is part of every patient's file and checked by the matron on a daily basis. Nurses are expected to note down which items they use in the care of a patient. Standard articles are cotton wool, (disposable and sterile) gloves and plasters, and more specific items include catheters, urine bags and naso-gastral tubes (see Appendix E). When discharged, a patient will be billed for this equipment. The system aims to balance the costs for the hospital: the more equipment needed, the more one has to pay. Some nurses might pity poor patients and charge them for fewer materials but the matron ensures the correct billing. Not charging patients has direct and negative consequences for the ward's status. New colleagues are instructed to understand that sufficient supply is one guarantor of appropriate nursing care.

In addition, nurses sell nursing aids that are necessary but not always provided. The most obvious examples are diapers for incontinent patients and blood-sugar strips for diabetic and newly admitted patients. Nurses buy the diapers and blood-sugar strips at the nearby pharmacy and sell them for ¢ 15,000 (€ 1.50) a time. That is a bit more expensive than the original price and they buy additional cotton wool or soap for the ward with any profits. The same goes for cool drinking water from the fridge. Patients and their relatives appreciate this service and willingly pay for it. On admission, patients are asked to pay an additional (voluntary) amount into the ward's funds to buy equipment that is needed. This money is kept by the nurse in charge and directly reinvested in diapers, blood-sugar strips and water, but also soap, spirit and cotton wool.

Donations are sometimes made. One example is a pledge to provide 200 sheets by the Catholic Archdiocese and four beds from an overseas NGO. If the supply of sheets worsens, the nurses appeal to visitors and patients' families. The text below appeared on a poster at the entrance to the ward requesting help.

> Special appeal: Dear valued visitor, it is our earnest desire to care for our patients in a healthy and conducive environment for their speedy recovery. We are compelled to make a special appeal to your for (1) one or two bed sheets for one bed or (2) more bed sheets for more beds or (3) material for bed sheets or (4) a token amount of money for the purchase of material for bed sheets. Measurement: 180 cm by 270 cm. We would cherish your contribution as a special gift to our ward K and our patients. God loves a cheerful giver. May God richly bless you! The Entire Nursing Staff.

After several weeks, sufficient donations had arrived and the pressure eased.

In extreme emergency situations, the nurses are all asked to donate money to buy soap and dressing materials for the patients. This happened a few times during the research period and all the nurses, nursing students and ward assistants contributed ¢ 10,000 (€ 1) to buy soap. While that action supported all the patients and nurses alike, there are also procedures to improve the situation of an individual patient. The nurses generally try to remain emotionally distant from their patients' well-being but some do evoke sympathy. In the case of an unemployed young woman who was admitted with a life-threatening allergic reaction[8] that needed specific and expensive skin treatment, the matron ordered all the nurses to contribute to her treatment. 'We will collect money from the staff and buy the dressing material ourselves. We leave it for two days before we renew it. Together with the gauze and bandages, each dressing is ¢ 100,000. All nurses will contribute and buy the next cream. I want this girl to go home.' After the girl's death a day later, one nurse said: 'The work of a whole morning is gone, and we wasted more than ¢ 200,000'. Patients needing costly chemotherapy or dialysis[9] face a dilemma. The costs present a problem and the nurses know that they cannot assist in financing such treatment. Due to the seriousness and advanced state of the disease and an inability to finance appropriate treatment or initiate palliative medication, an untimely and painful death for these patients appears the inevitable outcome.

The nurses' complaints and their inventiveness show the complexity of finding the right treatment in a culture where traditional and modern health settings exist alongside each other and nurses feel obliged to defend their work. Feelings of frustration are intensified by long working hours and, at least in the nurses' perceptions, very low salaries. This leads to financial struggles and tension in the nurses' personal lives and to low morale at work. Their dissatisfaction is vented at several levels: nurses are not present on their shifts because they are accompanying relatives to a polyclinic; some report late for work after a vacation; and others pursue their own affairs and run businesses such as cloth sellers or seamstresses or have a pharmacy nearby or work additional shifts at private clinics. Being organized in a professional union is one way of giving voice to their position. Working abroad in North America, Europe or Asia is a very attractive alternative for many young nurses. Idealizing the working conditions there and imagining high incomes overseas reinforces the limited and often uncritical reports from nurses who have already left. Nurses who stay in the system miss colleagues who go, especially as everybody is needed to keep the health system going. The older generation demands respect from younger colleagues but know that too much criticism might lead to an increased exodus of nurses. So nurses respond to demands by finding creative solutions, generating monies and exercising their power and authority over patients and their family members. Within the given structures, the ward turns out to be a place of

[8] Steven Johnson's Syndrome (or Toxic Epidermal Necrolysis) is a potentially fatal skin disease that usually results from an infection or an adverse reaction to a drug.

[9] In 2005, one dialysis treatment cost about € 100. Most patients were able to organize one treatment for acute kidney failure but were aware of the immense and unbearable financial burden if chronic kidney failure was diagnosed. Organizing regular dialysis several times a week is only possible for wealthy patients.

healing and treatment and at the same time a market place full of exchange and trade in material goods and immaterial ideas.

Discussion

The hospital represents Western-style healthcare delivery by promising biomedical diagnosis, modern technologies and state-of-the-art treatment. However, it soon becomes clear that hospitals are no isolated and replicable clones of such an imaginary system but are placed within a surrounding culture and economy. Ghana represents a developing country where tradition, cultural norms and modern concepts of healthcare shape and influence the health-seeking behaviour of its population. Traditionally, healing and caring were defined within the boundaries of balanced reciprocity and social interaction but through economic needs, globalization and the exchange of ideas and technologies, healthcare has been reshaped through increasing monetization to become a commodity. Patients need to take decisions on where to acquire help; while nurses represent and enforce the Western concept of hospital care. Both actors meet on the hospital ward, where working definitions of care and cure are presented and negotiated.

The unpredictability of the costs and the low standard of (working) equipment have consequences for the position of patients and the motivation of nurses. Patients are looking for medical treatment and healing and nurses are trained to deliver care. Even so, most nurses have firm religious convictions and are motivated by wanting to 'do a good deed', and they all know there will be times when job satisfaction is low and conflicts arise. A general statement is: 'We try our best, but our best is not good enough'. It seems difficult 'to enjoy nursing because we're just improvising'. Some nurses blame patients for postponing timely admission, being unprepared and putting themselves and their carers in a difficult situation. They accuse them indirectly of having waited too long or for having looked for treatment with traditional or religious healers before turning to biomedical healthcare. In addition, the reality on the ward does not fit with the expectations of a modern biomedical health centre that nurses envisage as their working environment when joining the profession. The hospital is no remote or separated space but is integrated in society both socially and economically. Nurses need to engage in various activities to organize monies and improve their working conditions. Being conscious agents activating personal skills in marketing contrasts with the idea of the serving and caring innocent nurse. Many nurses oscillate between the two approaches and blame the hospital management for being left to struggle alone.

How can the meaning of healing within the biomedical healthcare system in Ghana be understood? Since the introduction of this system, it has become a powerful actor that influences and guides the population in its health-seeking behaviour. It forms a complex whole combining cultural norms enriched by individual fears and expectations with the working reality of hospital wards and the financial implications of a hospital admission for patients and their families. Health workers and patients alike find themselves in this market place, needing to organize their strategies and mobilize their means to negotiate, defend and realize their position.

Patients are often unfamiliar with the hospital system and are overwhelmed by its organization and demands. On admission, they are intimidated by tits complexity and are unable to formulate their needs. The cost of an admission and the medications and examinations required are a burden on the whole family. Limited means can lead to delayed hospitalization and a break in treatment. This means for patients and their relatives that an illness and its treatment can unbalance the social and economic position of the whole family. The newly implemented health insurance scheme is supposed to act as an alternative to such current financial threats in the near future. But until it is fully functioning and has achieved an accepted new form of nationwide solidarity fitting the cultural understanding of support and reciprocity, the 'cash and carry system' will remain in place.

The financial risks and the resulting health-seeking behaviour have implications for the work of nurses. They are forced to use equipment delivered by the hospital and organized by the patients. Nurses feel unhappy with this part of the working routine and it undermines the motivation and enthusiasm of many health workers. Unclear about their expectations and maybe having been pushed into nursing by their family, they find themselves in the profession by chance rather than by choice. Once in a position in the health sector or on a hospital ward, nurses face situations that challenge them professionally and as individual members of society.

Acting against the spirit of the profession, nurses are using their creativity and entrepreneurial possibilities to deliver care, organize medications for needy patients and generate monies to buy necessary ward equipment. Being trained in Western standards of nursing and working in the West African reality of personnel shortages and with suboptimal hospital equipment, many nurses are developing feelings of frustration and disillusionment. Theoretically, they are part of the global biomedical family in a modern hospital building but, practically, the healthcare system with its hospitals, nurses and patients is situated and rooted within a society in which health and healing are complex systems. They are influenced and shaped by Western concepts but embedded in a culture of respect and reciprocity, family traditions and religion. Family solidarity, wide-ranging expectations and trading mechanisms are forcing patients and health workers to react as active members of the local and global market in the search for healthcare. Health and the treatment of disease are part of a wider exchange system.

Appendices

Appendix A The National Health Insurance Scheme (NHIS) in 2006

Registration fee	¢ 20,000[10]
Processing costs and card	¢ 10,000
Annual contribution	Free for children < 18 if registered with their parents
	Free for old persons > 70, the unemployed and 'core poor' (adults dependant on constant support from elsewhere)
	¢ 72,000 for students, apprentices and the 'very poor' (who can just meet their own needs)
	¢ 180,000 for middle-income workers and employed persons (who are able to meet their daily needs)
	¢ 480,000 for the rich and very rich (who are able to meet their needs and support others)
	2.5% of the monthly salary of civil servants and SSNIT contributors

[10] In 2005, ¢ 10,000 were equivalent to € 1.

Appendix B Statistics on Ghana

	2006	Past
Population	22,113 m	1960: > 6.7 m
Population in urban areas	46%	1970: 30%
Adult literacy rate	54%	1989: 32%
Primary-school enrolment	63%	1992: 73%
Gross national income per person	€ 380	1981: € 400
Government expenditure on health as % of budget	5%	1976: 10% 1980: 8%
Per capita expenditure on health	€ 17	
- private	68%	
- government	32%	
Life expectancy	Male: 58 years Female: 59 years	1957: 45 years 1970: 48 years
Infant mortality	68 / 1.000	1967: 250 / 1000 1988: 77 / 1000
Maternal mortality	540 / 100,000	c. 1990: 500-1500/ 100,000
Measles immunization coverage	83%	1994: 49.2%
AIDS prevalence	3.6 %	First cases in 1998
Access to safe water	Rural: 52% Urban: 88%	
Access to adequate disposal facilities	Rural: 62% Urban: 44%	
Access to pipe-borne (safe) water	Rural: 19% Urban: 80%	
Improved sanitation facilities	Rural: 10% Urban: 25%	1988: rural: 22% urban: 63%

Sources: WHO (2004); WHO (2006); Addae (1996); Twumasi (1979); Senah (1997); Nyonator (2004); Dugbatey (1999); Ghana MoH (2003).

Appendix C Facts on the healthcare system in Ghana

	2006	Past
Physicians	3,240	1957: 330 1960: 372
Nurses	19,707	1957: 800 1960: 1,684
Physician vacancy rate	47.3%	1998: 42.6%
Nurse vacancy rate	57%	1998: 25.5%
Hospital beds	>20,000	1960: 2,354
Physician : population ratio	1 : 6,790	1960: 1 : 18,000
Nurse : population ratio	1 : 1,116	1960: 1 : 4,000
Bed : population ratio	1 : 1,100	1 : 2,800
Access to health service within 30 minutes	Rural: 15-50% Urban: 50- 93%	
OPD visits per capita	0.50	
Hospital admissions	36 / 1,000	1996: 25 /1,000

Sources: WHO (2004); WHO (2006); Addae (1996); Twumasi (1979); Senah)1997); Nyonator (2004); Dugbatey (1999); Ghana MoH (2003)

Appendix D Patients on the ward by socio-demographic characteristics, 2005

	July	*August*	*September*	*October*	*November*	*December*
Age						
15-35	27	23	18	19	26	15
35-50	21	17	14	14	12	14
50-70	24	22	23	20	14	11
older	7	7	12	7	12	5
Profession						
trader	32	25	25	21	23	12
unemployed	14	12	15	8	17	13
shop/ seamstress	12	6	7	4	2	4
student	11	10	10	13	14	6
higher education	4	7	11	3	6	6
other, old age	7	8	3	8	12	4

Source: Ward statistic and data collected by the researcher

Appendix E Standard costs and expenditures in hospitals in 2005

Fixed costs	
Accommodation	¢ 5,000[11] daily
Food	¢ 12,000 daily
Sanitation	¢ 8,000
Documentation	6,000
Additional costs	
Development fund	10%
Spirit & disinfection	¢ 25,000 (for pharmacy)
Items used on demand	
Gloves	.¢ 1,000
Syringes & needles	¢ 1,000
Cotton balls	¢ 1,000
Sterile gloves	.¢ 5,000
NG tubes	¢ 4,500
Catheters	¢ 12,000
Urine bags	.¢ 7,000
Examples of final costs for hospital admission (excluding medication):	
up to 1 week:	¢ 160,000 - 538,000
1-2 weeks:	¢ 411,000 - 819,000
2-4 weeks:	¢ 767,000 - 1,680,000

Source: Information from the ward accountant and data collected by the researcher

Appendix F Costs for medical treatment and examinations

Tests and medication (not included on final bill)	
Blood test	¢ 20,000 - 60,000
EEG	¢ 75,000
CT scan	¢ 370,000
CT with contrast	¢ 700,000
Physiotherapy	¢ 15,000
Blood transfusion	¢ 58,000
Dextrose saline 500 ml	¢ 12,500
Normal saline 500 ml	¢ 8,000
Standard antibiotics 1g.	¢ 61,000 (given for at least 8 days)
Dialysis	€ 150
Chemotherapy	ca. € 150 per injection

Source: Information from the ward accountant and data collected by the researcher

11 In 2005, ¢ 10,000 were equivalent to € 1.

Appendix G Products sold by nurses

Water 500 ml.	¢ 300
Diapers	¢ 15,000
Blood sugar strips	¢ 15,000

Source: Data collected by the researcher

References

Addae, S. (1996), *History of Western medicine in Ghana 1880-1960*. Durham: Durham Academic Press.

Akiwumi, A. (1971), *Higher education for nurses*. Accra: Ghana Universities Press.

Akiwumi, A. (1995), *State registered nurses (SRN): 1945-1995*. Unpublished speech. Accra.

Andersen, H.M. (2004), 'Villagers.' Differential treatment in a Ghanaian hospital. *Social Science & Medicine* 59: 2003-2012.

Arhinful, D. (2003), *The solidarity of self-interest: Social and cultural feasibility of rural health insurance in Ghana*. Leiden: African Studies Centre.

Bierlich, W. (2000), Injections and the fear of death: An essay on the limits of biomedicine among the Damonga of Northern Ghana. *Social Science & Medicine* 50: 703-713.

Böhmig, C. (2010a), 'This is not what I expected – I want to go.' Krankenschwestern zwischen Erwartungen und Realität in einem ghanaischen Krankenhaus. In: H. Dilger & B. Hadolt, eds, *Medizin im Kontext: Krankheit und Gesundheit in einer vernetzten Welt*, pp. 139-160. Frankfurt a.M.: Peter Lang Verlag.

Böhmig, C. (2010b), *Ghanaian nurses at a crossroads. Managing expectations on a medical ward*. Leiden: African Studies Centre.

Böhmig, C. (2010c), 'There is somebody in heaven who takes care of you.' Nursing care and religiosity on a hospital ward in Ghana. *Medische Antropologie*, 22(1): 47-61.

Buor, D. (2004), *Accessibility and utilisation of health services in Ghana*. Utrecht: Nivel.

Curtin, P.D. (1992), Medical knowledge and urban planning in colonial tropical Africa. In: S. Feyermann & J. Janzen, eds, *Social basis of health & healing in Africa*. Berkeley: University of California Press.

de Witte, M. (2008), *Spirit media: Charismatics, traditionalists, and mediation practices in Ghana*. Amsterdam: University of Amsterdam, PhD thesis.

du Toit D. (1995), A sociological analysis of the extent and influence of professional socialization in the development of a nursing identity among nursing students at two universities in Brisbane, Australia. *Journal of Advanced Nursing* 21: 164-171.

Dugabey, K.L. (1999), National health policies: Sub-Saharan African case studies (1980-1990). *Social Science & Medicine* 49: 223-239.

Foucault, M. (2003) [1963], *The birth of the clinic*. London: Routledge.

Ghana Ministry of Health (2003), *Five-year programme of work 2002-2006*. Accra: Ministry of Health.

Gibson, D. (2004), The gaps in the gaze in South African hospitals. *Social Science & Medicine* 59(10): 2013-2024.
Hagopian, A. *et al.* (2005). The flight of physicians from West Africa: Views of African Physicians and implications for policy. *Social Science & Medicine* 61: 1750-1760.
Hawe, A.J. (1962), Looking back. *Ghana Medical Journal* 1: 15-18.
Holden, P. (1991), Colonial sisters: Nurses in Uganda. In: P. Holden & J. Littlewood, eds, *Anthropology and nursing*, pp. 67-83. London: Routledge.
Horton, R. (2001), Ghana: Defining the African challenge. *The Lancet* 358: 2141-2149.
Kisseih, D.A.N. (1968), Developments in nursing in Ghana. *International Journal of Nursing Studies* 5: 205-219.
Kleinmann, A. & S. van der Geest (2009), 'Care' in health care. Remaking the moral world of medicine. *Medische antropologie* 21(1): 159-168.
Korle Bu (2003), *80th anniversary. Souvenir brochure*. Accra.
Korle Bu (2006), *Newsletters*. Accra.
Martin, H.M. (2006), *Nursing contradictions: Ideals and improvisation in Uganda.* Diemen: AMB.
Melia, K.M. (1987), *Learning and working. The occupational socialization of nurses*. London: Tavistock.
Nukunya, G.K. (2003) [1992], *Tradition and change: An introduction to sociology.* Accra: Ghana University Press.
Nyanator, B. (2004), The health of the nation and the brain drain in the health sector. Paper at conference on migration and development in Ghana, Accra, 14-18 September.
Opare, M. & J. Mill (2000), The evolution of nursing education in a postindependence context – Ghana from 1957 to 1970. *Western Journal of Nursing Research.* Accessed 16 September 2003 at: www.library.uu.nl
Owusu, M. (1980), Handing-over notes by the director of nursing services. Unpublished article. Accra.
Patterson, K.D. (1981), *Health in colonial Ghana: Disease, medicine and socio-economic change, 1900-1955*. Waltham: Crossroads Press.
Schuster, I. (1980), Perspectives in development: The problem of nurses and nursing in Zambia. *Journal of Development Studies* 17(3): 77-97.
Senah, K.A. (1997), *Money be man. The popularity of medicines in a rural Ghanaian community.* Amsterdam: Het Spinhuis.
Senah, K.A. (2002), 'Doctor-talk' and 'patient-talk'. Power and ethnocentrism in Ghana. In: S. van der Geest & R. Reis, eds, *Ethnocentrism. Reflections on medical anthropology*, pp. 43-66. Amsterdam: Aksant.
Senah, K.A. (2004), In the mighty name of Jesus. Faith healing and health-seeking behaviour in Ghana. *Legon Journal of Sociology* 1(1): 59-70.
Sumani, M. (2005), *The role of the nurse in present day health delivery system.* Speech delivered on 10th anniversary of NTC Alumni Association, Accra, 3 November.
Takyi, B.K. (2003), Religion and women's health in Ghana: Insights in HIV/ AIDS preventive and protective behaviour. *Social Science & Medicine* 56(6): 1221-1234.
The Ghanaian Nurse (1997), *The House Journal of the Ghana Registered Nurses Association.* Accra.
Twumasi, P.A. (1979), A social history of the Ghanaian pluralistic medical system. *Social Science and Medicine* 13B(4): 349-356.
Twumasi, P.A. (2005) [1975], *Medical systems in Ghana*. Accra: Assembly Press.

van der Geest, S. (1997), Money and respect: The changing value of old age in rural Ghana. *Africa* 67(4): 534-559.
van Dijk, R. (1997), From camp to encompassment: Discourses of transsubjectivity in the Ghanaian Pentecostal diaspora. *Journal of Religion in Africa* 27(2): 135-159.
Vaughan, M. (1991), *Curing their ills. Colonial power and African illness*. Cambridge: Polity Press.
Ventevogel, P. (1996), *Whiteman's things: Training and detraining healers in Ghana*. Amsterdam: Het Spinhuis.
Vogel, R. (1999), *Health insurance in Sub-Saharan Africa*. Working Paper Series WPS 476. Washington: World Bank.
WHO (2004), *Country profile: Ghana*. Accessed 28 September 2004 at: www.undp-gha.org
WHO (2006), *World health statistics 2006*. Accessed 17 January 2007 at: www.who.int/whosis/core
Zaman, S. (2005), *Broken limbs, broken lives. Ethnography of a hospital ward in Bangladesh*. Amsterdam: Het Spinhuis.

4

Market forces threatening school feeding: The case for school farming in Nakuru town, Kenya

Dick Foeken, Wijnand Klaver,
Samuel O. Owuor & Alice M. Mwangi

School feeding has a direct and indirect impact on children's nutrition, and thus on their health. However the success of such programmes is determined by market forces, in particular the price of food at the market. Based on a survey of all the primary schools in Nakuru town, Kenya, this chapter shows that children in Standard 1 who received meal(s) at school were better off in nutritional terms. Yet many schools, especially government-run schools, did not provide this service, mainly because of a lack of school or parental funds. School farming can provide a solution: by producing some of the ingredients themselves, schools can sidestep the adverse effects of the market and make their feeding programme affordable for the school and parents. And although many schools in Nakuru did grow crops to support their feeding programme, major challenges in terms of land, water, support and leadership still have to be overcome. A few schools appeared to be performing very well in this respect and should be used as an example for others.

Introduction

School feeding – and the provision of lunch in particular – is generally considered a way of improving children's nutritional status, and thus their health and performance at school. However the success of school feeding is to a considerable extent determined by market forces as the ingredients for the meals have to be purchased at the local market. Costs have to be covered by parental contributions and parents will only be able to pay for their children's meals if food prices remain low. If these rise and parents are asked to contribute more, an increasing number will no longer be able to afford to pay for their children's school meals.

In an internal memo in 2007, the Municipal Educational Officer (MEO) in Nakuru town, Kenya urged government-run primary schools to find a way to provide lunch for all pupils and thus avoid the situation of some going hungry at lunchtime. In addition to the organizational problems, this is a challenging task for primary schools because of the initial high costs involved in setting up a well-equipped kitchen. The biggest challenge, however, lies in the steep rise in prices for staples over the last few years. For example, the price of maize and maize flour, which is the main ingredient in the Kenyan diet, rose by 130% in a one-year period between 2008 and 2009.[1] Schools are facing an uphill struggle in their attempts to comply with the MEO's memo, all the more so because government-run schools are known to be less affluent than private schools. It is, moreover, government schools that low-income households depend on for their children's education and these households are the ones that are increasingly less able to pay for school meals.

A possible solution lies in school farming, whereby the schools produce some of the ingredients themselves, mainly the staples and vegetables. School farming offers a way of sidestepping the adverse effects of market forces. In their 'School Meals Essential Package', the United Nations World Food Programme (WFP) and UNICEF consider school gardens as one of twelve interventions that can improve the health and nutrition of school-age children as part of the FRESH (Focusing Resources on Effective School Health) Framework (WFP/UNICEF 2004).

Health, school feeding and school farming are the 'ingredients' of this chapter, which discusses the extent to which school feeding contributes to pupils' general nutrition, and thus to their health. It also looks at school farming's contribution to school feeding and considers whether it can be extended to substantially contribute to school feeding but avoid the adverse effects of price increases at food markets.

School feeding and health

The relevance of the MEO's memo lies not only in the relationship between school feeding and educational objectives but also in how it affects children's nutritional status, and thereby their health and performance at school. The

1 See Oxfam (2009) and IRIN News: 'Kenya: Hungry and HIV-positive in Nairobi's slums', 10 March 2010.

school feeding programmes have thus focused on two major goals: education and food and nutritional security (Bennett 2003). The educational goals include higher enrolment levels, better school attendance, improved performance among children, as well as incentives aimed at addressing the gender imbalance in schools. The second set looks at improvements in the nutritional status of school children through increased nutritional awareness and improvements in the food security of their households and how school feeding acts as a food-based safety net.

From the literature it can be seen that primary schools that start offering lunch to pupils experience a surge in attendance among children from poor households who would have been unlikely to receive any lunch at all (WFP 2007). Studies of the physical and mental condition of children participating in school feeding programmes have shown encouraging results (Levinger 1986). For example, the nutritional state of children in Baroda, India improved significantly after the introduction of a lunchtime school feeding programme (Rajalakshmi & Vanaja 1967). Similar findings were recorded in Mafraq, Jordan (Hijazi & Abdulatif 1986). In the Philippines, Levinger (1986) observed that well-nourished children performed better at school than children on a poor diet. Similarly, Pollitt (1990) cited other studies (e.g. Wilson 1981; Moock & Leslie 1986; Simeon & Grantham-McGregor 1989) that also found a positive relationship between nutritional level and school performance. A recent meta-analysis of the international literature on school feeding found 18 well-controlled trials and studies on the basis of which it was concluded that school meals may have significant positive effects on growth and cognitive performance and thus may have physical, psychological and social benefits for disadvantaged children (Greenhalgh *et al.* 2007). Better-fed children are more likely to complete their schooling, which will, in turn, offer them greater opportunities in the labour market in the future.

The results of such studies show that school feeding falls within the ambit of at least two of the Millennium Development Goals, namely to eradicate extreme poverty and hunger, and to achieve universal primary education.[2] An increased 'market' for school feeding has been emerging and this is acting as a 'pull' factor for initiatives on the production side, be they in the form of school gardens or links with local producers or producer organizations. Several international initiatives that are promoting the link between local agricultural production and school feeding point to the developmental relevance of this topic (see Box 1).

---

[2] A prize-winning example of growing vegetables for school meals is the Ivo de Tassis Elementary School in Governador Valadares, Brazil. See http://www.idrc.ca/uploads/user-S/11456447921UA_4_Valadares.pdf, accessed on 12 August 2010.

This chapter presents a case study of school feeding programmes from Nakuru town, Kenya and looks at their potential benefit for children. An important consideration is the extent to which school farming contributes to school feeding. Based on a survey of almost all the primary schools in Nakuru, school feeding programmes, often in combination with school farming, now appear to be common practice in the town. The proposed causal chain is that an improvement in pupils' diets through school feeding alleviates hunger and nutritional deficiencies, which then leads to improved health and performance. One way of supporting school feeding programmes is through school farming and in the case of Nakuru town, this takes place within the limits of the built-up area and is thus a form of urban agriculture.[3] Some of the produce from school gardens can be used in the school feeding programme, which potentially constitutes considerable savings, especially in a context of rising food prices. If

Box 4.1 Programmes focusing on local agricultural production for school feeding

1. NEPAD's *Home Grown School Feeding Programme*[4] works in collaboration with the Millennium Development Task Force on Hunger, WFP, UNICEF and the FAO. This initiative links school feeding directly to agricultural development through the purchasing of locally produced food, school gardens and the inclusion of agriculture on school curricula.
2. The *School Feeding Initiative Ghana-Netherlands* (SIGN)[5] supports the US$ 212m Ghana school feeding programme (Government of Ghana 2006). The programme aims to stimulate local agricultural production by providing a stable market in the form of schools that buy produce for their feeding programmes, thus improving the nutritional status of all pupils.
3. The Gates Foundation provided the World Food Programme with a grant in 2008 to develop a framework for linking school feeding to local agricultural production. It also sponsored USDA/WFP missions to four countries (Ghana, Kenya, Mali and Rwanda) to assess potential links between school feeding and smallholder farmers (WFP 2009a).
4. The Gardens for Life programme has projects in India, Kenya, The Gambia and England. This is dealt with in Box 2 below.

---

[3] There is a rich literature on urban agriculture but studies on school farming in urban areas, despite its relevance, are almost non-existent. The only one in a developing country known to us is that in Cagayan de Oro, the Philippines (Potutan *et al.* 1999), while some basic data on school farming can be found in the aerial survey of Dar es Salaam from the late 1990s (Dongus 2000).

[4] See http://www.africa-union.org/root/UA/Conferences/2007/fevrier/REA/13-14%20 fev/NEPAD_Home_Grown_School_Feeding_Pogramme.doc, accessed on 12 August 2010.

[5] See http://www.sign-schoolfeeding.org/, accessed on 12 August 2010.

a variety of produce is grown (not only staples but also vegetables, fruit, legumes and nuts) or animals are kept, this also contributes to the promotion of sound food habits among pupils.

School feeding in Kenya

School feeding programmes were launched in Kenya in 1967 under the National School Feeding Council of Kenya (NSFCK) and peaked in 1986 when 60,000 pre-primary and primary school children in fifteen districts were involved. However as a result of financial constraints, activities had to be reduced and by 1996 only about 13,000 children in four districts were being reached. Two studies, one in Kirinyaga District (Pieters *et al.* 1977) and one in Nyambene District (Meme 1996; Meme *et al.* 1998), showed that children participating in NSFCK programmes were better off in terms of nutritional level and school performance than those not participating in a programme.

Providing a child with a daily nutritious meal at school is seen as a simple and effective way of improving school attendance and retention rates, and forms the backdrop of the global school feeding programme of the World Food Programme (WFP), which reached almost 23 million children in 68 countries in 2008.[6] One of these countries was Kenya, where school meals were provided to 1,211,000 children in 3947 schools in vulnerable areas (WFP 2009c: 45) in 29 districts and six Nairobi slums (cf. WFP 2007: 43).

An important recent development in Kenya was the political transition following the general election at the end of 2002. The provision of free primary education was one of the key policy changes that the new National Rainbow Coalition government implemented as soon as it assumed power in January 2003. This led to a massive influx of school children (VOA News 2003) and resulted in overcrowded classes in government-run primary schools, a shortage of teachers and school materials and, if in place, a school-feeding programme that could not cater for the large numbers of new pupils wanting school meals. School feeding in Kenya is included in the 2005 Sessional Paper on Education, which was approved by Parliament, and is one of the four components of the School Health, Nutrition and Feeding Programme. Finally, the 2008 National Nutrition and Food Security Policy has a section on school meals and calls for an expansion of the programme (WFP 2009c).

---

6 See: http://www.wfp.org/school-meals, accessed on 1 December 2009.

The Nakuru study

Nakuru town

Nakuru is in the middle of the Great East African Rift Valley, 160 km northwest of Nairobi. With an average annual rainfall of about 950 mm, it has a dry sub-humid equatorial climate (MCN 1999) with two rainy seasons: the long rains from March to May and the short rains from October to December. Over the past thirty years, the population of Nakuru town has increased fivefold from 47,000 in 1969 (Republic of Kenya 1970) to 239,000 in 1999 (Republic of Kenya 2000). Nakuru is currently the fourth largest city in Kenya after Nairobi, Mombasa and Kisumu.

Map 4.1 Nakuru town

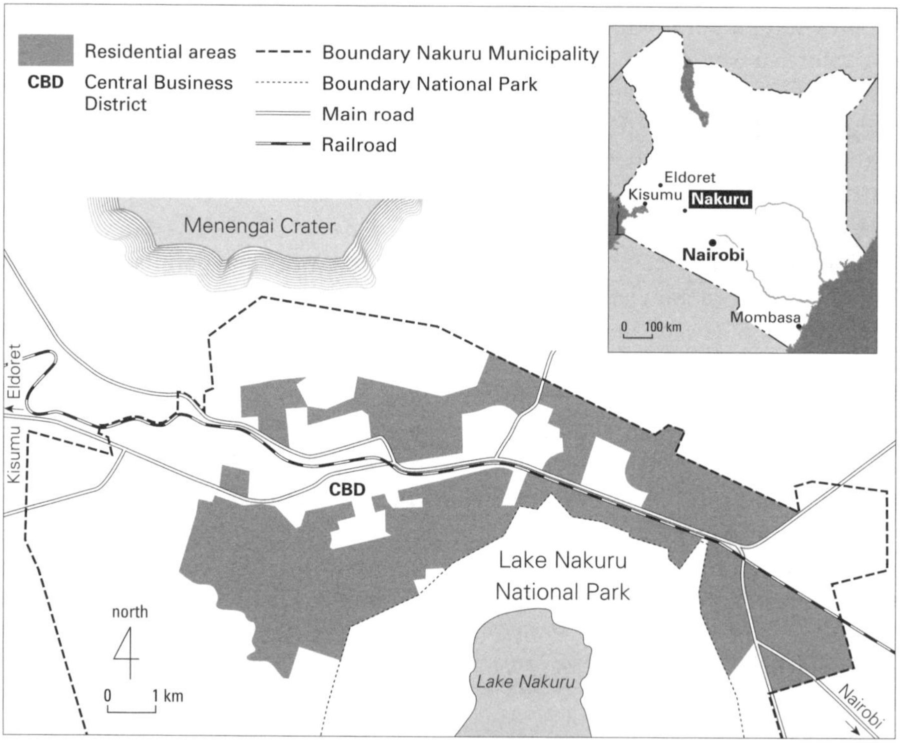

In 1997, the prevalence of absolute poverty[7] in Nakuru town was 41% compared to 30% in 1994 (Republic of Kenya 2001). In 2000, many households had to live off a monthly income of Ksh 5,000 (US$ 80) or less (Foeken & Owuor 2008), which translates to (much) less than the often-used definition of poverty of US$ 1 per person per day. Such households are not only unable to meet their basic needs but struggle to put food on the table on a daily basis. With recent steep increases in food and energy prices, the situation of such households has only worsened.

Methodology and study population

The findings presented in this chapter are based on a survey undertaken using structured questionnaires in 74 primary schools[8] in Nakuru in June 2006. Anthropometric measurements – height and weight – were taken from Standard 1 children in each school (if a school had several Standard 1 streams, one was selected at random) and their ages were recorded.[9] Additional information was obtained from observations in school compounds and interviews with local officials and school staff.

The 74 primary schools, ranging in size from about 40 to over 1600 pupils, can be categorized by type (day, boarding), by management (government,[10] private) and by kind (normal, special). Most of the primary schools were day schools (85%) or a mixture of day and boarding (11%). Three were boarding schools. In terms of management, two-thirds (70%) of the schools were government schools, while the rest (22) were privately run, i.e. by individuals (25%) or churches (5%). There were five government-run primary schools that catered for children with special needs, mainly deaf children and those with mental disabilities. Two of these also served as normal schools.

---

7 The absolute poverty line indicates a household's (in)ability to meet its basic food and non-food requirements. In 2000, it was estimated at Ksh 2,648 (approx. US$ 42) per month per adult in urban areas and Ksh 1,239 (US$ 20) in rural areas (Republic of Kenya 2001; SID 2004).

8 This was practically all the primary schools in Nakuru at the time. It was not possible to cover a few because of problems with cooperation or because the school was located in the rural southwestern part of the municipality.

9 The weight and height of 3145 pupils from 70 of the 74 schools were recorded. The ages of 318 pupils (10%) were not known. In one government school all the ages were missing, in five others 50-93% of the ages were missing, in another five 14-26% were not available and in eleven schools (nine government and two private) between 2% and 10% were missing. Anthropometrical indices of weight, height and body mass index by age could be calculated for 69 schools (for 41 pupils per school on average).

10 Also known as public schools.

School feeding in Nakuru

Table 4.1 shows that school feeding was quite common in Nakuru town, with a large majority of primary schools having a school feeding programme in 2006. In general, feeding programmes were more common among private and/or church-based schools (100%) than among government schools (69%).[11] The most common reasons mentioned among schools for *not* having a feeding programme were that parents were either not interested or could not afford it and/or the school lacked the necessary funds. Most of the respondents in the schools with no feeding programme said that the school intended to start one in the near future.

Table 4.1 Prevalence of school feeding in primary schools, by type of school management

	All schools (N=74)	Government schools (N=52)	Private schools[1] (N=22)
Schools offering school feeding	58 (78%)[2]	36 (69%)	22 (100%)
Schools offering school feeding to Standard 1 pupils	45 (62%)[2,3]	24[2] (46%)	21 (100%)[3]

Using Fisher's exact chi-square test, the differences between government and private schools are statistically significant (P<0.01).

Notes: 1) Including church-based schools.
2) Including one special government school where children do not sit in classes but in grades according to ability.
3) Relevant N is one less than indicated in the column heading because one private school starts with Standard 4.

Source: School Survey (2006), see Foeken *et al.* (2007).

Although some schools in Nakuru had a long history of school feeding,[12] most had only recently started: 33% between 2000 and 2003 and 45% since 2004 (55% and 27% respectively for private schools, and 19% and 56% respectively for government schools) By far the most commonly mentioned reason for starting the programme was to make pupils who lived far away stay at school at lunchtime (83%). In several schools, the reason given was that a feeding programme ensured that pupils got lunch (22%). Some schools started the feeding programme with the specific aim of helping those pupils (needy/poor/orphans) who would not otherwise eat at lunchtime (19%).

---

11 Private schools and church-based schools are grouped together as 'private schools'.

12 Not necessarily only boarding schools: one of the government-run primary day schools started its feeding programme in 1988.

All of the 58 primary schools that offered school feeding to pupils offered lunch and 41% provided tea at morning break. Breakfast and dinner were only served at boarding schools, and afternoon tea was not usual and was served in only 10% of primary schools.

What is more important, however, is who was eligible for the meal(s) and whether pupils benefit from the school feeding programme. In the schools where meals were served, almost all the pupils were in principle eligible but this did not mean that they all actually received lunch or a snack. In 40% of the primary schools *all* pupils were eligible, while in the majority of the schools (57%), only pupils whose parents could pay for school meals were entitled to them (Table 4.2). Payment was either included in the school fees or cash was handed over by the pupil on a daily, weekly or monthly basis. In ten primary schools, orphans and/or pupils from very poor households received free school meal(s) that were either subsidized by the fees of other pupils or were covered by sponsors or well-wishers. Government-run and private schools differed considerably in terms of children's eligibility for school meals. While in the large majority of the government schools only those able to pay were eligible, in private schools it was the other way round and all except three pupils were eligible for school meals. Providing free meal(s) for needy children only was done in 25% of the government schools with a feeding programme and in only one (church-run) private school.

In 41 of the 58 primary schools with feeding programmes, the number of meals being served at the time of the survey had not changed since the programme started. However, in all the other 17 schools, more meals were being provided than at the start of the programme. Moreover, 46 schools had ex-

Table 4.2 Pupils eligible for school feeding, by type of school management

Category of pupils	All schools (N=58)	Government schools (N=36)	Private schools (N=22)
All pupils	40%	11%	86%
Those able to pay	57%	83%	14%
Orphans/children in need	17%	25%	5%
Certain years only	5%	8%	0

Using Fisher's exact chi-square test, the differences between government and private schools are significant for 'all pupils eligible' and 'those able to pay' (both ($P<0.01$) and for 'orphans/children in need' ($P<0.10$), but they are not significant for the last category ($P=0.5$).

Note: N refers to the number of schools where pupils were eligible for school feeding. The percentages add up to more than 100% due to a partial overlap of those able to pay and the latter two categories.

Source: School Survey (2006), see Foeken *et al.* (2007).

panded their programme in terms of the number of pupils involved. On the other hand, the programme had decreased in four schools due to a lack of money as a result of cost cutting or parents who could no longer afford to pay.

School feeding in relation to nutritional status in Nakuru

Efforts were made in June 2006 to obtain the anthropometric measurements (body height and weight) and exact ages of Standard 1 children in all the schools. In principle, *all* children in the selected Standard 1 class per school were selected. All except five primary schools[13] (i.e. 69 schools) were covered and 54 schools were used for the analysis reported in this section.[14] The minimum age of the children was either five or six and the maximum varied between six and eleven. The majority of the children were between five and seven years old.[15]

Table 4.3 shows the results of the anthropometric measurements. Body mass index-for-age (BMIA) is a measure of concurrent (acute) malnutrition, i.e. the child is too light for his/her height and age and is denoted as being 'wasted'.[16] This was the case in almost 13% of the children and was slightly more common among boys than girls. About 3.8% of the children were severely wasted (2.5% of the girls and 5% of the boys). Height-for-age (HA) is a cumulative measure of chronic malnutrition, i.e. the child is too short for his/her age and is denoted as 'stunted'. Almost 14% of the children were stunted and 3.7% were severely so. Stunting was again much more common among boys than girls. Finally, weight-for-age (WA) is a combination of the previous two measurements and is an expression of the overall nutritional condition of a child ('underweight'). Almost 15% of all children were underweight, with incidences in boys being almost twice as high as among girls.

---

13 Two schools had no Standard 1, in two other schools it was not possible to measure the children and in one school children were measured but it was not possible to ascertain their ages.

14 Fifteen schools were excluded from the analysis. In eight schools (seven with and one without school feeding) Standard 1 was smaller than 17 pupils and in seven schools school feeding had only started in the year of study. For a detailed description of the anthropometrical data collection, see Foeken *et al.* (2007).

15 For more details on the anthropometrical analysis, see the Annex at the end of this chapter.

16 In the past, weight-for-height was used as a measurement of wasting but with the advent of new international child growth standards (WHO 2006, 2007), gross body proportion (ranging from thinness to overweight) in children older than five is expressed by calculating the child's body mass index (BMI: weight in kg divided by the square of height in metres) with reference to age-specific standard values.

Table 4.3 Percentages of children in Standard 1 being wasted, stunted and underweight, by sex

Anthropometric measurement[1]	N[2]	All children	Girls	Boys
Wasted (BMIAZ<-2)	2827/1397/1430	12.7%	11.4%	14.1%
Stunted (HAZ<-2)	2827/1397/1430	13.8%	11.5%	16.2%
Underweight (WAZ<-2)	2782/1382/1400[3]	14.4%	10.6%	18.2%

Notes: 1) For details about WHZ, HAZ, WAZ and <-2, see the Annex at the end of this chapter.
2) Number of children/girls/boys, respectively.
3) The WHO weight-for-age standards are given for children under ten, i.e. before the normal growth spurt in puberty occurs. For this reason, the WAZ could not be calculated for some Standard 1 children who were already 10-11 years old.

Source: School Survey (2006)

Initially two groups of primary schools were compared. The first group consisted of 27 'schools catering for school feeding for Standard 1' since 2005 or before and where (some or all of) Standard 1 pupils were eligible (see Table 4.4).[17] The second group of 'schools not catering for school feeding for Standard 1' (also 27 schools) did not have school feeding programmes or, if they did, they did not include Standard 1. For each school, the percentage of children who were 'wasted', 'stunted' and 'underweight' was categorized as being lower or higher than the overall median of the prevalence percentages (10.5%, 8.5% and 11.1% for wasted, stunted and underweight, respectively). For each sub-group in the sample, the percentage of schools in these two categories was calculated.[18]

Table 4.4 indicates that there is no significant relationship between school feeding and the percentage of children who are classed as wasted. In both groups, the percentage of schools with a prevalence of wasted children either lower or higher than the median for all children was close to the expected 50% mark. As far as the other two anthropometric measures – stunted and underweight – were concerned, there appeared to be a positive relationship between

17 Schools with fewer than 17 pupils in Standard 1 were excluded from this analysis. Three boarding schools without a day school were not included: one was a special school without classes, there were no measurements for another and one other had too few pupils to be included. Of the eleven boarding schools with a day school, five were not included in this analysis: one only had older classes, one was not measured and three had too few pupils. The other six mixed types of schools (i.e. both boarding and day schools) were included after statistical analysis showed that their results did not introduce any bias.

18 A further breakdown in four quartile categories was also analyzed (see Annex) but is not reported here.

Table 4.4 Relationship between school feeding and nutrition, in primary schools[1]

Anthropometric measurement	Categories[2]	Schools with school feeding for Standard 1[3] (N=27)	Schools with no school feeding for Standard 1[4] (N=27)
% of Standard 1 pupils classified as wasted	- up to 10.5% - more than 10.5%	44% 56%	52% 48%
% of Standard 1 pupils classified as stunted	- up to 8.5% - more than 8.5%	59% 41%	33% 67%
% of Standard 1 pupils classified as underweight	- up to 11.1% - more than 11.1%	59% 41%	22% 78%

The association by Fisher's exact chi-square test (2-sided) is significant for the % underweight (P=0.012) and almost significant for the % stunted (P=0.101), but far from significant for the % wasted (P=0.79). Deeper analysis based on the *quartile* values of the observed prevalence percentages confirms that the chi-square test on linear-by-linear association (2-sided) is significant for the % stunted (P=0.02) and the % underweight (P=0.01), but far from significant for the % wasted (P=0.90).

Notes: 1) For a detailed explanation on the method of analysis, see the Annex.

2) Cut-off values chosen are the median percentage (= second quartile) for all 69 schools with anthropometrical data.

3) These are the schools that have been offering school feeding since before 2006 and where all (12 schools) or some (15 schools) of the Standard 1 pupils were eligible. Seven schools where fewer than 17 pupils had been measured, three schools where no measurements were obtained, two schools with no Standard 1 and another seven schools that had just started their feeding programmes in 2006 were excluded from this analysis.

4) These are the schools either with a feeding programme but where Standard 1 pupils were not eligible (12 schools) and/or without a feeding programme for pupils at all (15 schools). One school with fewer than 17 pupils was excluded from the analysis.

Source: School Survey (2006), see Foeken *et al.* (2007).

school feeding and nutritional status. Among schools with school feeding, it was significant that there was a lower level of stunting and underweight than among schools where school feeding was *not* offered. To sum up, school feeding is associated with improved growth in stature (height growth), while body proportions (weight for attained height) are not different. As weight-for-age is the summary indicator of both dimensions of growth, the results for the percentage of those underweight reflect improved statural growth.

However, conclusions should be drawn with care. First, one major weakness is that the questionnaire used in the survey did not include a question to ascertain which of the Standard 1 children in the primary schools with school feeding were actually participating in the school feeding programme. Second, caution is also required regarding the causality between the two because there may have been less access to school feeding programmes in schools that had a higher number of malnourished (poorer) children.

To investigate actual enrolment in school feeding programmes, a comparison was made between 19 classes in which all the children were eligible for school feeding and 22 classes where school feeding was only provided to those able to pay and/or to selected destitute or very poor children (see Table 4.5). These data show a significant 'dose-response relationship'[19] among school feeding and attained weight and height: the larger the number of Standard 1 children receiving school feeding, the lower the percentage of children who were stunted and underweight. Surprisingly perhaps, this greater body size was inversely associated with body proportion (weight relative to attained height), expressed by wasting. One explanation may be that growth occurs in spurts (seasonal, pre-adolescent and in puberty), such that improved height growth may be at the cost of body weight, which leads to some degree of temporary thinning of the body (lower weight relative to height) before body proportions re-establish themselves (Hoorweg *et al.* 1995).

The second issue (the direction of causality) was investigated in three ways. First, to investigate the possibility of self-selection of school feeding programmes among schools with a larger nutritional need (i.e. the more disadvantaged schools), a comparison was made between the nutritional results of 15 schools *without* a school feeding programme and 12 schools *with* a school feeding programme but *not* covering Standard 1. This meant that any nutritional differences among the Standard 1 pupils could not be due to the school feeding programme *per se*. The results of both groups were very similar for all three anthropometric indices. Although the numbers are small,[20] there is no indication of a significant effect,[21] so the possibility of self-selection of schools is not supported.

A second possibility is that child growth results reflect differences in socio-economic background rather than school feeding and a third is that they might reflect conditions (other than school feeding) related to the management of the school (government versus private). This second possibility, which is related to the issue of the direction of causality, is explored in Tables 4.6 and 4.7 and the third in Table 4.8.

---

19 A 'dose-response relationship' means that the effect on an organism is greater as the level of exposure to a factor increases.

20 Thirteen schools with a feeding programme *not* covering Standard 1 and 15 schools without a feeding programme.

21 Fisher's exact chi-square test (2-sided) is not significant for the % wasted (P=0.45), the % stunted (P=1.00) and for the % underweight (P=0.36).

Table 4.5 Relationship between school feeding and nutritional status of Standard 1 pupils (results at school level)

Anthropometric measurement	Categories	Schools with school feeding for all Standard 1[1] pupils (N=19)[3]	Schools with school feeding for some Standard 1 pupils only[2] (N=22)[4]
% of Standard 1 pupils classified as wasted[5]	- up to 10.5% - more than 10.5%	32% 68%	59% 41%
% of Standard 1 pupils classified as stunted[5]	- up to 8.5% - more than 8.5%	68% 32%	50% 50%
% of Standard 1 pupils classified as underweight[5]	- up to 11.1% - more than 11.1%	79% 21%	41% 59%

Statistical analysis based on the *quartile* values of the observed prevalence percentages (thus capturing more information about the actual frequency distribution) reveals that the chi-square test on linear-by-linear association (2-sided) is significant (with inverse relationship) for the % wasted (P=0.07), and significant (with positive relationship) for the % stunted (P=0.01) and the % underweight (P=0.05).

Notes: 1) Due to low numbers, the results of seven schools were included in this analysis: one where school feeding started only in the year of study (2006) and six schools where the number of children measured was fewer than 17.

2) Due to low numbers, the results of seven schools were included in this analysis: six where school feeding started only in the year of study (2006) and one school where the number of children measured was fewer than 17.

3) 3 government schools, 16 private (of which 3 were church-run)

4) 19 government schools, 3 private (of which 1 were church-run)

5) The cut-off values chosen are the median percentage (= second quartile) for all 69 schools with anthropometrical data.

Source: School Survey (2006), see Foeken *et al.* (2007).

Table 4.6 shows that the occurrence of school feeding among Standard 1 primary-school children in Nakuru in 2006 is apparently related to the socio-economic area where the school is located. Roughly two-thirds of the primary schools in the low and low-to-medium income areas did not offer this facility against only one third of schools in the medium-to-high and high-income areas. This difference was, moreover, entirely attributable to a lack of feeding programmes among government schools. Incidentally, this points to an important unmet need for school feeding among government schools in Nakuru's lower-income neighbourhoods.

Table 4.6 Relationship between school feeding and socio-economic area[1]

Socio-economic classification[2]	No. of schools with school feeding and percentage of those that offer school feeding to Standard 1 pupils	Idem, government schools	Idem, private schools
Low & low-to-medium income areas	37% of 30	24% of 25	100% of 5
Medium-to-high & high income areas	68% of 28	50% of 18	100% of 10

The association by Fisher's exact chi-square test (2-sided) between the presence of school feeding for Standard 1 pupils and income level in the school's area (N=58) is significant (P=0.02). Within the government schools (N=43), the association is almost significant (P=0.109).

Notes: 1) The percentages refer to the number of schools with school feeding programmes; the schools with no school feeding are excluded from this analysis.

2) The classification of the socio-economic areas is from MCN (1999: Fig. 3.6).

Source: School Survey (2006)

Investigating the extent to which the effect of school feeding on height and weight growth may be attributable to background is hampered by the fact that this was a cross-sectional study and no anthropometric baseline data are available to measure the effect of one semester of school feeding on nutritional outcomes. In addition, the number of schools studied is quite small and makes assessing the interaction of three variables more difficult. However, an attempt was made to correct for the general income level of the households in the area as a possible confounder of the relationship between school feeding and child growth. To do so, the analysis of Table 4.4 was repeated by income level of the area for which the school caters. The results for schools in lower-income areas (see Table 4.7) show that the effect of school feeding on attained weight and height in the 27 schools in lower-income areas is at least as strong as the overall association across the income groups observed above (see Table 4.4): it is significant, even with the low sample sizes. Among the other 27 schools in the medium to higher income areas, the differences are not significant.

The third way that children's growth might reflect conditions (other than school feeding) concerning the management of the school (government versus private) was investigated among the 27 schools where all or some of Standard 1 benefit from school feeding. Table 4.8 shows that Standard 1 children in private schools tend to be less stunted and less underweight but somewhat more wasted than in government schools. The differences (although not statistically significant due to the small sample sizes involved) may be explained by the intensity

Table 4.7 Relationship between school feeding and nutrition in primary schools in lower-income areas only*

Anthropometric measurement	Categories	Schools providing school feeding for Standard 1 (N=9)	Schools not providing school feeding for Standard 1 (N=18)
% of Standard 1 pupils wasted	- up to 10.5% - more than 10.5%	44% 56%	50% 50%
% of Standard 1 pupils stunted	- up to 8.5% - more than 8.5%	67% 33%	22% 78%
% of Standard 1 pupils underweight	- up to 11.1% - more than 11.1%	78% 22%	17% 83%

* See notes for Table 4.4.

The association by Fisher's exact chi-square test (2-sided) is far from significant for % wasted; the associations for % stunted and for % underweight are significant (P=0.04 and P=0.01, respectively).

Source: School Survey (2006)

Table 4.8 Relationship between school feeding and nutrition according to school management (28 schools providing school feeding for Standard 1)*

Anthropometric measurement	Categories	Schools offering school feeding for Standard 1 (N=27)	Idem, government schools (N=14)	Idem, private schools (N=13)
% of Standard 1 pupils wasted	- up to 10.5% - more than 10.5%	44% 56%	57% 43%	31% 69%
% of Standard 1 pupils stunted	- up to 8.5% - more than 8.5%	59% 41%	43% 57%	77% 23%
% of Standard 1 pupils underweight	- up to 11.1% - more than 11.1%	59% 41%	43% 57%	77% 23%

* See notes for Table 4.4.

The association by Fisher's exact chi-square test (2-sided) of school management and child growth is not significant for % wasted (P=0.25). The associations for % stunted and for % underweight are almost significant (P=0.12).

Source: School Survey (2006)

of coverage: in 90% of government schools, *only* Standard 1 pupils who could pay or who were destitute or poor received school feeding, while in 86% of the private schools, *all* Standard 1 pupils were entitled to school feeding. The 'dose-response relationship' discussed above is apparent here too.

To conclude, school lunch was shown to offer positive nutritional benefits to Standard 1 children in Nakuru, with the effect being particularly notable in lower socio-economic areas where there is still a clear need for school feeding in government schools. The issue of access to school feeding does not only come into play at individual (pupil) level but also at school level. How do schools find the resources necessary to invest in this intervention? More specifically, how does school farming support school feeding? These questions are strongly related to the market issues described earlier and are the focus of the next section.

School farming in support of school feeding

One way of supporting school feeding programmes is by school farming. Products from the school farm can be used in the feeding programme, which offers economic advantages and precludes the need to buy ingredients at (much) higher market prices. A good example is the Gardens for Life project, a recent development in Kenya that combines school farming and school feeding (see Box 2).

Interestingly, two primary schools in Nakuru had started to participate in the Gardens for Life programme around the time of the survey, and crop cultivation became the pupils' responsibility as part of the Gardens for Life Club. Although the two schools also had a feeding programme, what they produced was not used in it but sold instead. This was mainly because harvests were very small, in one case due to labour constraints as almost all the work had to be done by pupils after school hours and, in the other, due to the lack of supervision by a teacher. At the time of the survey, the main benefits of the schools' crop cultivation activities were in the educational sphere. Nevertheless, both schools intended to expand the activity and support their feeding programmes. A year later, it was clear that crop cultivation in one of the schools had indeed improved considerably.

Albeit less common than school *feeding*, school *farming* appeared to be quite widespread in Nakuru town, with almost half of Nakuru's primary schools growing crops (Table 4.9). Keeping livestock was much less common but all the schools did so also practised crop cultivation. Crop cultivation was somewhat more common in government schools than private schools. It is interesting that while most private schools had a feeding programme for which all the pupils were eligible, only a third of these schools practised crop cultivation.

This may indicate the better financial position of private schools that allows them to buy food at the market.

Respondents were asked about the benefits of crop cultivation for their school and for the pupils. Benefits related to school feeding (Table 4.10) were considered first for the school itself and then for the pupils.[22] The products and the savings they bring for the schools are of benefit. The table shows that, based

Box 4.2 The Gardens for Life project

The Gardens for Life project is run by the Kenya Youth Education and Community Development Programme (and is also active in India, The Gambia and the UK). Its main objectives are to reintroduce agriculture into primary schools (since its exclusion as an examinable subject in 2000) as an essential and practical method of equipping children with easy and useful skills, and to encourage schools to grow crops for pupils' lunches.[23] The latter has two major benefits as it leads to an improvement in pupils' nutritional condition, which in turn increases their attention span and performance, and it drastically reduces the cost of providing school lunches. Moreover, the farming techniques used are as organic as possible, for example using kitchen waste to make compost, and new and nutritious crops are being introduced.

The programme started as a pilot project in 20 public schools in three districts (Nakuru, Laikipia and Nyandarua) and the results have been very promising. Nyandarua Boarding Primary School in Nyahururu town (750 pupils) saved KSh 200,000 on lunches in 2004 and introduced (home-grown) carrots, spinach and courgettes as daily supplements to the usual maize, beans and potatoes. Chemicals were rarely applied and natural methods were used to control pests and diseases instead. The one-acre plot even produced surplus vegetables that were sold to local communities as 'chemical-free' foods. Another school, Munyaka Secondary in Laikipia District, known as a 'slum school', saw a 38% increase in enrolment after its Gardens for Life project started. The school introduced radish, garlic, onions and beetroot, which are all known for their high vitamin contents. The students' health improved as a result of the quality of the meals on offer at the school. Students from poor families who were unable to pay school fees also benefited from the work-for-fees programme, in which they worked on the school plot to raise money to cover their fees. By doing so, pupils were able to stay at school to complete their education.

Source: http://www.edenproject.com/gardens-for-life/ and Kariuki (2005)

[22] As for the benefits for pupils, 'acquiring skills in farming' was mentioned by 74% of the respondents (with no difference by school management).

[23] Gardens for Life (http://www.edenproject.com/gardens-for-life/, accessed on 12 August 2010) is an initiative of the UK-based Eden Project that started in 2004. Its aims are to create school gardens to promote education for sustainable development and global citizenship. The latter was achieved through contact between the participating schools in the UK, India and Kenya (see Tearle 2006 and https://www.edennet.org/about/storysofar/). Soon after the project started in Kenya, the objective concerning school farming to support school feeding became increasingly important.

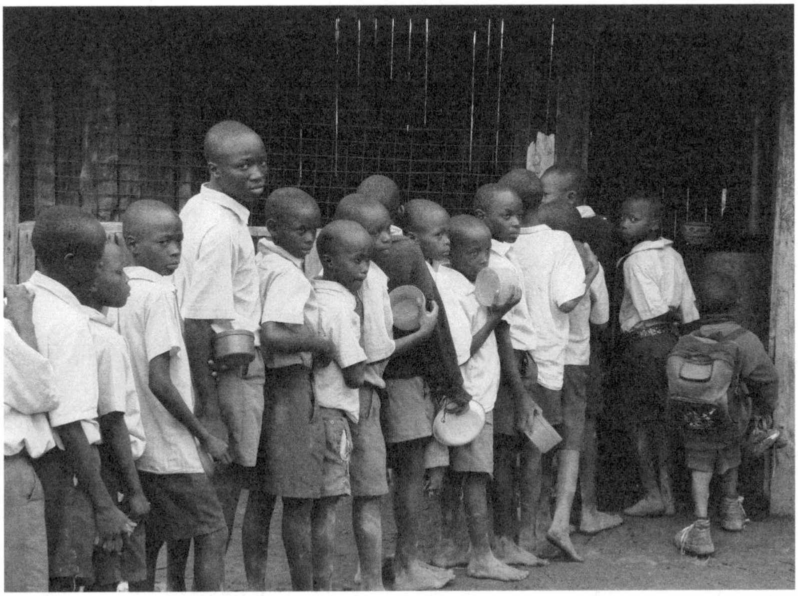

Photo 4.1 Pupils queuing for lunch at a government-run primary school in Laikipia District that participates in the Gardens for Life project [Photo: Dick Foeken]

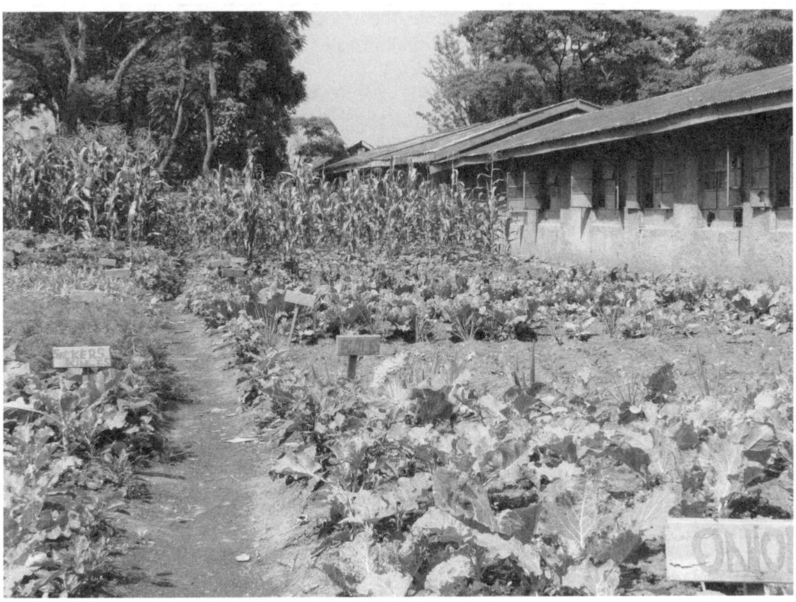

Photo 4.2 The well-tended *shamba* at one of the two government primary schools in Nakuru that participate in the Gardens for Life project [Photo: Dick Foeken]

Table 4.9 Prevalence of school farming in Nakuru town, by type of farming and school management

Type of farming	All schools (N=74)	Government schools (N=52)	Private schools (N=22)
Crop cultivation	46%	50%	36%
Livestock keeping	12%	10%	18%

The associations by Fisher's exact chi-square test (2-sided) are not significant (P=0.32 for crop cultivation; P=0.44 for livestock keeping).
Source: School Survey (2006)

Table 4.10 Most frequently mentioned benefits of crop cultivation for school feeding as perceived by the respondents, by school management

Benefit	All schools (N=34)	Government schools (N=26)	Private schools (N=8)
For the school:			
- it helps in school feeding programme	59%	46%	100%
- the school saves money on food	27%	15%	63%
For the pupils:			
- it supplements meals/lunches	50%	35%	100%
- orphans get lunch	6%	8%	0%

For the first three benefits mentioned in the table, the associations by Fisher's exact chi-square test (2-sided) are significant (P=0.01, 0.02 and 0.003 respectively).
Source: School Survey (2006)

on this information, the link between school farming and school feeding seems to be much stronger in private schools than in government schools.

One of the main objectives of the present study is to establish the contribution of school farming to school feeding and although it is difficult and time-consuming to measure this directly in terms of quantities of ingredients, there are various indirect (more qualitative) indicators that show strong links between the two. First, while half of the 57 primary schools in Nakuru with school feeding programmes appeared to be cultivating crops as well, these very schools represent the large majority (88%) of the 32 crop-cultivating schools, which indicates that farming was being practised to support feeding programmes. Government and private schools did not differ in this respect.

Second, the amount of each crop grown by schools and used for their feeding programme was established. And the same was done for milk produced by schools that kept cattle (Table 4.11).[24] For simplicity's sake, the answers 'all of it' and 'part of it' have been taken together. In general, more than half of the producing schools used part or all of each crop as well as the milk for their feeding programme. In a substantial number of primary schools, it can thus be inferred that part or all of the produce was sold (or given away).[25]

Table 4.11 Main self-produced ingredients used in school feeding programmes (no. of schools cultivating that crop and % using it in feeding programmes) and average length of time (in months) of use of self-produced ingredients for lunch and morning tea[1]

	Ingredient	Self-produced ingredients[2]		Average length of time[3]	
		N	%	N	months
Lunch	kale (*sukuma wiki*)	21	76%	15	7.4
	beans	11	55%	5	4.4
	maize	13	69%	8	6.6
	cabbage	6	67%	3	6.3
Morning tea	milk	6	67%	4	9.5

Notes: 1) Numbers are too small to compare government and private schools.
2) Numbers refer to schools producing this ingredient and the percentage indicates how many of them use it for their feeding programme, either 'all of it' or 'part of it'.
3) N refers to schools producing a particular ingredient *and* using it in their feeding programme *and* for which data were available (for one school, information on the duration was missing).

Source: School Survey (2006)

Table 4.11 indicates the length of time that milk and produce from the four most commonly cultivated crops could normally be used in the schools' lunch programme. For instance, the 15 schools cultivating kale (or *sukuma wiki*)[26] *and* using it for their lunch programme were able to use the crop, on average, for seven months of the year. Seven primary schools even produced sufficient kale

24 Only the results of the four main crops are presented here. For more details, see Foeken *et al.* (2007: 41, Table A3).

25 The figures in Table 4.11 should be viewed with caution as they are based on observations by respondents in hindsight and also because of the small number involved, which does not allow further disaggregation by school management. However, the figures do show a consistent pattern.

26 *Sukuma wiki* (Brassica oleraceae var. acephala) is the local name for a green, leafy vegetable in the cabbage family (kale). Literally it means 'to push the week', referring to its importance in the diets of subsistence dwellers due to its high yield and low price.

to last the whole year. Maize and cabbages lasted on average for slightly more than six months and beans for over four months. One school had enough self-grown beans for the whole year, while three schools realized the same for maize and one school for cabbage. A relatively small number of the primary schools (around 20%) used only some of their kale, beans and maize for their feeding programme; the explanation being perhaps the sufficiently large average harvests compared to the number of children they needed to feed.

Four of the six schools that kept cattle used their milk for feeding programmes. All used it for their mid-morning tea, three also for breakfast and two for afternoon tea. On average, the milk produced was able to cover their needs for almost ten months of the year (Table 4.11).

The potential of school farming in Nakuru town

Two success stories in 2006

One of the schools with a relatively high degree of self-sufficiency was a public day school with about 500 pupils in a medium-income area. It started cultivating crops (maize, beans, kale, cabbage and tomatoes) in 1995 and keeping livestock two years later. The work was done by hired labour using simple tools like *panga* and *jembe*, and the farming system was purely organic. Crops were irrigated during dry periods using rainwater from storage tanks. The harvest was almost entirely used for the school's feeding programme, with kale, cabbages and maize being produced in sufficient quantities to last the whole year. In addition, the school kept three cows to produce milk for mid-morning tea throughout the year. Since the start of its farming activities, the school had been a member of an NGO called SENVINET,[27] which was involved in activities such as tree growing, flower gardening, garbage management, grass planting, organic gardening (using tree leaves for mulching), advising on cattle keeping, and water catchment for irrigation purposes. The school started its feeding programme for which both pupils and teachers were eligible in 1990, although the

[27] SENVINET (Schools Environmental Network) was an important player in school farming in Nakuru. This local NGO's main objective was to work towards a sustainable environment and the control and management of HIV/AIDS by targeting children and youth, who it saw as the agents of change in society. SENVINET's members were mainly schools in the Nakuru municipality where it was trying to establish environmental awareness among pupils by promoting organic farming, tree growing and flower gardening. In 2005, almost half (45%) of the schools in Nakuru were members of SENVINET, the large majority (88%) of which were primary schools (data obtained from the SENVINET office in 2005). In late 2006, i.e. after the survey, SENVINET was forced to discontinue its activities following the withdrawal of its major partner and funder, MS Kenya (Nanna Jordt Jørgensen, former advisor of SENVINET, personal communication, 25 January 2010).

main beneficiaries were Standard 8 pupils who remained at school at lunch time. There were also some visually handicapped children at the school who were fed for free. The school provides breakfast, morning tea and lunch. The nutritional condition of the Standard 1 pupils selected was better than the average for all schools (8.1% wasted, 10.8% stunted and 2.7% underweight).

An even more successful example was a boarding school with about 170 pupils in a peri-urban area of Nakuru. The school only started in 2003 and in the same year began to cultivate crops, and to keep livestock too a year later. In 2006, six different crops were being cultivated on its two plots – one of 1.5 acres within the school compound and the other was a two-acre plot some 200 metres away. The school used both organic and chemical (fertilizer, pesticide, insecticide) inputs, and crops could be irrigated throughout the year if necessary thanks to a borehole. School staff did all the work with *panga* (large cutting tool, machete) and *jembe* (hoe). The school started to keep livestock in 2004, with the sole objective of making itself self-sufficient in food. At the time of the survey, the school had 14 cattle, 280 chickens and four goats. The cows produced sufficient milk for breakfast and morning and afternoon tea throughout the year and the chickens' eggs were used to feed pupils and staff. The school did not receive advice about cultivating crops and was not a member of SENVINET. Being a boarding school, it obviously had a feeding programme consisting of three meals a day including weekends. All the self-cultivated crops were used for the school's feeding programme and four of these (kale, spinach, onions and maize) were produced in sufficient quantities to last the whole year. Carrots normally lasted for six months and tomatoes for four. Some of the tomato harvest was sold to supermarkets as the school produced first-grade tomatoes in a greenhouse.[28] Food markets are clearly an obstacle for schools due to the high prices they ask for ingredients but they can also be an income-generating opportunity.

Challenges

The examples above show that school farming can indeed support a school's feeding programme and thus indirectly affect the nutritional condition and health of pupils. However to be able to fulfil the demands of the Nakuru Municipal Educational Officer to provide all pupils with lunch, the large majority of Nakuru's public primary schools will have to meet a number of fundamental conditions, four of which are briefly dealt with here: sufficient land, sufficient water, professional support, and leadership.

[28] No data on the nutritional condition of the 22 Standard 1 pupils were available because measurements were not recorded due to the pupils' tight schedule.

'Not enough land' was by far the most frequently mentioned answer for why non-crop-cultivating schools did not grow crops, while almost half of the schools that did cultivate crops saw having insufficient land as a serious constraint. Indeed, half of the non-crop-cultivating schools had a school compound of fewer than three acres (and some even less than an acre), so it was unlikely that there would be much space for a sizeable *shamba*. Yet four (29%) of these schools did actually grow crops and among these were two schools with a compound of one acre or less. There was even one school cultivating *sukuma wiki* on a *shamba* of only 400 m^2 and using it in its feeding programme throughout the year. There were also schools that had sufficient land but did not grow crops for reasons other than a lack of land, such as a shortage of capital, the fear of theft or crop destruction by animals. For instance, 60% of the schools had a compound of five acres or more. It is hard to imagine that the compounds of these schools could not provide the space needed for a *shamba* but 40% of these schools did not cultivate any crops. Finally, there were several schools that did grow crops but still had a compound of at least five acres left after deducting the size of the *shamba* from the size of the whole compound. In all, even though the compounds of some schools were (too) small for a *shamba*, the data suggest that a lack of land did not have to be a major constraint to starting or expanding crop cultivation for most schools. After all, the example of Nyandarua Boarding Primary School in Nyahururu – one of the schools participating in the Gardens for Life project – shows that even a plot as small as an acre can be very productive in terms of yield, feeding capacity and (saving) money.

Nakuru has a relatively dry climate so ensuring a constant supply of water is a problem, especially in the dry season, and most schools have to irrigate their crops. This was mainly done with water from municipal taps (which is not officially allowed), while some schools used collected rainwater too. Despite this, by far the most frequently mentioned problem regarding crop cultivation concerned the climate: the lack of rainfall, irregular rainfall and drought. Most schools faced problems with watering their crops and not all schools had their own borehole (only a few did), but collecting and storing rainwater in tanks – as was practised by several schools – shows that the problem can be solved.

This brings us to the importance of support. One of the schools with a well-functioning rainwater collection system had developed it with support from SENVINET but since this NGO has now disappeared, it is likely that a sudden vacuum in terms of support for school farming has arisen. The role of the extension officers from the Ministry of Agriculture (MoA) has been marginal, judging by the fact that only two respondents said that their schools had received assistance from them in 2005. It is very important that this vacuum be filled.

School farming is usually the responsibility of just one teacher, which means that the success of a school's farming activities is not only dependent on factors such as land, water and support but also on individual qualities like a teacher's organizational skills, enthusiasm and dedication. The first 'success' story described above illustrates this. During a visit to that public day school in June 2007, it appeared that over the course of 2006 (i.e. after the survey) the teacher in charge of the farming activities had been transferred to another school. It had taken some time before another teacher could be found to take over these responsibilities and the *shamba* had been noticeably neglected in the first half of 2007. The problem with sustaining school farming after the transfer of the teacher in charge of farming activities demonstrates how one of the key conditions for making school farming a success is the motivation, dedication and enthusiasm of the staff member involved.

The importance of good support and a dedicated teacher was confirmed by the former SENVINET advisor: 'In particular I have observed that the success of this type of activity often depends on the initiative of a few committed teachers as well as some kind of external back-up in terms of advice, encouragement and perhaps some limited financial inputs.'[29]

Conclusion

School feeding – and in particular the provision of school lunches – is high on the development agenda as it is linked to five of the Millennium Development Goals. It is of particular importance as providing lunch at school contributes to an improvement in children's health. The Nakuru study demonstrates that nutritional benefits, as shown by attained growth, were significant. The effect of school feeding was particularly strong in low socio-economic areas as well as in private schools. This implies that especially among government schools in the lower-income neighbourhoods, there is a large as yet unmet need for school feeding.

The Nakuru study also shows that urban school feeding was widespread but that many children whose parents could not afford it did not benefit from it. There were also schools however where all pupils received lunch on a daily basis at an affordable price. Some of these had been able to reach a relatively high degree of self-sufficiency in their feeding programmes through their school farming activities, thus providing their pupils with a decent lunch. Private schools perform better than government schools in this respect.

The explanation for these differences must partly be in the fact that private schools attract children whose parents can afford the (relatively high) cost of

---

29 Nanna Jordt Jørgensen, personal communication, 25 January 2010.

school meals. Lower-income households rely on government schools for their children's education. It is these children who would benefit most from school feeding but it is the government schools that suffer most from the adverse effects of market forces related to school feeding, such as rising food prices. However, some schools – and among them even a few government schools – have succeeded in sidestepping market forces through school farming, thus reducing their dependency on the market for ingredients. From a policy point of view, these schools – as well as those participating in the Gardens for Life project – can serve as an example for others regarding the integration of school farming and school feeding, and with the advantage of reduced dependency on the market.

Finally, the study shows that the majority of Nakuru primary schools do have some kind of school feeding programme and also the intention to expand their programme. Most of the schools without a programme were planning to start one in the near future. The Municipal Educational Officer even expected government-run primary schools to offer school lunches, which shows an interesting institutional development as schools are developing from being purely institutions of learning to institutions concerned with the health of their pupils too. The aim of providing school meals is to improve their children's nutritional intake, and by introducing school farming to support school feeding, schools are (potentially) able to act as a mitigating factor between the market (high food prices) and children's health.

Annex: Anthropometrical analysis

Classification of nutritional status

The children's nutritional status was classified according to WHO (2007) International Child Growth Standards. These provide figures for median weight, height and body mass index (BMI, i.e. weight in kg divided by the square of height in metres) for age[30] of normal healthy children, up to the age of 18 years (weight-for-age up to 10 years), and the equivalent values for ±1, 2 and 3 standard deviations (also known as Z-scores) from the median value. This expresses an observed weight or height in Z-scores of weight-for-age (WAZ), height-for-age (HAZ) and BMI-for-age (BMIAZ). Z-scores were classified according to the globally accepted cut-off points described by *Médecins sans Frontières* (Boelaert 1995) as shown below:

[30] The ages of the Standard 1 pupils were recorded in years attained. For comparison with the growth standards, six months were added to the recorded age in years.

Z-Score/Median based cut-off point for indicators of nutritional status			
Nutritional status*	Z-Scores		
	Severe malnutrition**	Moderate malnutrition**	Normal
WAZ, HAZ	<-3.00	-3.00 – -2.00	≥ -2.00

* WAZ = Weight-for-Age Z-score; HAZ = Height-for-Age Z-score. The same applies for BMIAZ.
** Together, 'moderate malnutrition' and 'severe malnutrition' are also denoted as 'global malnutrition', currently also denoted as 'global undernutrition', which should not be confused with overnutrition (Z-scores>+2.00).

The principle of this classification is that the range of values within 2 standard deviations above or below the reference median is considered to be the normal range of biological variation. Thus children growing normally are expected to have a nutritional status (in terms of attained body weight or height for age, or of body proportions) within the normal range. If a child has z-score below -2, it is considered to be underweight (in the case of WAZ), stunted (in the case of HAZ) or wasted (in the case of BMIAZ. If a child has a z-score above +2, this may indicate overnutrition, but that topic is outside the scope of this study.

Relationship between school feeding and nutrition

Based on the survey data, an attempt has been made to see whether there is a relationship between school feeding, on the one hand, and the average nutritional condition of Standard 1 primary school pupils, on the other. This is complicated and involved the following steps:

1. Two schools had to be excluded because they had no Standard 1. Two schools where no measurements could be done and one school where the ages could not be ascertained had to be excluded. This left 69 schools for further analysis. Another eight schools were excluded from some of the analyses because there were fewer than 17 pupils and this was considered too low to provide reliable estimates of the prevalence percentages of undernutrition among Standard 1 pupils in that school.
2. To qualify for 'school feeding: yes', schools had to meet the following conditions: (i) the feeding programme had to benefit the pupils (and not only staff and/or other school personnel); (ii) lunch had to be provided; (iii) the school feeding programme had to have been running since at least 2005 because otherwise the period between the start of the school feeding programme and the time of pupils' measurements (at the end of their first semester) would be too short to expect a measurable impact; and (iv) (some

of) the Standard 1 pupils had to be eligible for the school feeding programme. This last condition was difficult because the survey data did not show how many Standard 1 pupils actually *had* school feeding at school. In all, 27 schools met these conditions and were labelled as 'schools providing school feeding for Standard 1' in Tables 4.4 and 4.8 above.

3. Another 27 schools were labelled as 'schools not providing school feeding for Standard 1'. Fifteen were primary schools with no feeding programme whatsoever; the other twelve did have a feeding programme but did not qualify because Standard 1 pupils were not eligible.
4. To establish any possible relationship between school feeding ('providing school feeding for Standard 1' or not, as defined above) and the nutritional condition of the children, the question was whether schools offering school feeding for Standard 1 pupils had a lower percentage of undernourished children than those not offering school feeding for Standard 1.

For each of the anthropometric indicators (prevalence of being wasted, stunted and underweight, respectively), the schools in the whole sample were ranked according to their prevalence percentages and the quartile values Q1, Q2 and Q3 calculated. According to the definition of quartiles, a quarter of the total number of observations (schools) has a prevalence percentage below Q1, another quarter between Q1 and Q2, another quarter between Q2 and Q3, and the final quarter above Q3. To summarize the frequency distributions, categories were made according to these quartile values (depending on the anthropometric index in question) and the prevalence percentages in each category were counted and the frequencies obtained were expressed as percentages of the number of schools, so that the results could be presented in the form of tables. The tables in the main text are simplified versions that show the percentages of schools within only two categories of prevalence percentages:, namely lower or higher than the median prevalence percentage (i.e. Q2) of the index in question.

References

Bennett, J. (2003), *Review of school feeding projects*. London: DFID, Programme of Advisory Support Services for Rural Livelihoods.

Boelaert, M., A. Davis, B. Le Lin, M. Michelet, K. Ritmeijer, S. van der Kam & F. Vautier (eds) (1995), *Nutrition guidelines to facilitate the application of fundamental concepts and principles necessary for the assessment of nutritional problems and the Implementation of nutritional programmes in emergency situations*. Paris: Médecins Sans Frontières.

Dongus, S. (2000), *Vegetable production on open spaces in Dar es Salaam: Spatial changes from 1992 to 1999*. Dar es Salaam: Urban Vegetable Promotion Project.

Foeken, D., S.O. Owuor & A.M. Mwangi (2007), *School farming and school feeding in Nakuru town, Kenya: Practice and potential*. Leiden: African Studies Centre, ASC Working Paper 76. https://openaccess.leidenuniv.nl/dspace/handle/1887/13008.
Foeken, D. & S.O. Owuor (2008), Farming as a livelihood source for the urban poor of Nakuru, Kenya. *Geoforum* 39(6): 1978-1990.
Government of Ghana (2006), *Ghana School Feeding Programme. Programme document 2007-2010*. Accra: Government of Ghana.
Greenhalgh, T., E. Kristjansson & V. Robinson (2007), Realist review to understand the efficacy of school feeding programmes. *British Medical Journal* 335: 858-861.
Hijazi, S.S. & D. Abdulatif (1986), The nutritional impact of a school feeding programme in Mafraq, Jordan. *Journal of Tropical Paediatrics* 32(4): 174-180.
Hoorweg, J., D. Foeken & W. Klaver (1995), *Seasons and nutrition at the Kenya Coast*. Aldershot: Avebury.
Kariuki, J. (2005), Schools in novel farm project. *Daily Nation*, 13 April 2005. http://www.nationmedia.com/ dailynation/printpage.asp?newsid=46980.
Levinger, B. (1986), *School feeding programs in developing countries: An analysis of actual and potential impact*. Washington, DC: Bureau for Food and Voluntary Aid.
Levinger, B. (1996), *Nutrition, health and education for all*. Newton, MA: Education Development Center. Accessed 9 January 2003 at: http://www.edc.org/GLG/NHEA.
Meme, M.M. (1996), *Nutrient intake and nutritional status of children in a school with and without a feeding programme in Nyambene District, Kenya*. Nairobi: University of Nairobi, Applied Nutrition Programme, MSc Thesis.
Meme, M.M., W. Kogi-Makau, N.M. Muroki & R.K. Mwadime (1998), Energy and protein intake and nutritional status of primary school children 5 to 10 years of age in schools with and without feeding programmes in Nyambene District, Kenya. *Food and Nutrition Bulletin* 19(4): 334-342.
Moock, P. & J. Leslie (1986), Childhood malnutrition and schooling in the Terai region of Nepal. *Journal of Development Economics* 20(1) 33-52.
MCN (1999), *Strategic Nakuru Structure Plan. Action plan for sustainable urban development of Nakuru town and its environs*. Nakuru: Municipal Council of Nakuru.
Oxfam (2009), Urban poverty and vulnerability in Kenya. Oxfam GB Briefing Note, 10.
Pieters, J.J.L., J.P.C. de Moel, O. van Steenbergen & W.J.M. van der Hoeven (1977), Effects of school feeding on growth of children in Kirinyaga District, Kenya. *East African Medical Journal* 54: 624-629.
Pollitt, E. (1990), *Malnutrition and infection in the classroom*. Paris: UNESCO.
Potutan, G.E., E.M. Imam, R.J. Holmer & W.H. Schnitzler (1999), *School gardens of Cagayan de Oro contributing to food security. Initial observations*. Mimeo.
Rajalakshmi, R. & K. Vanaja (1967), Chemical and biological evaluation of the effects of fermentation on the nutritive value of foods prepared from rice and grains. *British Journal of Nutrition* 21: 467.
Republic of Kenya (1970), *Kenya population census 1969, vol. 1*. Nairobi: Government Printer.
Republic of Kenya (2000), *Economic survey 2000*. Nairobi: Government Printer.
Republic of Kenya (2001), *Poverty reduction strategy paper for the period 2001-2004*. Nairobi: Ministry of Finance and Planning.
SCN (2004), *Contribution to the Millennium Development Goals. Report of the thirty-first session at the United Nations and UNICEF, New York, 22-26 March 2004*.

United Nations System Standing Committee on Nutrition. Accessed 1 December 2009 at: http://www.unscn.org/files/Annual_Sessions/31st_SCN_Session/31st_session_REPORT.pdf.

SID (2004), *Pulling apart: Facts and figures on inequality in Kenya*. Nairobi: Society for International Development.

Simeon, D.T. & S.M. Grantham-McGregor (1989), Effects of missing breakfast on the cognitive function of school children of differing nutritional status. *American Journal of Clinical Nutrition* 49: 646-653.

Tearle, P. (2006), *Gardens for Life: Pilot. Final evaluation report.* Accessed 15 January 2010 at: https://www.edennet.org/evalresearch/final-eval-complete.pdf.

VOA News (2003), Kenya's schools try to accommodate free education. Nairobi, 3 February. Accessed 19 March 2003 at: http://www.insnews.org/world/focus/2003/02/kenya.free.education.

WFP (2007), *Food for education works. A review of WFP/FFE programme monitoring and evaluation 2002-2006*. Rome: World Food Programme. Accessed 1 December 2009 at: http://www.schoolsandhealth.org/sites/ffe/Key%20Information/Food%20for%20Education%20Works%202006.pdf.

WFP (2009a), *Feed minds, Change lives: School feeding: highlights and new directions*. World Food Programme. Accessed 1 December 2009 at: http://home.wfp.org/stellent/groups/public/documents/newsroom/wfp204709.pdf

WFP (2009b), *Our work: School meals*. World Food Programme. Accessed 1 December 2009 at: http://www.wfp.org/school-meals.

WFP (2009c), *Learning from experience: Good practices from 45 years of school feeding*. World Food Programme. Accessed 4 June 2010 at: http://home.wfp.org/stellent/groups/public/documents/newsroom/wfp204664.pdf.

WFP/UNICEF (2004), *The essential package. Twelve interventions to improve the health and nutrition of school-age children*. Rome: World Food Programme & UNICEF. Accessed 22 February 2010 at: http://documents.wfp.org/stellent/groups/public/documents/newsroom/wfp212806.pdf.

WHO (2006), *Child growth standards for children 0-5 years*. Geneva: World Health Organization.

WHO (2007), *Standards for school age children and adolescents*. Geneva: World Health Organization.

Wilson, A. (1981), Longitudinal analysis of diet, physical growth, verbal development and school performance. In: J. Balderston, A. Wilson, M. Freire & M. Simonen (eds), *Malnourished children of the rural poor*, pp. 39-79. Boston: Auburn House Publishing Company.

5

Dashed hopes and missed opportunities: Malaria control policies in Kenya (1896-2009)

Kenneth Ombongi & Marcel Rutten

This chapter discusses the fight against malaria, a disease that kills some two million people, mainly young children, in Africa every year, and the attempts that have been made to overcome it since the arrival of the British in Kenya in the late 19th century. Early efforts were characterized by a lack of knowledge and funds. Whenever funding was available, the choice as to where anti-malaria programmes were to be implemented was marred by politically, economically and even racially motivated arguments. Specialized traditional medicine was driven underground but seems to have re-established itself nowadays due to urbanization and, until recently, a lack of cheap modern drugs. This is also offering new business opportunities for individuals marketing themselves as herbalists and for (multinational) companies patenting new drugs derived partly from indigenous knowledge. Access to anti-malarials might appear to be in the hands of market forces and the ability to pay determines one's chances of being cured. However, international donors, includeing those in the private sector, have finally joined the fight in recent years with the delivery of free drugs, impregnated nets and the possibility of a vaccine in the near future.

Introduction

> The world has started a war against malaria, a war we can all win. We have a grand alliance, called Roll Back Malaria. And on the first World Malaria Day, we have presidents and basketball players involved. This is the only war the leaders can win, and they have to win this war against malaria. (Senegalese singer Youssou N'Dour, 25/4/2008)

Malaria[1] in Africa accounts for an estimated 90% of the 300-500 million cases of the disease that occur globally each year. It is responsible for 10% of Africa's disease burden and for 1 in 4 deaths among children under the age of five (Siso 2007). A child dies of malaria every 30 seconds. And when adults or their children have malaria, they cannot generate an income or produce the food they and their countries need, which makes malaria a major cause of poverty and widens the gap in prosperity between countries.[2] Finding a cure for malaria is essential to Africa's development.

Malaria is caused by a parasite that is transferred in the bite of an infected *Anopheles* mosquito.[3] *Plasmodium (P.) falciparum* is by far the deadliest of the four human malarial species. *P. malariam, P. ovale and P. vivax* are less severe although *vivax* is the most common. Complications from the *P. falciparum* variety include acute anaemia and cerebral malaria (WHO 2009).[4]

In Kenya, 70% of the population live in malarial areas (Republic of Kenya 2001a) although the pattern and severity of the disease varies in different parts of the country. Kenya has 63 malaria-endemic districts, with 16 highland malaria epidemic-prone districts and 8 arid and semi-arid districts with an unstable malaria epidemiological pattern. Efforts to control the disease in these different epidemiological zones have involved a variety of interventions. The above eco-

---

1 The disease's name comes from the Italian *mal'aria* meaning 'bad air'. In Rome, where malaria raged for centuries, it was commonly believed that the air in swampy areas was a breeding ground for the disease. Some scientists even believe that one in every two people who have ever lived have died of malaria (Finkel 2007).

2 The 2005 Abuja Declaration notes that 'malaria has slowed economic growth in African countries by 1.3% per year as a result of which GDP for African countries is now 37% lower than it would have been in the absence of malaria'. Others, however, question these findings (Ashraf *et al.* 2008).

3 This mosquito has long legs and dappled wings, is of the genus Anopheles and is the only insect capable of harbouring the human malaria parasite. Only female mosquitoes are a danger as they depend on protein-rich haemoglobin to nourish their eggs. The mosquito oils the bite area with a spray of saliva containing one-celled malaria parasites, known as plasmodia, which originate in the mosquito's salivary glands. Typically, a couple of dozen slip into the bloodstream but it takes just a single plasmodium to kill a person (Finkel 2007).

4 Following an *Anopheles* mosquito bite, the sporozoites, the infectious form of the malaria parasite enters the liver cells within minutes, takes on a new form and multiplies. When the liver cells rupture, blood stage parasites – known as merozoites – are released. Each merozoite invades a red blood cell and multiplies. The red cell ruptures to release more merozoites. This stage causes the disease and, too often, culminates in death. Some merozoites change into gametocytes that can be eliminated by a drug or taken up by the bite of a mosquito. In the mosquito's stomach, these gametocytes fertilize new eggs full of sporozoites, which will ultimately be injected into another human with the next bite (MVI/PATH n.d.).

logical zones are classified as follows: *high malaria risk areas* are lakesides, coastal, highland and arid areas (Categories 1-4), and *low malaria risk areas* include highlands within Central Province (Category 5).

In 2009, 4.3 million people (10.6% of Kenya's population) were living in areas of very high transmission intensity. There is a strong suggestion that more and more regions of Kenya have low, stable endemic conditions, notably along the coast (Snow *et al.* 2009). It is not clear whether the provision of treated nets, new drugs and better environmental management have caused this decline, as the downward trend seems to have started before these measures were implemented. Other causes could be changing weather patterns and improved socio-economic conditions. Still, an estimated 6,000 primgravid Kenyan women suffer from malaria-associated anaemia each year and 34,000 children under the age of five die from malaria. When a family member gets malaria, household resources are needed to transport the patient and to pay for the consultation and for drugs. In Kenya, it is estimated that 170 million working days are lost each year due to malaria. School attendance is also disrupted with approximately 4 million school days being lost annually as a result of malaria, which can rise to 10 million in years with epidemics (KGF 2 2002). This disease burden has a draining effect on Kenyan health resources as 30% of all outpatient appointments and 19% of inpatient admissions are due to malaria (Republic of Kenya 2001a). In recent years, new ways have been sought to increase spending on public health globally and leaders of the G8 countries acknowledged the need for resources in their meeting in Okinawa, Japan in 2000. This was welcomed by African leaders at a summit held in Abuja, Nigeria in April 2001 that resulted in the establishment of the Global Fund to Fight AIDS, Tuberculosis and Malaria (GFATM) in early 2002. It provides a quarter of all international financing for AIDS globally, two-thirds of tuberculosis funding and three-quarters of the money being used in the fight against malaria.[5]

Besides these resources, progress is being reported in understanding and finding a cure for the disease. At the same time, new medicines able to cure or control the devastation were soon priced beyond the reach for those who most needed them. This fuelled a global movement to reduce the cost of essential

---

[5] The World Health Organization (WHO) has made the reduction in cases a top priority. Bill Gates, who has called malaria 'the worst thing on the planet', has donated hundreds of millions of dollars to the cause through the Bill and Melinda Gates Foundation (Finkel 2007). For example, the Gates Foundation has been working in collaboration with the Institute for One World Health, the first non-profit pharmaceutical company in the US, to produce a cheap synthetic artemisinin-type of anti-malarial drug.

Map 5.1 Malaria endemicity in Kenya

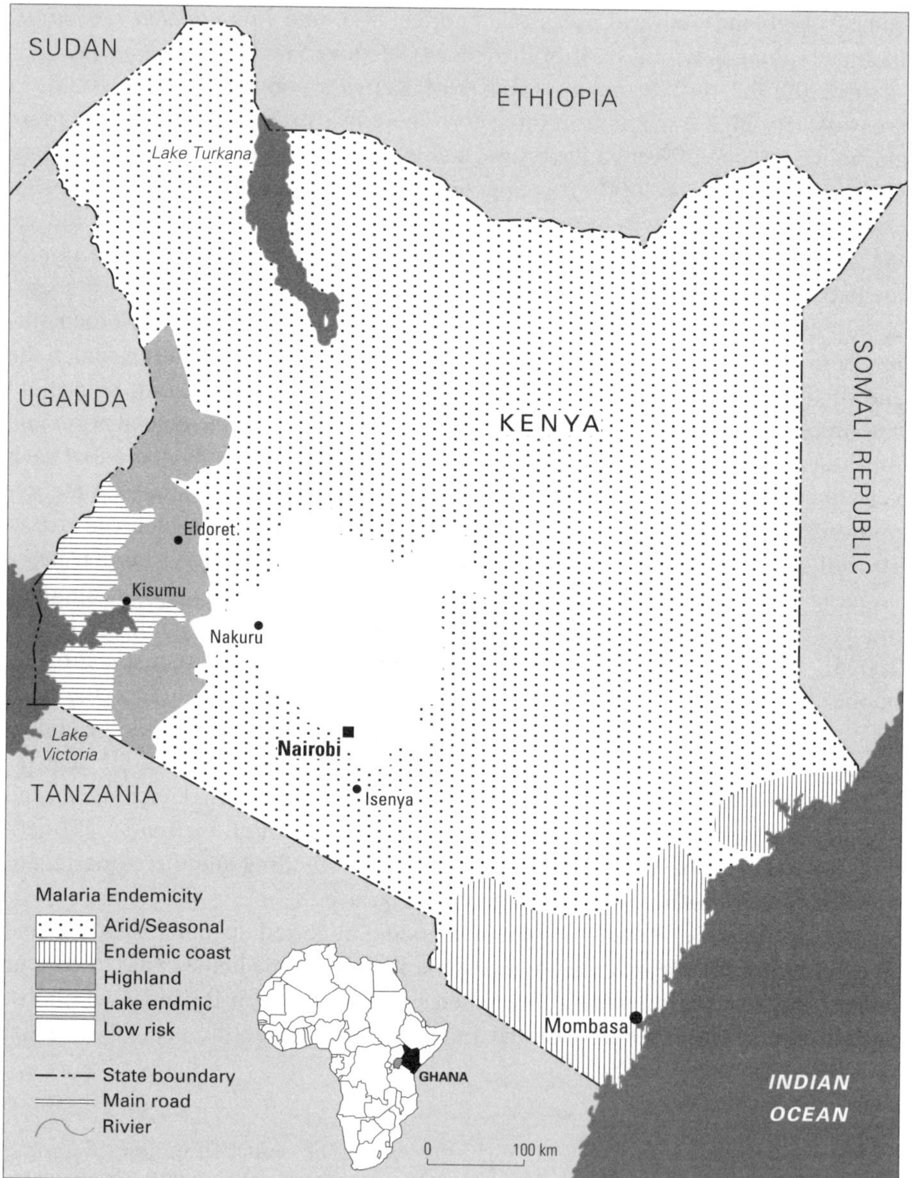

Source: Adapted from PMI (2009)

medicines, backed by an appeal that such commodities be seen as global public goods rather than commercial products (GFATM 2009).

Here we attempt a historical exposition of malaria control policies in Kenya from the late 19th century onwards. This longduree analysis of forces at stake in the fight against malaria is the background deemed necessary to understand the circumstances, knowledge and means that could be effective in defeating the disease. Attention will be devoted to processes of location and group-specific policies, commoditization and public-private counterforces in this enduring fight in the world, and in Kenya in particular. The questions posed in this chapter will, therefore, centre on which regions in Kenya that have suffer(ed) most from malaria. Which anti-malarial measures have been available and put in place? Which factors explain failures and successful interventions, if any? Who were the beneficiaries of these measures? Is malaria still the largely intractable, most important killer in Kenya? What treatment is provided by traditional healers to prevent and cure malaria? Which perceptions towards malaria are present among the African population now and in the past? Will bio-science provide the final blow for this disease or are we right in concluding that while the rest of the world seems to be basking in the power of bio-medicine to eradicate vector-borne diseases, the story of malaria control in Kenya smacks of dashed hopes and missed opportunities over the years?

Colonial policies to control malaria in Kenya: The early years (1896-1926)

Malaria control before World War I

During the early colonial years in Kenya, the fight against malaria was primarily in urban areas. The majority of the British, who the malaria campaign aimed to protect, settled initially in the emerging urban areas, while most of the Kenyan towns developed following the policy of the management of Uganda Railways. Malaria remained a public health threat in Mombasa, along the coast, in Kisumu and at Lake Victoria throughout the first quarter of the twentieth century. Even the mild malaria situation in Nairobi, the colonial capital, attracted official attention because of its perceived threat to European residents.[6]

While contagious diseases, such as plague, tended to dominate African and Indian areas in Nairobi, the increase in malaria was notable among Europeans. In Kisumu and Mombasa, where locals demonstrated some level of tolerance to the disease, Europeans suffered immensely. Urban officials, eager to protect Eu-

[6] Much of the material here is taken from K. Ombongi, *Urban malaria control in Kenya* (forthcoming).

ropeans, adopted racially selective sanitary practices that provided the context in which malaria control activities were to be conceived and executed during Kenya's colonial era.

The early control of urban malaria revolved around traditional methods of town sanitation.[7] The 'sanitation syndrome' had been perfected in the campaign against epidemic plague between 1900 and 1915[8] and represented a triumph of environmental determinism over bio-medicine. This was reflected in the over-emphasis on general sanitation *vis-à-vis* laboratory-based medicine.

The overemphasis on environmental management, as a method of choice in the fight against malaria, was not unique to Kenya. This was commonplace in the malaria-prone British African territories at the beginning of the twentieth century (Dummett 1968: 158-159). Sanitation, as a strategy in the fight against malaria, received a boost when it became accepted that mosquitoes played a role in the transmission of the disease after Ronald Ross's work of 1897 (Ross 1910: ix). The need for good sanitation remained deeply embedded in the early colonial administration's psyche and it was only gradually that quinine prophylaxis and more scientifically informed vector-based measures were used.[9]

Environmental management however had its apparent limitations so the colonial urban authorities were forced to adopt social control of, as opposed to social provision for, its growing African and Indian population as a strategy in its attempts to control malaria (Hake 1977: 40). The key mechanisms of social control included legislation and racial segregation.

The content, target and application of urban malaria legal policies were informed by the imperial notions of African and Indian hygienic 'backwardness' and vector prevention measures. The earliest rules to control mosquitoes appeared in Nairobi with 'The Nairobi Township (Suppression of Mosquitoes) Rules, 1911'. The timing of the rules was determined by reports of 'many cases of malaria amongst Europeans' (MD 1911: 12) and they forced the sanitary inspector to check households regularly and issue warning notices to those that tolerated mosquito propagation.

---

[7] Other strategies against malaria, such as the use of quinine, a primordial anti-malarial, were not officially emphasized. Quinine was sparingly used and mainly for prophylactic purposes.

[8] The phrase 'sanitation syndrome' is borrowed from Swanson (1997) in which she discusses the significance of sanitary measures in the configuration of urban power relations in apartheid South Africa. Plague and smallpox epidemics were common in Nairobi, Mombasa and Kisumu between 1900 and 1915.

[9] The first widely known malaria remedy was the bark of the cinchona tree, a close cousin of coffee, and was discovered in present-day Peru and Ecuador. Local people called the remedy *quina quina* (bark of barks), which was later distributed worldwide as quinine (Finkel 2007).

In Mombasa such a legal framework was necessitated by the 'complete apathy of the coloured population' and the 'habits of the natives' (MD 1910: 28). The authorities had contemplated a 'Mosquito Ordinance' as early as 1908 but this was 'deferred pending the education of public opinion' (MD 1908: 33). The intended education programme was frustrated by the use of earthen vessels and shallow wells for domestic water, which forced the authorities to adopt the Mosquito Suppression Rules in 1912 (MD 1912: 14-15).

Racial segregation became another measure of social control adopted in urban centres against malaria and was in keeping with the interests of white urban residents. 'The Public Health Ordinance of 1913' was the first statute to institute racial segregation on health grounds in Kenyan towns.[10] However, *de facto* steps in that direction were evident in Nairobi, Mombasa and Kisumu from the turn of the twentieth century onwards (KNA/DC/NBI.1/1/1:6; KNA/PC/NZA/1/4: 2; Curtin 1985: 610).

The use of racial and residential segregation as a measure to control malaria was a product of the colonial distortion of late nineteenth-century developments in immunology. The concept of 'health disease carriers' was pioneered in 1884 by Friedrich Loeffler, a German bacteriologist, while studying diphtheria. In 1893 Robert Koch, another German scientist, discovered that cholera could be spread the same way, by carrying bacteria (Leavitt 1992: 610-615). By 1900, Koch had firmly established that people in malarial areas acquired gradual immunity to infection and became 'health disease carriers' of plasmodia, the protozoan parasite that causes malaria (Dummett 1968: 171-172). Although Koch's discovery proved that immunity to malaria was individual and not racial, skin colour became an important issue when determining health policy in urban Kenya.

The legal and social control measures of the first two decades of the twentieth century notwithstanding, an upsurge of malaria, particularly among Europeans, was increasingly evident (KNA/DC/NBI.1/1/1: 15; MD 1908: 1-2, 26) due to the emerging social geography of colonial towns. Beneath the new urban order was the unanticipated (dis)order of matters as a result of African mobility in the wake of colonialism. While African mobility bred the 'Black Highlands' (squatter areas) on the edges of the so-called White Highlands, it led in urban centres to what Hake (1977: 9) called the 'two-faced city'. The city presented

---

10 The promulgation of this ordinance followed the visit to Kenya of W.J. Simpson, a professor of hygiene at Kings College, London, who was detailed by the CO to advise on the colony's sanitary policy. On the basis of his findings, he recommended the formalization of racial residential zoning on health grounds (*The Official Gazette*, 15/10/1913: 875-8; MD 1913: 18, 34).

both 'a modern front to the world' and a 'backyard' of a 'self-help city',[11] 'a shanty town, where reside (sic) ever-increasing number of [African] migrants, hawkers and odd-job men'. This led to networks that were important for urban epidemiological change and sustained a two-way migration, 'straddling', to a much wider rural catchment that accounted for the rising rates of urban malaria (Lonsdale 2002: 207-222).

Malaria control during and after World War I

World War I was, in a sense, both a bane and a blessing for urban malaria control in Kenya. While in the short term the war disrupted routine anti-malarial sanitary measures, it shifted the paradigm of malaria policy in fundamental ways in the long term. Massive labour demands and mobility during the war disrupted existing labour-intensive sanitary work against malaria (Clayton & Savage 1974: 81-91). However, it also induced new malaria epidemiological patterns. Colonial officials readily implemented measures, such as the mass administration of quinine, which would have been unimaginable before the war (MD 1914: 31-32; 1915: 32; 1916: 15).

After the war, 'laboratory medicine' enthusiasts believed that the general health of the African population infringed upon that of Europeans and government personnel and that Africans also needed official medical services for the common good of the colony. Public health education was touted as the basis of more racially inclusive measures to control malaria in urban areas. The disease came to be seen as the function of 'dirt and dearth' (MD 1922: 65; KNA/PC/NZA/1/20; MD 1925: 69).

In addition to the new concerns for native health, the campaign against malaria in the post-World War I period underwent other dramatic developments, such as making increased use of the Nairobi Medical Research Laboratory (NMRL). During the war, the laboratory was important in the microscopic diagnosis of malaria through 'blood films' (NMRL 1915: 56). And in the 1920s, with a new laboratory and an entomologist, basic research became a significant

[11] The three towns had 'self-help cities'. In Kisumu, Nyalenda & Manyatta estates were began in 1914 outside the town boundary and housed Africans who were not provided for by the administration. These areas soon became popular with low-income earners in the town. Later, railway and harbour workers were among the first Africans in Kisumu to receive permanent housing on Ubari Estate. In early Kisumu, Europeans lived in the higher Millimani area, the Indians lived in town and the Africans lived along the labour lines and landhies,on Ubari Estate and in the slums of Nyalenda and Manyatta, and a number commuted to town from their rural homesteads. African 'villages' developed on the outskirts of Nairobi in areas such as Pangani and Pumwani. Before World War I, there were five African villages within Nairobi (Kasoa 1989: 22, 87-88; Hake 1977: 24, 38).

part of vector-based sanitary works in urban Kenya (KNA/PC/NZA/3/45/6, 1925-29: 8-10; MD 1923: 28).

Colonial policies to control malaria in Kenya: The intermediate years (1939-1950)

World War II provided a major breakthrough in the control of malaria globally as a result of an increase in new drugs and residual insecticides. New strategies facilitated a large-scale rural malaria campaign that was to be a significant feature in policies to control malaria in the 1950s. The prospects of success in fighting malaria, which the war period offered in the short term, were disappointing in the long term. The war years set in motion the prolonged use of drugs and insecticides that would ultimately lead to the development of vector and parasite resistance.

Vector control in urban Kenya during World War II

The outbreak of World War II exacerbated a resurgence in malaria to the levels that Nairobi had experienced in the 1920s and in the second half of the 1930s. This upsurge culminated in an epidemic in 1940 and impacted on the military malaria programmes in determining the course of malaria control campaigns throughout the war.

Towards the end of 1939, there was an increased risk of malaria transmission in Nairobi due to military activity, increased rural-urban population movements and vector-conducive weather conditions.[12] The authorities responded to the epidemic along traditional lines of vector destruction but with a vigour generated by the war.[13] At the same time, the government fostered interdepartmental coordination in the organization and execution of activities to fight malaria in Nairobi.[14]

The epidemic of 1940 ignited the *ad hoc* reorganization of the anti-malaria service in Nairobi that involved the military, Nairobi Municipal Council (NMC) and various government departments. What the city lacked in organization and finance in the pre-war years, it was able to make up for with increased funds and military and civilian labour during the war period. The military unit res-

---

12 Commissioner for Local Government, Lands and Settlement to Town and District Clerks, 19/02/1940, p. 1, KNA RN/13/12; Nairobi Native Affairs Department Annual Report 1939, p. 1, KNA RN/13/12.

13 Commissioner for Local Government, Lands and Settlement to Town and District Clerks, 19/02/1940, p. 2, KNA RN/13/12.

14 Town Clerk to Councillor E.E. Biss (Member of the Public Health Committee), 4/4/1940, KNA RN/4/10.

ponsible for malaria engaged in anti-malaria work with such discipline and regularity that the media attributed the drastic reduction in incidences of malaria in 1941 to their efforts.[15]

The enormous expansion of vector control by environmental sanitation in Nairobi came with new challenges in terms of the high demand for sanitary labourers.[16] Consequently, bush clearing, the canalizing of streams, the draining of swamps and the use of larvicides, which had been put in place by the military, disintegrated after their withdrawal in 1946.

Although the malaria situation in Mombasa and Kisumu on the eve of the war had been quite different from that in Nairobi, similar policies were followed there too. Although Mombasa and Kisumu did not experience the epidemics prevalent in Nairobi,[17] the three cities were equally important as military mobilizing centres and required intense malaria control programmes to protect the military.[18] In the early war period, the cities depended on vector control by routine environmental sanitation and the use of larvicides but a shortage of labour affected the effective application of these strategies. The introduction of synthetic drugs and Dichloro-diphenyl-trichloroethane (DDT), a residual insecticide, ended dependency on labour-intensive larvicidal and environmental sanitation control methods from 1946 onwards.

Malaria control by drugs and insecticides during and after World War II

Before World War II, Paris green and pyrethrum predominated as larvicidal and fumigating agents for controlling mosquitoes in Kenya. Quinine was the dominant drug for malaria therapy and prophylaxis. The introduction of DDT during the war revolutionised vector control, and the invention of quinine substitutes did so for the malaria pharmacopoeia throughout the world. In Kenya these new anti-malaria 'tools' became available towards the end of the war and influenced malaria control policies more in the post-war era.

At the outbreak of the war, no malaria drugs were being produced in Kenya and the colony, like other British territories, was heavily dependent on imports

---

15 East African Standard, 7/07/1942: 3.

16 *Ibid.*: 3-4; Town Clerk's annual report of anti-malaria work in 1945, KNA RN/11/5, pp. 5-6.

17 *Mombasa Times*, 7/11/1935, p. 5. In the 1930s it was common knowledge within medical circles that mosquito proliferation in Mombasa had declined alongside a general improvement in the health of the town. Ironically however, 'A not insignificant amount of malaria still occurs ... and periodically assumes larger proportions'. This is the malaria that was usually referred to as 'residual malaria'. See Wiseman *et al.* (1939: 1).

18 Coast Province senior MO to Mombasa Fortress Commander, 2/2/1940, KNA/BY/13/170; Kisumu Municipal Board Annual Report (1942: 7).

for the supply of quinine. In 1939 it dawned on the Kenyan authorities that they should regulate quinine distribution more strictly as the war could dramatically affect their demand and price.[19] To guard against the possibility of hoarding by unscrupulous traders out to take advantage of the war conditions, the government immediately increased the price of quinine from cost price to a level at which one could not make a profit in the event of re-sale.[20]

In no time at all, the escalation of the price for quinine became obvious, particularly in view of Kenya's reliance on imports from the Dutch colony of Indonesia. In 1942 the Japanese overran the Indonesian island of Java, cutting off Europeans and most of their colonies from the leading producer of quinine.[21] In Kenya, as in the rest of East Africa, this led to strict attempts to economize on existing quinine stocks and, on the other hand, efforts were made to produce quinine locally. However, attempts by East African governments to grow cinchona trees and establish a quinine manufacturing plant in Dar es Salaam, Tanzania, did not result in much success.[22]

The end of Javanese quinine supplies prompted developments in Europe and America that dramatically transformed the contemporary malaria pharmacopoeia. Research concerns in the UK focused on the development of synthetic anti-malarials. Mepacrine, one of the earliest products, was developed by Imperial Chemical Industries (ICI) in Manchester and proved successful as a suppressive in field trials in 1943-44 among Australian volunteers (Bruce-Chwatt 1988: 44). It replaced quinine among the Allied forces in the malarial war theatres in South-East Asia and the southeastern Pacific. The drug reached Kenya in 1945 and was quickly put on the market to replace the dwindling stocks of quinine.[23] However, mepacrine did not gain local popularity due to its toxicity and skin paling. In 1946 ICI released another drug, paludrine, which was better accepted because of its low toxicity, had no staining effect on the skin and caused no gastro-intestinal upsets in comparison with mepacrine and

---

19 *Ibid.*: 2.

20 Chief Secretary to DMS, 6/11/1939; Extract from *Official Gazette*, 7/11/1939 General Notice, KNA/BY/14/50.

21 Colonial Office Memorandum, 1/4/1942, p. 1, KNA/BY/14/49.

22 See Chief Secretary Tanganyika to Chief Secretary Kenya, 24/3/1942; Chief Secretary to DMS, 25/11/1943; Secretary E.A. Production and Supply Council to Chief Secretary, Entebbe, 2/12/1943; Secretary of Governors Conference to Under Secretary of State for Colonies, 15/07/1943, KNA/BY/14/49.

23 *East African Standard*, 10/5/1945 and DMS general notice draft to the Chief Secretary for publication in the *Official Gazette*, 12/4/1945, p. 1, KNA/BY/14/28.

quinine.[24] In Kenya, paludrine field trials started in November 1946 on the Buret Tea Estate in Kericho and in a Kisumu jail to observe its prophylactic value compared with mepacrine.[25] By the end of the experiment, paludrine had failed to provide full protection, compared to mepacrine which suppressed malaria, but the Director of Medical Services (DMS) was optimistic 'that paludrine given more frequently might produce better results'.[26] Later this was proved in an experiment carried out in Nairobi.

Other anti-malarials developed directly or indirectly as a result of the war included chloroquine and pyrimethamine.[27] Chloroquine quickly gained acceptance because of its low toxicity and more therapeutic effect than many of the other contemporary anti-malarials. Pyrimethamine development was a joint Anglo-American venture between 1949 and 1950 and clinical trials conducted in Lagos, Nigeria, and The Gambia produced good results (Coatney 1963; McGregor & Smith 1952; Bruce-Chwatt 1988: 44-45). Chloroquine and pyrimethamine became the mainstays of large-scale malaria programmes in Kenya in the 1950s and 1960s. Indeed, chloroquine would hold sway as an effective first-line malaria therapy and suppressant in Kenya, as in the rest of Africa, until the late 1970s when plasmodia resistance broke its dominance.[28] Pyrimethamine, like chloroquine, was less toxic than many contemporary anti-malarials and provided an effective prophylactic tool in rural Kenyan malaria control programmes in the 1950s.

In addition to synthetic drugs, the introduction of DDT revolutionalized the control of malaria in the post-World War II period. DDT was invented in 1941 by a Swiss chemist, Paul Muller, and was commercially manufactured in the

---

24 Imperial Chemical (Pharmaceuticals) Ltd, 'Paludrine in the chemotherapy of malaria', KNA/BY/14/13 and Sales Manager Imperial Chemical to DMS, Kenya, 17/06/1946, KNA/BY/14/13.

25 'A field trial of paludrine and mepacrine in malaria control', p. 1, KNA/BY/14/13.

26 DMS to Chief Secretary, 20/11/1946, KNA/BY/14/13.

27 During World War I, Java and its valuable quinine stores fell into Japanese hands. German troops in East Africa suffered heavy casualties from malaria as a result and the German government asked Bayer Dye Works to find a quinine substitute. In 1934 German scientists synthesized resochin but it was considered to be too toxic and was forgotten until the outbreak of World War II when, due to the German invasion of the Netherlands and the Japanese occupation of Java, the Allied forces were cut off from quinine supplies. This stimulated a renewed search for other anti-malarials in the UK and the US. After the Allied occupation of North Africa, French soldiers raided a supply of German-manufactured Sontochin in Tunis and handed it over to the Americans. They made slight adjustments to it and this new formulation was called chloroquine. It was later found to be identical to the older and supposedly toxic resochin. See: http://www.malariasite.com/malaria/history_treatment.htm

28 For an analysis of the development of resistance to chloroquine, see Muhindi (1993).

UK and the US in 1943. The first DDT trials in Mombasa started in May 1945, with the aim of controlling anopheline breeding in a 600-yard strip by spraying the area weekly. The results were disappointing due to technical difficulties that inhibited precision in spraying and the high costs involved. In the eyes of the medical authorities, the DDT fiasco in Mombasa was compensated for by success in the Kisumu trials in the same year. They gave 'a very dramatic reduction in the anopheline population followed immediately on the beginning of air-spray with D.D.T'.[29] Encouraged by this success, the medical authorities expanded malaria control programmes of mass drug administration and insecticide spraying. This continued into the 1950s.

Colonial policies to control malaria in Kenya: The late years (1950-1963)

In the late colonial period between 1950 and 1963, the Kenyan authorities applied two large-scale methods to control malaria. One was the combined use of synthetic drugs and residual insecticides, while the other was the biological technique of fish culture, which was mainly tested in Nyanza Province. The former was used continuously and offered good results. The latter had unexpected consequences and was deemed a disaster. Many of the anti-malarials and insecticides common in the 1950s became available during the war and were considered useful among civilians in the post-war era. They extended malaria control to rural areas and previously neglected suburbs in towns but the prolonged use of malaria drugs and insecticides gradually stimulated parasite and vector resistance, which complicated the campaign.

Drugs and insecticides in rural areas

The rural malaria control policy in the 1950s focused on irrigation and settlement schemes, using drugs and pesticides to reduce malaria transmission in both endemic and epidemic localities that were usually inhabited by non-immune populations. These malaria control schemes added a preventative dimension to the countryside, which had previously been dominated by self-medication or hospital treatment. However these curative anti-malaria measures remained important in the rural areas in the 1950s.

The development of drugs and pesticides had instilled hope of controlling malaria in the late 1940s. In 1950, the WHO malaria conference in Kampala, Uganda discussed the opportunities that these new tools offered in the fight against malaria in Africa (WHO 1951: 4). Debate there centred on two diver-

[29] Nyanza Province Annual Report 1945, KNA PC/NZA/1/40.

gent views; one group of malariologists supported the feasibility of malaria eradication in Africa, while another opposed it. The former argued that developments in chemotherapy and insecticides could enhance prospects of malaria eradication in Africa as they had done elsewhere in the world.[30] The latter doubted whether the continent's infrastructure would allow eradication.[31] Rural malaria control in Kenya in the 1950s tended towards 'control' rather than eradication and embraced the Kampala recommendations such as statistical improvements, training courses and interdepartmental collaboration, which inclined more towards a long-term policy of control than to immediate eradication. The Kenya government, however, rejected Kampala's call to undertake immediate anti-malaria measures regardless of local immunity. This recommendation, in the government's view, undermined the control policy dictated by the degree of malaria endemicity in various parts of the colony and was believed to have a bearing on people's immunity or tolerance.[32] On the application of residual insecticides, which according to Kampala could 'bring about a very large reduction in transmission of *gambiae* malaria' (WHO 1951: 47), the Director of Medical Services advocated caution: 'Residual insecticides, though effective are relatively expensive and total application in rural Kenya may be prohibitively high. Any scheme for residual insecticidal impregnation must be certain of continuation if disaster later is to be avoided.'[33] It was such arguments, in addition to economic considerations, that determined the course, scale and pace of large-scale malaria control schemes in the countryside in the 1950s.

The Uasin Gishu integrated malaria control project was one such scheme. It cut across the African reserves and the European settler area, involving the mass administration of drugs and insecticides, and local as well as international collaboration. The government undertook the project for three reasons. One was that Uasin Gishu was economically significant as the heart of the European farming region and thus the lifeline of the colonial economy. The second was that the area had 'unstable' as opposed to endemic malaria, whose transmission was easier to interrupt, and thus was typical of the areas to which the government had resolved to confine malaria control measures. Thirdly, cost sharing with local farmers solved the problem of financial paucity. Initially, the medical

---

30 For example, it was clear by then that the use of residual insecticide spraying had 'resulted in excellent malaria control in parts of Venezuela, British Guiana, Brazil, Argentine, Peru, Italy, Mauritius, Ceylon, India, and elsewhere' (WHO 1951: 10-11).

31 See Grewal (1996) & Malowany, Dobson & Snow (n.d.).

32 For the recommendation on the control of malaria regardless of local immunity, see WHO (1951: 45-46).

33 DMS to Director East Africa Malaria Unit, 20/12/1951, pp. 1-2, KNA Health/3/90.

administration made attempts to mobilize Uasin Gishu farmers by attributing low farm productivity to ill health due to malaria. The enthusiasm of European settlers for such a scheme was aroused and they were prepared to accept a project of this nature at their own expense. Mass treatment with pyrimethamine was successful in 1953 and 1954 but when dieldrin became available in 1955, it replaced this prophylaxis as a malaria control strategy in Uasin Gishu. The Kenya government, Uasin Gishu farmers, the United Nations International Children's Emergency Fund (UNICEF) and the WHO jointly funded the dieldrin hut impregnation scheme, which significantly reduced the *Anopheles* mosquito.[34] In 1957 because of the rising vector resistance, dieldrin spraying was replaced with 'a [malaria] case-detection and surveillance programme'.[35] The struggle to keep the district free of malaria by prophylactic chloroquine was the concern of the medical authorities from 1963 onwards.

In the 1950s, official efforts to control malaria extended beyond the European areas and adjoining African reserves. Irrigation and settlement schemes for Africans, which proliferated in this period, became the focus of the malaria control policy. Usually made up of non-immune people, the irrigation and settlement schemes became patches of epidemic malaria within areas of high endemicity. By the mid-1950s, Kenya had four major irrigation schemes: Mwea-Tebere and Yatta in Central Province, Perkerra in Rift Valley, and Hola in Coast Province.[36] Before irrigation, these areas had had a similar malaria ecology, characterized by high endemicity with occasional epidemics.[37] The introduction of 'wet cultivation' exacerbated malaria transmission because of the proliferation of mosquito breeding, and the resettling of non-immune people in these areas also worsened the situation as it increased the prospects of outbreaks of malaria. In March 1955, Mwea-Tebere had seven acres of land under rice cultivation and it was estimated that ultimately 70,000 acres could be available for paddy production.[38] The scheme was earmarked for the resettlement and employment of landless Africans released from Mau Mau detention camps as well as Africans who had remained loyal to the colonizers. However, protecting

---

34 Armed with the twin weapons of chloroquine and DDT, the WHO launched the Global Malaria Eradication Programme in 1955 to eliminate the disease within ten years. More than a billion dollars was spent, tens of thousands of tons of DDT were applied each year and chloroquine was widely distributed in what was probably the most elaborate international health initiative ever undertaken (Finkel 2007).

35 Ministry of Health and Housing annual report 1964, p. 49.

36 MD annual report 1956, p. 14 and Minutes of the 26th meeting of the Joint Irrigation Committee, 24/11/1956, KNA BY/13/300.

37 For the malaria ecology of the Mwea area, see Embu MOH to DMS, 20/1/1956, KNA BY/13/300.

38 Central Province PMO to DMS, 19/3/1955, KNA BY/13/300.

'imported loyalists and their families'[39] presented challenges. The authorities resolved to use chemoprophylaxis only in a way that would help immigrants develop immunity and if it was essential.[40] Financial constraints limited official efforts against malaria in Mwea-Tebere, unlike in Uasin Gishu where the government mobilized wealthy farmers to finance anti-malaria measures. Funding for the control of malaria came predominantly from official sources.

In the Shimba Hills, a settlement scheme in Kwale to the south of Mombasa, local officials resorted to the use of prophylactic drugs when residual insecticide spraying failed to offer protection to non-immune African settlers from central Kenya and Machakos.[41] In 1957 the authorities had used gammexane to curb malaria transmission in an impending epidemic, but to no avail. They quickly changed to using mass pyrimethamine treatment and achieved a sharp drop in the parasite rate from 40% to 15%.[42] The 1957 treatment set in motion a trend in which the authorities undertook annual drug distribution in the settlement to reduce malaria transmission. By 1962, the difficulty of completely eliminating malaria from an endemic area like the Shimba Hills had become clear to the authorities. Nevertheless, malaria had 'been adequately controlled and there is no doubt that this has added to the popularity of the scheme'.[43] The Shimba Hills project, unlike those in Mwea-Tebere and Uasin Gishu, depended only on the mass administration of drugs and illustrates how the contemporary malaria control policy hinged upon the use of synthetic drugs and residual applications of insecticides selectively applied from one area to another.

Drugs and insecticides in urban malaria control

The urban malaria control policy in Kenya in the 1950s was one of change and continuity in intensity, scale and strategy. In Kisumu and Mombasa, the authorities largely sustained malaria control programmes inherited from the war period. The Kisumu authorities used two techniques, hut spraying and swamp oiling, indiscriminately among Africans in and outside the municipal boundary. When DDT became available in Kisumu in 1946, the authorities used it for vector extermination in African huts until 1954 when its success rate against mosquitoes became doubtful. By 1956, dieldrin had been adopted as the first-

39 'Loyalists' refers to Africans who supported the government during the Mau Mau revolt.

40 DIBD senior medical entomologist to Embu MO, 25/1/1956; Central Province entomologist to Central Province PMO, 5/1/1956 and EMBU MOH to DMS, 30/1/1956, KNA BY/13/300.

41 Ministry of Health and Housing Annual Report 1962, pp. 23-24.

42 MD Annual Report 1957, p. 20.

43 Ministry of Health and Housing Annual Report 1962, pp. 23-24.

line pesticide as it required one instead of two sprayings a year, like other pesticides. In this lakeside town in the 1950s, vector control by environmental sanitation was the order rather than the exception. Constant reclamation of lake-shore land and the clearing of 'floating islands' were strategies unique to Kisumu over the years because of its proximity to the lake.

Mombasa had low rates of malaria as a result of the collaborative efforts of military and civilian staff after the war.[44] At the beginning of the 1950s, however, there were indications that this state of affairs could change due to the municipality's high rainfall and the increased re-infection of Mombasa Island from the mainland. This ended the easily controllable malaria situation on Mombasa Island offered by its relative isolation from the immediate hyperendemic hinterland. In response, the health authorities not only intensified control on the island but also anti-malaria services to outlying areas on the mainland. In 1952 the Mombasa Municipal Board extended its anti-malaria programmes to include those one mile outside the municipal boundary because it had been realized that *anopheles* easily crossed over from the mainland to infect the town residents.[45]

The Nairobi situation was different. Malaria control programmes had broken down at the start of the 1950s due to dwindling numbers of staff working on the control of malaria. The city[46] engaged the services of Bagster Wilson, the Director of the East African Malaria Unit, who helped to revitalize malaria control programmes in the early 1950s.[47] With only occasional malaria transmission creating complacency, Nairobi was different from other towns. However, all three towns – Kisumu, Mombasa and Nairobi – shared in efforts to extend the anti-malaria campaign to extra-municipal areas as a protective strategy against re-infection of areas within their municipal boundaries. The towns had a history of malaria control measures confined to the central areas and European quarters but by the 1950s this policy was no longer effective. The authorities realized that for anti-malaria measures in the inner areas of towns to be successful, control was necessary in the outlying suburbs. The availability of residual insecti-

44 In the post-war period, the Mombasa Municipal Board oversaw malaria control within the municipality and the army malaria control unit covered military bases in the town. In 1951, the government transferred malaria control on the military bases to the provincial medical office because the army detachments had been reduced too much to 'justify the retention of a Military Malaria Control unit to cater for the needs of the few army installations that will be left'. See Coast Province senior medical officer to Chief Secretary, 15/3/1951, KNA BY/13/176.

45 MD Annual Report 1952, p. 7.

46 Note that Nairobi ceased to be a municipality in March 1950 when it became a city.

47 For example, see Nairobi MOH Annual Report 1951, p. 28; Nairobi MOH Annual Report 1957, p. 33.

cides facilitated the extension of malaria control services to the peri-urban areas. Residual insecticide spraying, unlike the traditional larvicidal oiling and the use of Paris green, was less expensive and laborious.

Biological malaria control trials and fish farming in Nyanza

Official attempts to control malaria by larvivorous fish took place in Nyanza Province in the 1950s, although such efforts had been tried earlier in the 1930s.[48] However, the haphazard promotion of domestic fish farming by the Division of Fisheries against the wishes of the Nyanza medical officials made the fish pond project a disaster concerning malaria. The ponds induced mosquito breeding and demonstrated how easy well-intentioned colonial development projects led to mistakes due to minimal inter-departmental collaboration.

Initially the experiment aimed to test the potency of two tilapia species and *Astatoreochromis alluaudi* for weed and snail destruction respectively. In the proposed biological malaria control programme, scientists intended to interstock the larvivorous *gambusia* with a weed and snail-eating species of fish.[49] The argument was that *gambusia* and the snail-eating species could control malaria and bilharzia respectively and the weed-eater would check vegetation growth in ponds.[50] Of all the species tried, only the weed-eating species, *tilapia zillii*, showed good results. However, domestic fish ponds for commercial purposes gained popularity among local people in a short time. Instead of opposing the construction of ponds, the medical officials promoted the 'containment policy' that sought to control the spread of fish ponds to areas of low malaria endemicity unaffected by fish farming.[51] However, these efforts achieved little and the practice spread to the highlands more quickly than envisaged.[52]

If rampant fish pond proliferation in Nyanza undermined vector control by biological means in the late 1950s, resistance to drugs and insecticides gradually undermined malaria control by chemical methods. As early as 1953 there were reports of resistance to paludrine and pyrimethamine in Kisumu and Uasin Gishu.[53] In 1955 public health officials noted mosquito resistance to DDT in

48 Note that colonial Nyanza included the current Nyanza and Western Provinces.

49 Notes on a meeting with Dr Hickling, CO chief fisheries advisor 20/2/1952, KNA Health/3/90; Nyanza PMO to DMS, 20/10/1954 and the minutes of the meeting on fisheries in Nyanza Province, 6/9/1955, p. 2, KPRC ND/1/3.

50 Snails are as essential to bilharziasis (schistosomiasis) as mosquitoes are to malaria. The disease is contracted when schistosoma larvae released by snails penetrate the human skin contacted with infected water.

51 Fish ponds and their attendant health hazards, Medical Department memo, p. 2, 13/5/1959, KPRC ND/1/3.

52 Nyanza PMO to South Nyanza/Kisii MOH, 18/5/1961, KPRC ND/1/3.

53 Kisumu Municipal Board Annual Report 1953, n.p. MD Annual Report 1954, p. 20.

Kisumu and resolved to use dieldrin in their hut impregnation trials instead.[54] In 1956-57 there were reports of fly and mosquito resistance to dieldrin in Kisumu and Uasin Gishu respectively, which prompted calls for a return to DDT in the former and the setting aside of a pyrimethamine reserve to curb an anticipated epidemic in the latter.[55] The situation in Mombasa regarding dieldrin's potency towards mosquitoes was no better and the authorities in Mombasa replaced dieldrin with DDT in their hut impregnation in the mainland areas of the town in 1960.[56]

The prolonged use of drugs and insecticides gradually dashed the very hopes of success against malaria they had initially created. Nevertheless, these strategies were the most important of the combination of factors that provided a conducive environment for the expansion of malaria control in the 1950s and 1960s. This expansion needed other factors such as interdepartmental, regional and international collaboration besides colonial health infrastructure to regulate and determine its course. The simmering parasite and vector resistance somewhat constrained it and indicated what lay ahead in independent Kenya's anti-malaria campaign: a collapse of drug and insecticide control strategies and an upsurge in epidemic malaria with a vengeance never seen before.

The years after independence (1964-present)

Growing worries about synthetic drug resistance

Post-independent Kenya has witnessed new challenges in fighting the malaria menace, especially since the late 1970s. A study conducted in southwestern Kenya by Froeling & van Haften (1983) revealed that drug regime resistance of *P. falciparum* was clearly recognized for chloroquine and mefloquine. Fansidar, a widely used drug that combines sulphadoxine and pyrimethamine also showed rapidly decreasing affectivity in curing malaria, down from 35% in 1978 to 3% in 1980. Nyamongo (1997) reported that poverty in the 1990s forced people to use a drug with the highest resistance (Malaraquin), which was also the cheapest available. A lack of government finance to fight malaria and the growing adaptation of mosquitoes to the poisons used to kill them further exacerbated the situation.

Kwendo & Muganzi (1996) show figures for malaria cases of out-patients in hospitals in 1980, stressing the high level of incidences (over 34%) for the

---

54 Minutes of monthly meeting of Health Committee, Kisumu Municipality, 15/8/1955, KNA DC/KSM/1/16/37.

55 Minutes of the monthly meeting of Health Committee, Kisumu Municipality, 12/11/1956: 5-6, KNA DC/KSM/1/16/44 and MD Annual Report 1957, p. 20.

56 Mombasa MOH Annual Report 1960, p. 30.

Nyanza and Western regions compared to the Rift Valley region (around 15%). Epidemic malaria has increased in frequency and severity among the densely populated and economically important areas of Kenya since the late 1980s, following a period free of major malaria epidemics between the 1950s and the late 1980s. Likewise, the arid areas of Kenya experience rainfall-driven (El Niño) epidemics (Rep. of Kenya 2001a: 32). Several authors have suggested that the higher incidences of malaria reported in the 1980s and 1990s might be due to other causes. For example, Verhoef (2001: 178) hinted that HIV-1 infection might have led to an increased frequency of malaria although more research is needed to confirm this claim. Others have pointed to environmental changes, notably water development, as causing increased incidences of malaria. Thitai (1991) mentioned that irrigation schemes and hydropower reservoirs along the Tana River had created more breeding habitats for malaria vectors and changed the disease prevalence from seasonal to perennial, which led to higher mortality rates.

The issue of population growth, migration, water development and climate change might explain the rising chances of disease transmission as seen in areas that had been relatively free of malaria. For example, the 1940 disaster apparently went unnoticed in Kajiado District to the southeast of Nairobi.[57] Lately, the area has witnessed a rising growth in population, an increased development of shallow wells, boreholes and water pans as well as slightly higher rainfall regimes. Information from a public and a private hospital in the area shows that in 2008 malaria was the single most important reason for visiting the public hospital (47.2%), followed by respiratory disease (36.6%). The same picture emerged in 2009. In the private hospital, data concerning malaria tests for the 2007-2009 period showed that out of 552 malaria blood tests, a total of 184 scored positive (33.3%). This outcome might also explain why, in addition to financial costs and accessibility (transport, opening hours), local people take an intermediate treatment step first by visiting local herbalists.[58]

Perceptions and practices towards malaria

Siso (2007) conducted a survey to establish people's perceptions and practices concerning malaria in a high-incidence region in southwestern Kenya. Until the 1980s, the Nyamira region had limited exposure to malaria, which resulted in

---

57 KNA/KJD Annual Report 1941.

58 One of the authors witnessed the treatment of malaria by the traditional healer portrayed in the photo. The patient, a school teacher, had contacted the healer but was directed to a clinic where he tested positive and was provided with free drugs. After 10 days he still felt ill and returned to the healer. He paid Ksh 50 for treatment that was meant to 'empty the stomach' and treat malaria. (The local names of the drugs used were *oloisuki* and *oltepilikwa*.)

low immunity levels. The local people differentiated between cerebral malaria, recognisable by patients becoming violent and falling into a comma, and uncomplicated malaria, indicating that in the former case immediate assistance should be sought from formal health practitioners. Malaria had reportedly affected every household and incidences of malaria were linked to mosquitoes and periods of high rainfall but also to eating sugary foodstuffs, pollen, unbilled water and dirtiness. A majority (79.2%) would primarily acquire painkillers and Fansidar drugs, although 41% of respondents indicated that Fansidar was becoming less effective. Some had lost any hope of a cure unless a vaccine could be found.

Self-medication was seen first aid, to be followed up with proper treatment at the hospital. The difficulty of diagnosing malaria is another reason for delaying seeking professional help, as are a lack of money and the weekend closure of government health facilities. However, young children are directed to (private) hospitals as quickly as possible.[59] Siso (2007) also found that people resorted to traditional remedies (20.8%) and self-medication using Neem and other shrubs and trees whose leaves and bark are boiled and whose juices are drunk. Kenyans, especially those living in rural areas, are generally knowledgeable about the specific medicinal values of different trees, shrubs and herbs. And certain individuals in society are considered to be specialists who should be consulted for more complicated diseases. Let us briefly consider these traditional herbalists in relation to malaria.

Traditional treatment of malaria: Is ethnobotany the final answer?

Basic indigenous ethnomedical knowledge is present among most (rural) Africans (Kokwaro 2009). The curative abilities of plants and trees are part of people's appreciation of the rich biodiversity of the African landscape. For wounds, colds and fevers many know which roots, barks or herbs to use and some people specialize in the provision of herbal medicines, collecting plants, sometimes from afar, and preparing medicines for sale and use. Usually, as a Kenyan journalist stated: 'These practitioners have continued to shroud their trade in mysticism so that the isolation and extraction of the bark or the leaf of a medically-useful tree remains a secret that is normally passed on to a selected few within their family largely through word of mouth' (*Standard* 3/4/2006). The trade went underground during the colonial period when white missionaries and

---

[59] Local chemists and pharmacies are the leading channels for the distribution of consumer healthcare products. Medical assistance for young children among the poorest 20% of the Kenyan population is sought in public (47%), private (including NGOs and other non-profit players) (47%) and other (6%) facilities (see Ruiters & Scott 2009: 9).

colonial government officials engaged in open demonization of the practice. However, there is ample evidence today that more than a century after the scramble for Africa, the use and trade in herbal medicine is becoming more entrenched (*Standard* 3/4/2006).

In the mid-1990s, Ibrahim *et al.* (1998) conducted a survey among herbalist in Arusha town, concluding that many of these were female Maasai with an average age of 42. The few men herbalists found were much younger and new to the business. Poverty was their main reason for resorting to the profession of herbalist. On the demand side, they are finding a rapidly urbanizing environment that is creating a concentrated demand in towns for medical plants found only in the rural setting. Nowadays, Maasai herbalists are reportedly operating not just in their area of origin but as faraway as Sudan, Uganda and Zambia. The effects of Structural Adjustment, the distrust of modern medicine because of troublesome side effects, high costs and fake pills, a deterioration in public health services and a more welcoming attitude towards herbal products have all helped to boost the commercialization of this indigenous knowledge.

An African herbal antimalarial meeting held in Nairobi in March 2006 to discuss the use of plant products for the control of malaria illustrates this renewed interest in herbal knowledge. However, it also brought to the fore some contentious issues linked to the role of different players in the fight against malaria. Africans aired their frustration at the failure of multinational drug companies to confront the malaria pandemic in Africa. Worries were also expressed about the replacement of drugs like Fansidar and Metakelfin with Coartem, the only WHO-recommended artemisinin-based combination therapy (ACT), which is manufactured by Novartis Pharmaceuticals (*Standard* 1/5/2006). Coartem was said to be too costly for ordinary Kenyans but this was mainly due to the fact that the production of ACTs did not meet global demand because of a lack of its key ingredient, artemisinin from the Chinese plant artemisia annua (sweet wormwood). The global production of ACTs stood at only 25 million of the 130 million doses required each year to combat malaria throughout the world (*Standard* 1/5/2006). Dependency on the international donor world, in particular the Global Fund, for the financing of drugs and the training of healthcare workers was also mentioned. Others, however, stressed that artemisia was rapidly put under cultivation in various parts of Kenya and that herbalists have been administering the herb to malaria victims. There are artemisia plantations in Kiambu near Nairobi, in parts of Kajiado District and in the Rongai area of Nakuru in Rift Valley Province. The way the herbalists provide the anti-malarial drug is by boiling the leaves in 'tea', although WHO officials have pointed out that this is not ideal and is potentially even dangerous because it is, first, a monotherapy running the risk of the malaria germ developing resistance and, second, difficult to apply in the right concentration.

Many governments are in a process of recognizing herbal medicine and their practitioners. In 2006, for example, the Kenyan government drafted a policy on traditional medicine and medicinal plants. The government aims at the proper and regulated use of herbal medicine in the country, in particular with respect to the conservation of medicinal plants, equitably sharing their benefits, enhancing production and domestication, while ensuring the safety and efficacy of the products. However, while supporters welcome a policy framework that should stop bio-piracy by multinational pharmaceutical companies at the expense of local herbalists, the latter have been lobbying to stop the draft policy being passed in Parliament. They fear that the government's move is simply to pay testimony to the growing realization that the commercialization of indigenous ethnobotany knowledge might bring in a billion-dollar industry. Critics fear that this could be at the expense of herbalists, as has happened with traditional medicines (e.g. those derived from *Prunus Africanus*) in the fight against cancer which did not benefit the local people in Madagascar, Cameroon and Kenya, the home of the plant, due to external patents (*Standard* 3/4/2006).[60] This also counts for related industries as in food supplements and appetite suppressants. Supporters of the policy though also point to the need for regulation to protect patients and the environment. For example, reports are increasingly claiming that 'growing numbers of quacks infiltrate the herbal business in an attempt to profit from the ethnobotany interest' (*Standard* 20/5/2007). Forest departments complain that people residing in urban slums de-bark trees in nearby forests for their herbal practices and that this is causing rare species to die out.

The search for African anti-malarial plants is progressing rapidly. Research reports for Tanzania and DRC are forthcoming and, in Kenya, Orwa *et al.* (2008) mention the use by traditional healers of Orange climber, a medical plant (*Toddalia asiatica*), for treating malaria. Its therapeutic values, however, were not fully clear. By contrast, a study conducted by Koch *et al.* (2005) among three Maasai herbalists reported that 21 species of plants were being used to treat malaria, of which over half tested antiplasmodial, and all but one displayed selectivity for the malaria parasite *Plasmodium falciparum*. These results, it was concluded, supported the Maasai herbalists and justified ethnomedical inquiry as a promising method, specifically in anti-malarial therapy. So far though, these traditional medicines do not seem to posses the same qualities as the group of artemisinins that have proven to be highly effective, albeit costly and

[60] A report by the Edmonds Institute and the African Centre for Biosafety entitled 'Out of Africa: Mysteries of Access and Benefit Sharing' details how the commercialization of traditional knowledge systems, including herbal cures, by multinational drug and cosmetic companies is raising ethical issues, especially in the absence of profit-sharing agreements (*Standard* 20/5/2007).

difficult to produce (Lovgren 2005). Optimism about bringing down prices has been aired recently by a gene-modification project aimed at producing high-yielding seeds of artemisia annua suitable for the East African environment. The plants will be grown in Kenya, Madagascar and Uganda and are intended to reduce costs by a factor of 30 (*Standard* 31/8/2010). The alleged coming together of 'modern' and 'traditional' medicines in the fight against malaria is clearly illustrated in the opinions and practices of two Maasai individuals (see below).

Modern medicines	*Traditional medicines*
Peninah is a retired nurse at Isenya Health Centre. She stresses the difficultty in diagnosing malaria as it shows similar signs to typhoid and food poisoning. Her advice is to always go first for a blood test and afterwards, if necessary, to take an anti-malarial. Unfortunately there is no proper health education which increases the risk of drug resistance as people take anti-malarial drugs too soon. Nets are handed out free for the under fives and pregnant women. Some of the traditional herbs are good, or at least not harmful. Expensive modern drugs make people choose self-treatment although they may seek advice from herbalists. They might also take preventive measures, like burning dry cow dung or rubbing certain leaves onto the skin as a repellent. Fortunately, the malaria mosquito is mainly active in a limited period (the early morning when people cover themselves up well due to chilly temperature). She believes that malaria is under-recorded because when people die at home from it, the cause of death given is often vomiting or diarrhoea.	Julius started as a veterinary specialist. He travelled to several places in Kenya and Tanzania and discovered that the same types of herbs were used to cure specific diseases, e.g. malaria. Some of these qualities were not known by his own people, the Maasai of Namanga, on the Tanzania border. However, he believes that there is no complete cure available for malaria from traditional medicines, they only reduce the severity. Malaria in dry, hot places is known to be more deadly and there is certainly no treatment for cerebral malaria (which goes to someone's head) and he refers these patients to hospital. Malaria is a tricky disease, especially in children as they cannot describe their symptoms. The right dose of herbs when treating children is also difficult to assess so he refuses to treat children. For adults he uses a mixture of three drugs. Sometimes he adds Aloe Vera, but it has side effects. Before treatment, he wants to know the patient's history of symptoms. He also looks in their eyes to differentiate flu from malaria. Even the kind of fever, he claims, is different. Some patients first go to hospital and then come to him for traditional drugs. Malaria is the fourth most frequent disease he treats, after typhoid, brucellosis and respiratory diseases.

Source: Interviews (2/2/2010)

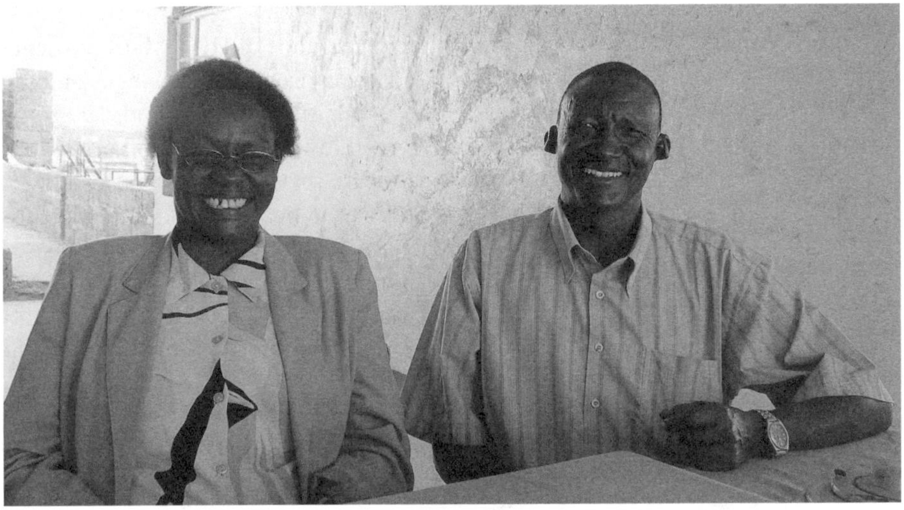

Photo 5.1 Distant relatives: modern nurse Peninah and traditional healer Julius [Photo: Marcel Rutten]

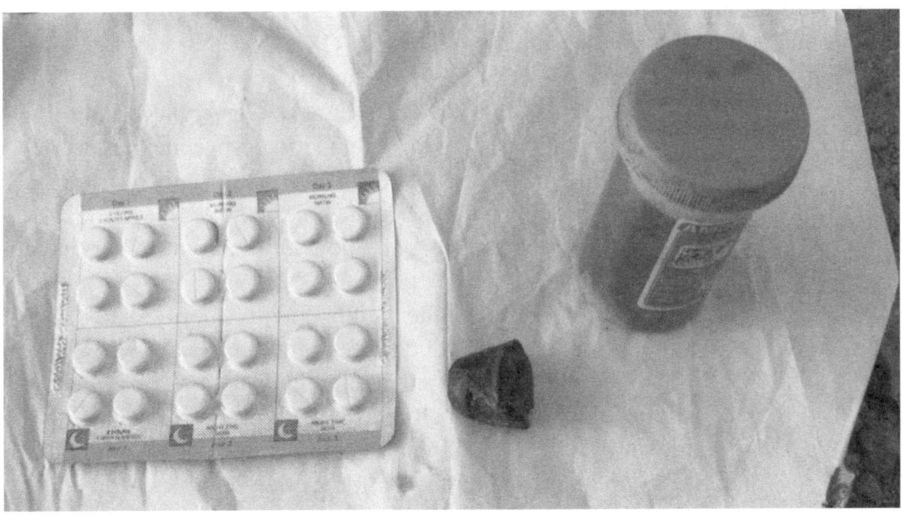

Photo 5.2 Modern (zero cost) malaria drugs and traditional malaria medicines [Photo: Marcel Rutten]

The 21st century: The start of the final battle?

The deteriorating situation in Kenya with the emergence of HIV/AIDS, growing anti-malarial drug resistance, population growth, environmental changes and the bad economic situation, which was exacerbated in the 1980s and 1990s by Structural Adjustment Programmes coupled with lower levels of donor support, led to major challenges in the country's healthcare services. No significant staff recruitment occurred for almost a decade and public healthcare facilities perennially lacked essential medicines and efficient microscopy and diagnostic tests.

Following the Kenyan government's signing of the Abuja Declaration on Roll Back Malaria (RBM), a National Malaria Strategy (2001-2010) was developed to guide the country to meet RBM targets. The Division of Malaria Control (DOMC) was set up to coordinate and provide technical leadership in implementing this strategy. The core strategies adopted were (i) vector control using Indoor Residual (Household) Spraying and Insecticide Treated Nets (ITNs); (ii) Anti-malarial Combination Therapy (ACT) and improved laboratory diagnosis; (iii) information, education and communication for behaviour change communication, health system strengthening strategic actions, as well as effective monitoring and evaluation; (iv) the management of malaria in pregnancy; and (v) epidemic preparedness and response. These targets were to a large extent anchored around 60%, i.e. with 60% of vulnerable children and pregnant mothers sleeping under an insecticide treated net (ITN); 60% of children with a fever in the previous two weeks accessing effective treatment within 24/48 hours of the onset of symptoms; and 60% of pregnant women accessing intermittent presumptive treatment (IPTp) with sulphadoxine-pyrimethamine (SP) during their second and third trimesters. These were useful indicators for the DOMC to track progress through national household sample surveys, annual sentinel district surveys in the community and audits at the point of service delivery (Republic of Kenya 2009).

Malaria treatment failure prompted the authorities to adopt ACT. Recent studies have shown that more than 40% of children failed to clear their infection by Day 28 (KGF-8). Since 2004, arthemether-lumefantrine (AL) has been selected to replace sulphadoxine-pyrimethamine (SP), showing resistance as the first line anti-malarial drug while quinine is recommended for uncomplicated *falciparum* malaria in pregnancy and for children weighing less than 5 kg. Quinine is also used for severe and complicated malaria.

In addition, preventive measures are increasingly geared to the Long Lasting Insecticide Treated Nets (LLITNs). Experts say malaria infection can be cut by at least half with the use of bed nets, since mosquitoes generally bite at night (Lovgren 2005). Table 5.1 illustrates ITN coverage during two surveys in 2001 and 2003, suggesting no or minimal gains, and shows the gap that needs to be filled to achieve the 60% coverage set as a target for RBM.

Table 5.1 Comparison between KDHS 2003 findings and 2001 RBM sentinel baseline data on ITN coverage in Kenya (%)

Indicator	KDHS 2003	Baseline 2001
Children under 5 sleeping under a mosquito net	15	14
Children under 5 sleeping under ITN	4	4.3
Pregnant women sleeping under a mosquito net	12	15.3
Pregnant women sleeping under an ITN	3	4.5
Households owning at least one net	22	21.2
Households owning at least one ITN	8	5.6

Source: KGF-2

The coming to power of President Kibaki in 2003 resulted in an increase in Kenya's overall health budget. The amount rose from 4% in 2004/2005 to 5.6% in 2005/2006, 9% in 2006/2007 and 11% in 2007/2008.[61] There are plans to reach 15%, in line with the Abuja Declaration but external funding will continue to be required for the foreseeable future (KGF-8). The main development partners in addressing malaria in Kenya include the World Bank, UNICEF, the WHO, the EU, the ADB, some individual countries, notably the US and the UK, and various NGOs. The largest contribution is being made by GFATM (Snow *et al.* 2009: 125) that rewarded Kenya's applications in 2002 and 2004.[62]

Working towards reaching the Millennium Development Goals, existing and new funding partners have begun to increase investment in malaria control in Kenya. For example, the President's Malaria Initiative (PMI) began supporting Kenya in October 2007 and aims, with its partners, to reduce malaria-related deaths by 50% by ensuring 85% coverage of highly effective prevention and disease management strategies (PMI 2009).[63] Malaria drugs (Artefan) contain-

61 In 2008/2009 the funding allocated to malaria control was 4.8% of the MoPHS budget and annual increases in public spending on health have continued to fall short of international expectations (Snow *et al.* 2009).

62 Other applications were rejected based on Kenya's dismal track record in managing previous funds, especially in the field of HIV/AIDS. In September 2010, the Global Fund released US$ 39 m to combat malaria as part of Round 4 grants.

63 In June 2005, the US government announced a US$ 1.2 billion initiative to scale up malaria prevention and treatment interventions in Sub-Saharan Africa. The President's Malaria Initiative (PMI) began in three countries in 2006: Angola, Tanzania, and Uganda. Since 2007 twelve more countries were added (Malawi, Mozambique, Senegal, Rwanda, Benin, Ethiopia (one region), Ghana, Kenya, Liberia, Madagascar, Mali and Zambia). Funding began with US$ 30 m in 2006 and will reach US$ 500 m in 2010. Efforts will be coordinated with the Global Fund to Fight AIDS, Tuberculosis, and Malaria, Roll Back Malaria, the World Bank Malaria Booster Program and the non-governmental and private sectors (PMI/MOP 2009).

ing arthemeter and lumefantrine, which is produced by Ajanta Pharma in India, became available free of charge through the Ministry of Health. There was also improved access to ITNs in 2007 (49%) and 2009 (54%) and the percentage of children under five who received treatment with an anti-malarial within 24 hours had reached 16% in 2007, up from 11% in 2003 (*Ibid.*).

Evaluation of the DOMC in 2007-2009 indicates that deaths from malaria are declining in many areas of Kenya, particularly at the coast and in selected areas of the Kenyan Highlands. Yet in most areas the decline began prior to the rapid scaling up of malaria interventions, such as ITNs, and before the launch of the new case-management strategy including Arthemether-Lumefantrine drugs. This reduction was probably caused by other factors, such as improved economic status, health awareness and the increased availability of curative services. And there is little evidence of a reduction in hospitalization for malaria at sites around Lake Victoria where transmission remains high and despite increases in intervention coverage, changes in the burden of the disease are far less evident (Snow *et al.* 2009: 17).

In 2009, Kenya launched its second National Malaria Strategy for the period 2009-2017. It has an increased scope compared to its predecessor, with a notably ambitious vision for a 'malaria free Kenya' (DOMC 2009b). However, to move to a diagnosis-based case-management strategy in all age groups in all parts of Kenya will require a huge effort on the part of the DOMC and its partners to ensure a paradigm shift away from the popular dogma among many Africans that all fevers are malaria. Also, the range of anti-malarial products on the Kenyan market remains extensive and less than half are registered with the Pharmacies & Poisons Board.[64] Ensuring that artemisinin monotherapies remain off the market and other products are registered and quality assured demands increased investment in minilab technology and the ability to sample effectively and appropriately. Moreover, as in the early 1960s, there are still not enough qualified professionals to deliver quality healthcare.

As well as the search for effective drugs, other groups are continuing to try to prevent outbreaks of malaria. For example, the Kenya Red Cross Society (KRCS) is piloting the Home Management of Malaria (HMM) project in 108 villages in the coastal areas of Malindi and Lamu to help geographically isolated communities overcome the challenges of fighting malaria. Besides the provision of free access to arthemether-lumefantrine for children under five, this includes training and equipping selected locals with treatment tools to manage

---

[64] 187 innovator brands, branded and non-branded anti-malarial products were identified in the public, private, mission and commercial sectors (covering 40 unique product formulations). Only 42.6% were registered with the PPB, 42.2% were not registered and registration status could not be verified for 15.2% (Snow *et al.* 2009).

home treatment and the prevention of malaria. The project is a joint effort of the Ministry of Health and the KRCS with technical and financial support from the WHO and the Canadian Red Cross (*Standard* 31/8/2010).

All of the above-mentioned weapons needed to win the war against malaria may become redundant if the battle against either the mosquito and/or the parasite can be won. The latest development in this respect is an effective malaria vaccine. This is still a huge challenge. The polio virus, for example, consists of exactly 11 genes; *Plasmodium Falciparum* has more than 5,000 (Finkel 2007). At least 90 teams around the world are working on some aspect of a vaccine. One experimental vaccine (RTS,S), which was developed in a partnership between the pharmaceutical company GlaxoSmithKline and the US Army, was tested in Mozambique and proved effective at protecting as many as 50% of children against the disease for six months (Lovgren 2005). Kenya is among the countries selected for these trials. Another group, headed by Stephen Hoffman at an American company called Sanaria (healthy air), is also in the process of developing a vaccine. Having failed to produce an effective vaccine while working at the Naval Medical Research Center, he is convinced they are nearing success (Finkel 2007). The new method uses radiation to weaken the parasites. When injected, these only cause a mild immune reaction. In theory, this is just enough to keep a person free of malaria.

Conclusion

This chapter has examined malaria control patterns in Kenya over the last century. Initially confined to the emerging major towns of Nairobi, Mombasa and Kisumu, numerous factors have determined ways of controlling malaria, including the prevailing theories of malaria, historical legacies from metropolitan practices, pragmatic responses to realities on the ground and an element of management by crisis, which was manifested by the panic measures taken by the colonial regime. It is, however, important to note that these factors operated within the framework of urban, social and economic circumstances embedded in various forms of domination and the power of the colonizer over the colonized, at least until the early 1960s.

Kenya's early urban malaria control activities pointed to one basic conclusion: a disease policy at the crossroads. First, there was the transition at the medical level from the romantic notions of urban cleanliness at a time when few Europeans were affected by malaria to a more medical approach, as indicated by the use of quinine and rudimentary research as rates of European malaria infection grew in the post-World War I era. Secondly, there was the transition at the political level that involved change from an over-emphasis on coercion based on puritanical and cultural chauvinism to a greater reliance on persuasion, racial inclusion, albeit minimal, and public education based on modern institutional and legislative frameworks.

Underlying these transitions lay factors that made malaria fairly intractable and often required *ad hoc* measures. These defined and interrupted transitions until 1926 when an all-out malaria epidemic ravaged Nairobi and the outlying areas of Central Kenya and the northern Rift Valley, which were hitherto believed to be free of malaria. The epidemic threatened the safety of potentially successful agricultural areas and caused alarm and panic within the colonial administration. It facilitated the extension of malaria control services to the African reserves and European-settled areas away from Nairobi, Mombasa and Kisumu as it threatened the African labour force and subsequently settlers' incomes.

World War II revealed new global elements in the fight against malaria: the supply of quinine to Kenyan patients and Allied forces, which was produced in Indonesia and on which so many were dependent, was interrupted when Japan invaded Java. This triggered local regulations to ensure the economic and fair use of quinine and aimed to guarantee availability first and foremost for soldiers. The expansion of anti-malaria measures during the 1950s was a spin-off effect from the war period and chloroquine and DDT were made available in a WHO-sponsored Global Malaria Eradication Programme that aimed to eradicate the disease worldwide within ten years. Chemical vector-based measures did indeed prove effective mechanisms that reduced malaria transmission in Nairobi in this period. Warning notices to residents who allowed mosquito to breed on their premises were also issued. At the end of the 1950s, malaria had ceased to be a major health problem in Nairobi according to contemporary medical opinion.

In a sense, therefore, the large-scale malaria control schemes vindicated the argument of malariologists who opposed a policy based on malaria eradication in Africa because of practical considerations, such as finance and infrastructure. These anti-malaria schemes also illustrated how although the reliance on drugs and insecticides in the 1950s reduced the dependence on other vector control strategies, such as the use of larvicides and environmental sanitation, as some scholars have argued, this was not entirely the case in Kenya.[65] The urban

[65] See R.M. Packard, 'No other logical choice: global malaria eradication and the politics of international health in the post-war era', p. 13, paper presented at a conference on strategies against malaria: eradication or control? at the Foundation Marcel Centre des Pensieres, Annec, France, 17-21 April 1996. Packard argues that 'Reliance on DDT and declining popularity of other forms of malaria control left public health workers in developing countries vulnerable to the emergence of anopheline resistance, which began to be observed as early as 1951 in Greece'.

authorities used the new and old strategies either interchangeably or simultaneously depending on local conditions to maximize their potency.

Developments in the 1950s campaign against malaria in Kenya questioned the common argument that the WHO's global malaria eradication policy actually eradicated malariology because the authorities came to believe that they possessed a magic bullet in insecticides (DDT in particular) and that further costly research was no longer needed.[66]

Post-colonial developments, especially those of a more recent nature, stress that the fight against malaria is yet to be won. Increased resistance to the drugs available, notably chloroquine, until the 1980s created worries from an ethical as well as an economic point of view. Kenya, like most other African countries, lacked the capacity to produce effective anti-malarial drugs. Its socio-economic level of development likewise created severe obstacles or even promoted the presence of mosquitoes through irrigated water development projects. The international community too seemed to have lost interest in developing an effective anti-malarial drug until the turn of the century. The anti-malarial characteristics of a Chinese herbal plant, artemisia annua, that has been effective for over 2000 years, and the coming together of private-public funds to freely provide a package of anti-malarial tools, including insecticide treated nets, training and free drugs, are reasons for this renewed global assault, this time of a more varied nature. However, commercial interests might still block a full-fledged approach to stemming malaria. The high demand for artemisia has pushed up prices and it is still to be seen if the Chinese government will share the best artemisia plants with the wider world. Local plantations of artemisia have started in Kenya and other African countries that, besides providing job opportunities, are meant to boost the supply of ACTs and lower prices, ultimately subsidized and provided at no cost for malaria patients at public and private-non-profit health centres, as is the case today in Kenya. The cheap synthetic production of artemisinin-type anti-malarial drugs will also help in this respect.

The positive experiences with artemisia have started a run on indigenous African herbal knowledge, which has risks and opportunities for the African population and their economies. Will Africa provide its own non-resistant anti-malarial drug in the near future? And who will be the beneficiaries of these developments? The fact that African research institutes are increasingly joining hands with their Western partners might be just a first small step in the right direction. Recently, outside assistance to add to Kenyan attempts to control the disease has increased as a result of more global funds being made available from a number of new initiatives such as Roll Back Malaria and the Global

---

66 *Ibid.*: 3.

Fund to Fight AIDS, Tuberculosis and Malaria. However, high-quality national plans are needed to qualify for this financial assistance and other challenges, such as higher population densities and the still weak institutional infrastructure of the health sector, will add to this financial burden. Renewed hopes for a vaccine are high though.

References

NB: Unless otherwise stated, all the archival references listed below are from Kenya National Archives (KNA), Nairobi, & the Public Record Office (PRO), London.

KNA/DC/NBI.1/1/1, *Political Record Book*, Nairobi District, 1899 to 1915.
KNA/Health/1/6081, MOH Nairobi, Annual Report, 1906 & 1909.
KNA/KJD, Kajiado District Annual Report 1941.
KNA/PC/CP.4/2/1, Annual Medical Report, Ukamba Province, 1907-1908, p. 29, in Ukamba Province Annual Reports, 1906-1915.
KNA/PC/NZA/1/1, Nyanza Province Annual Report, 1905-1906.
KNA/PC/NZA/1/10, Nyanza Province Annual Report, 1914-1915.
KNA/PC/NZA/1/3, Nyanza Province Annual Report, 1907-1908.
KNA/PC/NZA/1/4, Nyanza Province Annual Report, 1908-1909.
KNA/PC/NZA/1/7, Nyanza Province Annual Report, 1911-1912.
KNA/PC/NZA/1/9, Nyanza Province Annual Report, 1913-1914.
KNA/PC/NZA/1/20, Nyanza Province Annual Report, 1925.
KNA/PC/NZA/3/45/6, Annual Report of Medical Officer of Health, Kisumu, 1925-1929.
Nairobi Medical Research Laboratory (NMRL) 1914-1920 & 1922-24 in Colony and Protectorate of Kenya, Medical Department Annual Reports, PRO CO 544/1-13 & 544/16-17.

Anderson, D.M. (2000), Master and servant in Colonial Kenya, 1895-1939. *Journal of African History* 41: 459-485.
Ashraf, Q., A. Lester & D. Weil (2008), When does improving health raise GDP? Working Paper 2008-7, Brown University, Department of Economics.
Bruce-Chwatt, L.J. (1988), History of malaria from prehistory to eradication. In: W.H. Wernsdorfer & I. McGregor, *Malaria: Principles and practice of malariology. Vol. 1*, pp. 1-59. Edinburgh: Churchill Livingstone.
Clayton, A. & C. Savage (1974), *Government and labour in Kenya, 1895-1963*. London: Frank Cass.
Coatney, R.G. (1963), Pitfalls in a discovery: The chronicle of chloroquine. *American Journal of Tropical Medicine and Hygiene* 12: 121-128.
Curtin, P. (1985), Medical knowledge and urban planning in tropical Africa. *American Historical Review* 90(3): 594-614.

Dummett, R.E.D. (1968), The campaign against malaria and the expansion of scientific medical and sanitary services in British West Africa, 1898-1910. *African Historical Studies* 1: 153-197.

Finkel, M. (2007), Stopping a global killer: The rapidly spreading disease affects more people than ever before. But until recently, the outcry has been muted. *National Geographic Magazine* (July).

.Froeling, A. & M. van Haften (1983), An in vivo and in vitro study of the resistance of Plasmodium Falciparum to Chloroquin and Mefloquine in south-west Kenya. Unpublished Working Paper Medical Studies, Leiden University.

Grewal, N. (1996), The rationality of the malaria eradication programme in sub-Saharan Africa and why it failed. Unpublished MSc Thesis, University of Oxford.

Hake, A. (1977), *African metropolis: Nairobi's self help city*, London: Chatto & Windus for Sussex University Press.

Headrick. D. (1981), *Tools of empire: Technology and European imperialism in the nineteenth century*. New York: Oxford University Press.

Ibrahim, F. & B. Ibrahim (1998), The Maasai herbalists in Arusha Town, Tanzania. *GeoJournal* 46: 141-154.

Kasoa, M. (1989), Political and administrative factors influencing Kisumu the Municipal Council in Service provisions - Housing, Water and Health. Unpublished MA dissertation, University of Nairobi.

Koch, A., P. Tamez, J. Pezzuto & D. Soejarto (2005), Evaluation of plants used for antimalarial treatment by the Maasai of Kenya. *Journal of Ethnopharmacology* 101: 95-99.

Kokwaro, J. (2009), *Medicinal plants of East Africa*. Nairobi: University of Nairobi Press.

Kwendo, O. & Z. Muganzi (1996), Infant mortality differentials in western Kenya (1979-1989). *African Anthropology* III(2): 55-67.

Leavitt, J.W. (1992), 'Typhoid Mary' strikes back: Bacteriological theory and practice in early twentieth-century public health. *Isis* 83(4): 608-629.

Lonsdale, J. (2002), Town life in colonial Kenya. In: A. Burton (ed.), *The urban experience in Eastern Africa 1750-2000*, 207-222. Nairobi: British Institute in Eastern Africa.

Lovgren, S. (2005), Malaria aid, research ramp up to tackle Africa crisis. *National Geographic News* (21 July).

Malowany, M., M. Dobson & R.W. Snow (n.d.), Malaria control in East Africa: The Kampala conference and the Pare-Taveta Scheme; a meeting of common and high ground. Unpublished paper for Wellcome Unit for the History of Medicine, Oxford University.

McGregor, I.A. & D.A. Smith (1952), Daraprim in treatment of malaria: A study of its effects in falciparum and quartan infections in West Africa. *British Medical Journal* (April): 730.

Muhindi, D.W. (1993), A comparative study of the efficacy of halofatrine and chloroquine in uncomplicated malaria at the Kenyatta National Hospital. Masters of Medicine Dissertation, University of Nairobi.

Nyamongo, I. (1997), The malaria cognate: Folk classification of illness among the Abagusii of Kenya. *African Anthropology* IV(2): 27-37.

Orwa J., I. Jondiko, R. Minja & M. Bekunda (2008), The use of *Toddalia asiatica (L) Lam. (Rutaceae)* in traditional medicine practice in East Africa. *Journal of Ethnopharmacology* 115: 257-262.

President's Malaria Initiative (PMI) (2009), Malaria Operational Plan (MOP) KENYA FY 2010. http://www.fightingmalaria.gov/countries/mops/fy10/kenya_mop-fy10.pdf

Republic of Kenya (2001), *National Economic Survey 2001*. Nairobi: Ministry of Planning and National Development.

Republic of Kenya (2001a), *National Malaria Strategy 2001-2010*. Nairobi: Ministry of Health, Division of Malaria Control.

Republic of Kenya (2004), *Kenya Demographic and Health Survey (KDHS) 2003*. Nairobi.

Ross, R. (1910), *The prevention of malaria*. London: Dutton.

Ruiters, G. & B. Scott (2009), Commercialisation of health and capital flows in east and southern Africa: Issues and implications. EQUINET Discussion Paper 77, Institute of Social and Economic Research, Rhodes University.

Siso, J. (2007), Malaria focused ethnographic study of community perceptions and practices in Rigoma Division, Nyamira District, Kenya. *Mila* (8): 17-26.

Snow, R.W., E. Okiro, A. Noor, K. Munguti, G. Tetteh & E. Juma (2009), *The coverage and impact of malaria intervention in Kenya 2007-2009*. Nairobi: Division of Malaria Control Ministry of Public Health and Sanitation.

Swanson, M.W. (1977), The sanitation syndrome: Bubonic plague and urban native policy in the Cape Colony, 1900-1909, *Journal of African History* 3(xviii): 387-410.

Thitai, W.N. 1991, Water resource development and malaria in Kenya: An environmental perspective. In: American Association for the Advancement of Science, *Malaria and development in Africa - A cross-sectoral approach*, pp. 205-216. Washington DC: AAAS.

Verhoef, H. (2001), Iron deficiency and malaria as determinants of anaemia in African children. PhD Thesis, Wageningen University. Veenendaal: Universal Press.

WHO (1951), *Malaria conference in equatorial Africa. Technical report no. 38.*

Wiseman, R.H., C.B. Symes, J.C. McMahon & C. Teesdale (1939), *Report on a malaria survey of Mombasa*. Nairobi: The Government of Kenya.

Websites

IRIN (PLUSNEWS) 10 November 2009: KENYA: Government protests Global Fund rejection (extracted 12 November 2009 from http://www.irinnews.org/report.aspx?ReportId=86969).

GFATM 2009 http://www.theglobalfund.org

KGF 2 - The Global Fund to Fight AIDS, Tuberculosis and Malaria *Kenya Global Fund Round 2 Proposal* 27th September 2002

KGF 4 - The Global Fund to Fight AIDS, Tuberculosis and Malaria *Kenya Global Fund Round 4 Proposal* 2004.

KGF 7 - The Global Fund to Fight AIDS, Tuberculosis and Malaria *Kenya Global Fund Round 7 Proposal* 2007.

KGF 8 - The Global Fund to Fight AIDS, Tuberculosis and Malaria *Kenya Global Fund Round 8 Proposal* 11th August 2008

Malaria Vaccine Initiative http://www.malariavaccine.org/
WHO (2009) WHO Malaria Fact sheet No 94, 1998 updated January 2009. http://www.who.int/mediacentre/factsheets/fs094/en/print.html

6

The market for healing and the elasticity of belief: Medical pluralism in Mpumalanga, South Africa

Robert Thornton

The demand for healing appears to produce a kind of 'market for healing'. It is often not possible, however, to evaluate healing's effectiveness, utility or economic efficiency (value for money). The market for healing is governed less by price than by a parallel market for belief. In the Umjindi (Barberton) Municipality in Mpumalanga Province, South Africa, medical choices are made on the basis of belief systems since the effectiveness of therapies is itself contingent on belief (the placebo effect). As beliefs change to accommodate the choice of therapies and because the perceived effect of therapies often influences belief, markets for belief and healing are closely related. But not all healing in this market produces health. Healing also offers protection from other people, from other healers and from other therapies and their effects or side effects. Since few therapies in this market produce reliable results, belief allows clients to evaluate the moral states of being rather than the mere evidence of efficacy as they search for healing. Belief in a therapy allows clients to evaluate their choices and participate in healing with a greater sense of certainty. In short, what a person believes is thought to influence how and whether s/he can be healed and to what extent the therapy has been effective.

Belief and the market for healing

I argue in this chapter that people who experience illness, and even those who do not, seek healing in a way that is like acquiring goods at a market: they seek knowledge about what is available, evaluate the goods on the basis of some criterion, make selections and pay a price. I use the term 'market' in its most general sense, as a social space in which many kinds of healers offer an array of medicines and therapies to potential clients who acquire these goods as healing, protection and relief from suffering, disease, misfortune or loss. In the market for healing, however, the value of the goods – healing, health, success and protection – is determined largely by the belief that the client holds in the therapy. It is as if this were a double market: a market for healing and a market for belief. In practice, the economic price of these goods is relatively inelastic, but since belief is the condition for the efficacy of healing, and vice versa, it is the quantity and quality of belief itself that is more elastic than price.

The market of healing is not an economic market because choices are not made on the basis of an economic rationality. Instead, belief in the efficacy of a therapy functions as the primary criterion for selecting it in this market. It is belief *in* the therapy that most people believe makes therapies of all kinds effective. Belief also allows clients/patients to evaluate the efficacy of therapies and is the price of being healed, while it is also the condition for healing's efficacy. You get what you believe in, and you must believe in being healed.

Therapies also have prices but differentials of price are usually very small, and people do not select therapies based on price. A traditional healer, prophet (faith healer), massage therapist or herbalist sets their price according to what a bio-medical general practitioner would charge for a first consultation or a visit to the surgery. As in any market, healing is a good that has a price and a cost; specialists supply services for those that require them (demand) with some risk to both client and practitioner. Many types of medical and healing systems are available to all or most patients/clients. While the therapies offered in this 'market for healing' are owned by specific practitioners and their knowledge is jealousy guarded, there is little or no formal regulation of this market, no contracts or means of enforcing them. It is therefore an incomplete or partial market that does not fully conform to the theoretical ideal of the market (Fafchamps 2004). It is, however, a space in which choices are made and information circulates and where few political or institutional constraints interfere with the client's choice of therapies. In this way it is a 'free market'. Unlike most economic markets in the developing world, transaction costs are very low: everyone has some knowledge of most therapies and therapeutic systems; and more information is not difficult to obtain. (On the other hand, there are no contracts,

Map 6.1 South Africa, showing research location

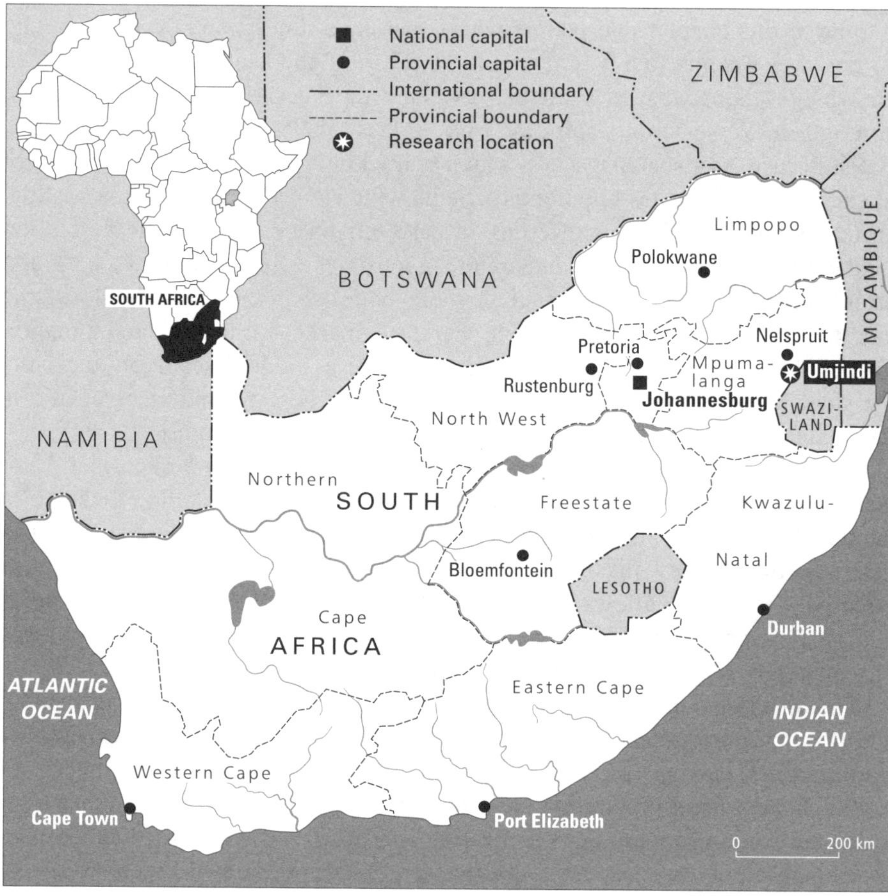

so there are none to enforce.) The market for belief ensures this as to subscribe to a therapy, one must believe in it, and to believe is to hold at least some knowledge of it.

The market for belief appears to be efficient. Everyone professes some belief and every belief seems to be related to therapeutic options and protection from illness or misfortune. Everyone spends a good deal of time discussing their beliefs, going to church, attending healing sessions be they Christian, traditional African, New Age or others such as spas, self-help groups, seminars or healing workshops where knowledge circulates and options are discussed. People clearly invest a great deal in the maintenance of their beliefs, in convincing others or in being persuaded themselves.

When we talk about 'healing' we mean many things. As a category it is only definable in terms of what Wittgenstein (1953: §65) called a 'family resemblance' category. The elements of categories of this sort have overlapping resemblances like the features of members of a family: no element exhibits all features, and all share only some features with others. Members of such categories are nevertheless recognized as being 'of the same sort'. Bodies and minds are healed in different ways by different means including rituals, song, prayer, dance, massage and medication. Herbal or pharmaceutical methods are used to accomplish 'healing' but the ways in which they heal have little in common. Healing may consist of correcting 'balances' of forces or 'energies' within the patient; it may result from the elimination or attenuation of disease and reduction in pain or discomfort from many causes, or it may simply make suffering more bearable (Geertz 1973; Segar 2009). Healing here takes many pathways but not all of them lead to health.

Whether of not healing has occurred and what has actually been healed – the body, mind, social relations, spirit or blood – often remains ambiguous but it is recognized as healing. Ambiguity is a necessary and unavoidable property of healing (Waldram 2000). Conceptualizing this inconsistency of belief and practice in terms of the market, rather than in term of institutions and structures, allows a clearer vision of this reality.

There is another reason to use the notion of 'market' rather than a 'medical culture' or medical system. People in Umjindi, and in South Africa more generally, do not insist on, and one rarely finds, logical or formal consistency in belief systems, especially as these relate to health and healing. It is not possible to imagine this as a cultural system – a self-contained sub-set of mutually reinforcing concepts and values with internal consistency – but it is instead more like a cultural bazaar where the value and commensurability of independent systems are on display, available for the taking and make no claims to cultural coherence.

Medical anthropologists often treat ethno-medical systems as if they are internally coherent structures of meaning within definable boundaries of the community of practice. By treating healing as a market, I am moving away from the more usual metaphors of healing as a search, a gift or as the receipt of specialized services. A search has a goal; a gift is received as such, and a service is expected and rendered, all with a degree of internal consistency of rights and obligations or rules. A market, on the other hand, has options and risks, gains and losses, and outcomes are not guaranteed. In the case discussed here, any therapeutic or medicals intervention does not necessarily lead to better health, a cure or even reduced suffering.

Contrary to expectations, bio-medical practitioners or 'Western doctors' (though in this case almost all are African and have trained in South Africa, elsewhere in Africa or internationally) are generally – or are believed to be – little better than other options, including traditional healers. There is – or it is *believed* that there is – little objective differentiation between bio-medical and alternative therapies. In other words, in people's experience, there is often little perceived difference between the success of one form of healing compared to others.

Methods of healing are not entirely independent of each other. Many types of therapies implicate or entail each other. Thus, the unpleasant side effects of antiretroviral medication (ARVs) or TB medication are frequently mitigated by traditional medicine consisting of herbs and teas or the 'magic' of *muti*. People spread the risk of commitment to one therapy by initiating others. A more or less elastic belief system permits this: beliefs change to fit the therapy, and thereby enable it. For instance, one might seek Christian faith healing if traditional healing or patent medicines do not work. People who go to bio-medical doctors also heal themselves with other New Age systems such as Reiki, reflexology, crystals, patent medicines, home cures and other options. In all cases, it is held that therapies only work if one believes that they will work.

While we can characterize this as a situation of medical pluralism, we could better think of it as complex system of multiple therapies in which different medical systems function as different modalities in a common system. Here I try to show how the competing truth claims or claims to therapeutic efficacy play out in the reality of a market for healing. How has this market for healing come about? How does it function? I claim that this question cannot be answered simply in terms of a cost-benefit assessment of therapeutic efficacy or value for money but can best be understood in terms of a market for belief.

The research site: Barberton/Umjindi Municipality, Mpumalanga Province

The approach and data presented here are based on long-term ethnographic fieldwork in Umjindini Municipality, an administrative district established in 2001 in Mpumalanga Province, South Africa.[1] Barberton, the administrative and historical centre of the municipality, was established in 1884 as the principal mining centre of the old Zuid Afrikaansche Republiek (Transvaal Republic). Today, it is sustained by farming, gold mining, forestry and government services as it lies close to Nelspruit, the province's burgeoning capital, and houses many civil servants as well as a large population of employees of the two large government prisons in the town. Barberton has a stable population of White,

1 My research comprises participant observation, historical research, oral histories, questionnaires and other modalities and has been conducted intermittently in this town and surroundings from 1998 to the present (2010).

Black, Coloured and Indian people, roughly in proportion to South Africa as a whole, who live largely, but not exclusively, in respective neighbourhoods where their families have lived in since the town's foundation. There are also significant immigrant populations from China, Pakistan and surrounding African countries such as Mozambique and Zimbabwe. Most White, Indian and Coloured people speak Afrikaans and/or English, although perhaps 10-20% also speak SiSwati (Swazi). The Black Africans mainly speak SiSwati (Swazi) but most also speak English and/or Afrikaans too. Many also speak other Bantu languages such as SePedi and/or Shangaan (XiTsonga). Relative to the rest of South Africa and despite its diversity, the municipality's political history has been remarkably peaceful even in the apartheid period and during its decline and fall. With the exception of the predominantly Muslim Indian group, most of Barberton's population is nominally Christian.

Barberton is in some ways a classic 'small town.' The shops on the main street are owned by Indian and Chinese immigrants, as well as by Black and White South Africans. The small centre dating from the late 19th century has Indian, Coloured and Black townships to the northern downhill side, while mountains with their game reserves and over 1000 now-abandoned gold mines and prospecting claims rise immediately to the south of the town. In the main, almost all the population are comfortably off, with a standard of living that is well above most other African countries and comparable to the poorer EU countries. The economy is only partly legal and formal and a large proportion of the economy comes from illegal gold mining and smuggling marijuana from Swaziland and cigarettes from Mozambique. There is also the informal, cash-only trade in other things. Indeed, the town is jokingly described as a small drinking town with a gold-mining problem.

The main formal industries in Barberton – mining, timber, forestry and prisons – are tough industries. Despite its political quietness, there are high levels of violence, drinking and alcoholism and many people carry visible scars from interpersonal and domestic violence or other traumas on their faces and elsewhere on their bodies. Observation, stories and court cases at the tribal court, which have been collected over ten years, suggest that both men and women are likely to engage in and to initiate violence. HIV prevalence is one of the highest in the world and TB, including multiple drug-resistant TB (MDR-TB), is also extremely prevalent with high levels of HIV and TB co-infection. Barberton hosts a specialized TB treatment facility. Diabetes and obesity are prevalent too, especially among Blacks[2] and Afrikaans-speakers (mostly Whites

---

[2] I use here the 'canonical' colour/racial terms that are used by most South Africans: Black, White, Coloured and Indian. I do not define them except to say that these are

and Coloureds). Witchcraft accusations are common but almost never result in violence against suspected witches, and they are strongly downplayed and discouraged by the leaders of the traditional court where they are most commonly heard. On the other hand, malaria and other common tropical diseases, such as diarrhoea, are largely absent, and public life in the streets, shops and at work is generally congenial and friendly, with no obvious tensions between people.

Medical pluralism in Umjindi

Social diversity is matched by a diversity of options for healing the many illnesses and diseases that afflict the people of Umjindi Municipality. A 'Doctor Mukasa' who runs a shop in central Barberton, for instance, offers healing or cures for 'court case, Drop (Gonorrhoea), Bring back lost love, Tuberculosis (TB), and penis enlargement'.[3] Dr Mukasa's menu of services points to the primary causes of morbidity in Barberton: TB, HIV/AIDS, sexually transmitted infections and violence arising from jealousy over 'lost love' and lovers' quarrels. While seeming initially to be a random list, Dr Mukasa's treatments are a good indicator of what ails Barberton. The protection he offers in the case of 'court case' often has to do with issues of violence arising from 'lost love', as well as from accusations of witchcraft or other 'undue influence' among 'co-wives' (usually a mix of girlfriends and/or wife/wives) or competing boyfriends/husbands, as well as conflict between generations over rights and obligations of kinship. Gonorrhoea is one consequence of the complex sexual networks in Barberton, but so is the desire for a bigger penis. Dr Mukasa's treatments are symptoms of Barberton's Zeitgeist.

Most of Barberton's medical doctors have a favourable attitude towards traditional healers (Green *et al.* 2003). Within 500 metres of the city centre one can consult several healers like Dr Mukasa, five or six medical doctors and a similar number of *sangomas*. There are psychologists and dentists, chiropractors and homeopaths as well. There are seven centrally located churches and around 40 formally constituted churches with buildings and staff in the municipality. All the churches offer healing services of various kinds. In addition to pharmaceuticals, South African pharmacies sell a wide range of traditional and natural or homeopathic medicines and substances. Some, such as 'blue stone' (copper sulphate crystals) and oils (almond, olive, glycerine) are used by *sangomas* and other healers such as massage therapists and aroma therapists. Packaged herbs

---

somewhat arbitrary categories. The labels are those that people in Barberton use colloquially too.

3 This shop was operating in early 2010 and had been for at least a year prior to this.

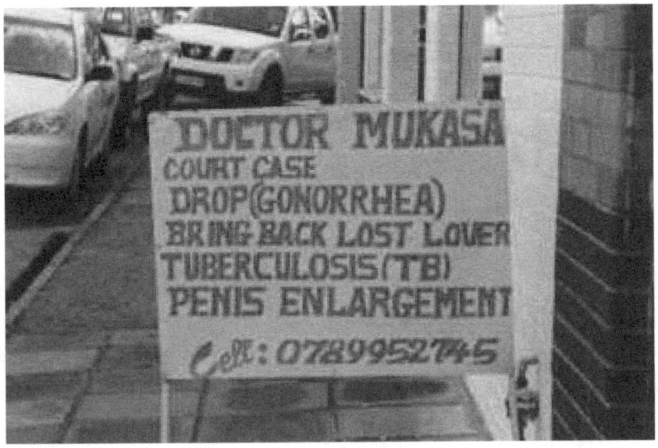
DOCTOR MUKASA
COURT CASE
DROP(GONORRHEA)
BRING BACK LOST LOVER
TUBERCULOSIS(TB)
PENIS ENLARGEMENT
Cell: 0789952745

Photo 6.1 Sandwiched between a beauty shop and a furniture repair shop in central Barberton, Dr Mukasa offers a range of healing services attuned to the people's needs [Photo: Robert Thornton]

like Echinacea and St John's Wort and dietary supplements are also sold in large quantities. Patent medicines such as Lennon's Dutch Medicines are an important retail item in South African pharmacies and most small general dealers and *spaza* (informal) shops in the townships. These natural, packaged, 'cure anything' remedies such as Borsdruppels, Witdulsies, Behoedmiddel, Haarlemensis and Duiwelsdrek are marketed by Aspen Pharmacare, South Africa's largest producer of generic antiretroviral medications for AIDS. In addition, the Chinese merchants offer traditional Chinese medicines, and the Pakistani immigrants' shops offer a range of Indian home remedies. New Age healing services are offered on flyers in hairdressers, on the street and in local newspaper advertisements, including aroma therapy, 'energy therapy', massage and reflexology. Almost everyone seems to be aware of the healing power of crystals, water and candles, and of prayer and holy water, as well as other healing practices such as eating clay, fasting, and smoking marijuana. Finally, there is a reasonably well equipped and well staffed government hospital in addition to private and public clinics.

While there are many options in this broad market for healing and a steady demad due to the relatively high disease burden for this fairly prosperous community, not all of this is aimed at healing. Much attention is directed at protection. Christian churches vigilantly guard their members against witches and evil spirits. In this time of immune deficiency – everyone knows this phrase, even those who do not listen to the rest of the HIV/AIDS prevention messages – and co-infections, people talk constantly of 'building up their immune system' and do so by means of drugs (ARVs), chemicals (e.g. 'blue stone', copper sulphate), commercial herbs (Echinacea), baths using herb-infused water, steam or smoke, body rubs and consulting *sangomas* and many types of other healers. Thieves, smugglers and illegal miners also guard themselves similarly. People talk of increasing their immunity to witches and point to White people in the community who appear to have neither deaths from AIDS nor witchcraft. In this context, all healing is protection since disease is always sent from some other source and to heal is also to protect from such influence. But protection is also healing since the failure of protection (from evil or viruses) brings illness and makes it worse. One's health improves as one's defences improve. Even as almost everyone refuses to admit the vast prevalence of HIV or to admit someone has it or has died from it, the idea that AIDS is the failure of protection (immunodeficiency) accords as well with the indigenous theories of illness as it does with the bio-medical, while not being wholly true of either.

Exploring the options in the market for healing

When Susan (not her real name), one of my research collaborators in Barberton fell ill, she entered the local market for healing. At first, she consulted widely among traditional healers but eschewed clinics and Christian faith healers. She expressed concern that we (she and I) had not yet done a *pahla* – formal recognition of the spirit by calling it and making a small offering of beer and snuff – for a local healer with whom we had worked on previous projects, and who had committed suicide a year previously. She frequently told me that she was afraid her health would be affected by this neglected duty but I continued to neglect it due to the pressure of other work. I was not aware of how ill she was becoming, or how ill she feared herself to be. Several months previously her health had seen a serious and rapid decline. Her two sons had come to visit her from Johannesburg to perform a healing ritual with her that involved sacrificing a goat and a cleansing ritual for all of them including vomiting, emetics and, especially, reconciliation among all the kin and friends who attended the ritual. Late in 2009, however, she lost weight precipitously and eventually became too weak to stand alone. By the time I came to assist her, she had been in and out of the local government hospital but had refused treatment. She feared that the hospital drip would cause further illness. I took her back to hospital where a government-employed Tunisian doctor saw her. His English was poor but he eventually diagnosed her with active TB. She was sent for HIV counselling and testing at a separate facility, and was diagnosed as HIV positive. The night she was admitted to hospital her temperature was over 40°C according to her chart, and her blood pressure was 95/65; she was dehydrated and close to death.

It emerged that she had also been to see several local bio-medical practitioners and had been self-medicating with a range of other drugs that she had acquired from other people. These included a number of TB-specific antibiotics, other antiprotozoal and antibiotics, as well as a range of herbal and commercial products. Some, such as Ilvitrim, is widely used in South Africa for treating opportunistic infections amongst AIDS patients, especially TB and others, such as Flagyl/metronidazole, for treating infections commonly associated with AIDS. An anti-inflammatory, such as Naproxen (a.k.a. Aleve, Midol), and other strong painkillers had also been used, probably from local pharmacies but not on prescription. Ciprofloxacin, however, is considered to be a second-line TB treatment and should only be used when drug resistance is beginning to manifest. Using it inappropriately, as she was doing, is likely to increase drug resistance. (Indeed, the efficacy of this drug has decreased markedly due to abuse of this sort and it is no longer used in many cases.) Local GPs had given her vitamins and other substances such as sea salt. Pyridoxine (vitamin B6), however, is also used in TB and AIDS treatment to alleviate neuropathy. One GP had diagnosed high blood pressure, according to her, even though her blood pressure was dangerously low when she was admitted to hospital. Despite telling her that she had high blood pressure, that doctor had not prescribed any appropriate hypertension medication.

Over 16 medications had been prescribed or acquired for self-medication including the following.

- From government clinics but not prescribed directly for the patient (Susan):
  Ilvitrim (sulphamethoxazole 400 mg and Trimethoprim 80 mg), prescribed for J. Ngobeni and issued by a government clinic
  Metronidazole (brand name: Flagyl) 200 mg, prescribed for J. Ngobeni, Mpumalanga Provincial Clinics 'Pre-pack'
  Flagyl tablets (generic: metronidazole), (large white, scored, no other identifying marks; '1 Tablet 2 Times a day') in a generic prescription plastic packet, neither patient nor issuer was identified
  Ciploxx 500 (Ciprofloxacin 500 mg) in trade-marked box with package insert, 'Cipla Live Sciences', expiry date 6/2012; 10 tablets in original packaging, all but one taken
  Naproxen 200, in a generic plastic packet from a pharmacy but no identification of the pharmacy, patient or prescribing doctor
- Other pharmaceuticals:
  Nucotrim tablets (co-trimoxazole 480 mg), Gulf Drug Company, in a blister pack, not otherwise identified

- From Dr A, MB Ch B (Wits):
  Multivitamin (small bi-convex orange tablets)
  Salterpyn (large light-green tablets)
  Vit-B-Complex (small bi-convex black tablets)
  Betacin (small yellow gelatine capsules)
- From Dr B, MB ChB (NUI) [National University of Ireland], LRCS & PI (Eire) (Licentiate of the Royal College of Surgeons):
  Sea salt
  UHC 20
  B6 [pyridoxine, one of the B vitamins]
  Folic 15 (small yellow scored tablets)
  (unreadable writing on packet), 10 small green gelatine capsules
  Voltrol (?) 15 (small yellow tablets without markings)

Susan seemed to have been aware that she might have TB and/or HIV and/or AIDS but had resisted a formal diagnosis and had refused hospitalization. She had refused to go to government clinics that I had suggested many times, possibly because she feared or already strongly suspected what the diagnosis would be. It is significant that although both the GPs she consulted apparently held appropriate bio-medical degrees, according to their stationery and printed medication packets, their diagnoses were entirely incorrect and their treatment inappropriate and ineffective.[4] Susan felt that she was getting better on traditional medications, with prescribed rituals and herbal concoctions from local street vendors and pharmacies. Only the government hospital, which was under-resourced in all ways and relying on foreign staff, managed to save her life with a correct diagnosis, care and appropriate treatment. Ironically, the patient had refused this option. Six months later after treatment for TB, but prior to starting ARV treatment, her weight had increased 20 kg from 34 kg to 54 kg, and she felt better despite still being quite ill. She spent much more time with traditional healers as her condition improved, however, seeking purification from the polluting effects of Western medicine. She frequently expressed uncertainty about whether she was better or not. She never discussed her HIV positive status and as her TB improved, she started to smoke and drink again, effectively denying the threat that HIV still posed.

This case is far from unusual. Even in a life-threatening situation such as this, people continue to shop around and often select ineffective and dangerous healing treatments while refusing effective ones. It is clear, too, that the bio-medical practitioners here were no more effective than most of the others (excluding the foreign-staffed government hospital) or were of no use at all. More-

[4] Wood & Lambert (2008: 220-221) documented a similar case of a private doctor's incompetence in the Eastern Cape, South Africa.

over, these practitioners were among the best known and most widely consulted in Barberton. The effectiveness of bio-medicine, therefore, is often no better than the many other healing methods. We often assume that the superiority of bio-medicine is obvious but in this market and in this population, there is often little difference in effectiveness, real or perceived. Scepticism is an essential skill for shoppers in this market.

The role of belief in assessing healing efficacy

However we understand or define healing, it is a 'good' that all humans desire and for which they are willing to pay. The cost of healing – what people are willing to pay – is extraordinarily difficult to assess and payment almost never takes the form of a single 'price'. There is a universal and stable demand for healing, here as elsewhere, and there are myriad specialists who provide the various services. There is a demand for it, a supply of healing in the form of therapies and medications, with a cost that is, in principle, measurable. Unlike the economic market, the costs of healing, its benefits, the nature of supply and demand and their relation to price are not measurable in ordinary currencies of trade. (What is the 'supply' of ancestors who can be supplicated? How can the 'demand' by ancestors to inhabit a living body or the quantum of evil in a spirit be measured?)

Accordingly, we call this a non-economic market – that is, a range of choices with costs, prices, inputs and outcomes – but judgements are not made on the basis of relative utility or value for money. Choices are made on the basis of belief, even though belief itself is not stable. People change their beliefs to access therapy and abandon beliefs if it fails. It is as if the economic rationality of the market changes the premises of its reason with each purchase.

The role of belief in healing has long been known but it is only recently that research has shown that the so-called placebo effect (the quantum of healing achieved by physiologically ineffective or inefficient therapies) is a genuine psychobiological event attributable to the overall therapeutic context, and that such effects can be robust in both laboratory and clinical settings (Finniss *et al.* 2010; Amanzio *et al.* 2009). While belief might account for a placebo effect, the placebo effect is not sufficient to account for the complex interaction of belief and therapy in this market.

People seek healing whether they are ill or not and continue to seek healing after being healed, and even if they have not been healed. When a client pays a bio-medical doctor for treatment or purchases pharmaceuticals or when actuaries assess risk and demand health, bio-medicine has a price and definable outcome because hospitals, pharmaceuticals, equipment, doctors, adjunct personnel and the patients are all highly regulated and bureaucratically controlled. This is not a free market: it intersects powerfully with politics, ideology and the state, professional organizations and other institutions. For the many other types of healing that are on offer in a town such as Barberton, this is not the case. Results are unpredictable and most things are negotiable. In such an environment, the primary problem for a potential client is how to evaluate the options that are available.

Healing, whether it be bio-medical, traditional, by means of faith, herbs or other means, offers its services through a complex organizational grid that regulates the types and costs of healing that are available. It is not enough simply to assess which healing mode or method is best or most effective, even if this kind of evaluation can be made at all.

Of course, medical doctors and formal pharmacies also have membership organizations that prescribe elements of their practice and provide credentialing and the regulation of pricing and practices. The same is true of traditional healers, though to a lesser extent and more informally (Thornton 2008). Traditional healers primarily refer patients to each other and share their knowledge through restricted groups of healers in *mpande* (schools). Access to all of these services is, therefore, partly controlled by formal institutions or complex networks of knowledge.

The primary challenge for any client such as Susan or others is to find ways to assess the effectiveness of these modes and methods of healing, given that none of them are obviously superior in practice, and that all have both a price and a risk attached to them.

A *sangoma* succinctly stated this quandary. She had been discussing with me what many traditional healers, along with the general public, often suspect or declare: 'healing is fake'. She believed that only 'the mind', as she put it in English, could heal the body. '(Biomedical) Doctors have a lot to fear from us, and that is why they do not like us,' she said. She had up to this point been engaged in a diatribe against both traditional healers and medical doctors. I asked her what she meant. How could traditional healers be a threat to doctors when she was telling me that most of them were 'fakes'? 'Because most of them are no better than we (*sangomas*) are,' she concluded. 'Haven't you noticed?' (Gogo A, 4 April 2010).

Healing as spiritual protection and a cultural revival

It is not only persons who seek healing and protection in this market. Businessmen, chiefs and groups of all kinds also do. Individuals speak of 'boosting their immune systems' in the same breath as talking about how best to protect themselves against witches; both are elements of healing as a response or prophylaxis. AIDS, clearly and correctly understood as a failure of the immune system, is taken to be evidence (or perhaps a complex metaphor) for a more general need for protection of all kinds. Healing is protection and vice versa, as AIDS campaigns seem to attest.

The large congregation of Zionists has gathered in the garden of Chief Kenneth Dlamini of the Emjindini Tribal Trust. The members of the Zion Church of Christ, one of the biggest churches in South Africa,[5] have come to bless the upcoming *ummemo* in October 2009. This will be only the third Ummemo that Chief Kenneth has hosted at the Royal Kraal of Emjindini since this chiefdom was re-established on restituted land in the late 1990s. The *ummemo* is an annual celebration of the chiefship. In the past, members of the chiefship gathered together on this day to offer service to the chief and to be seen and blessed by him. Today, it is part of a movement to revitalize older Swazi traditions. As in medicine, modernity and tradition compete with their offerings and potentials on display without a clear hierarchy of values. The diversity in the market for healing mirrors and is conditional on the inchoate and emerging political culture.

Chief Kenneth wants it to be a success. He has invited the members of the local ZCC to hold weekend services at his place. The local members of the ZCC are augmented strongly by ZCC members from many other churches, some as far away as Bushbuckridge in Limpopo Province and others from Elukwatini and Nelspruit in neighbouring municipalities and districts. They come from within a radius of perhaps 150 km and all have been summoned by the regional elders to participate in the blessing of Emjindini, Chief Kenneth and the *ummemo* that will take place in two weeks' time.

The congregation is divided into male and female sections. All wear different versions of the ZCC uniform. The elder males are dressed in what looks to be a version of the uniform of the South African Police Service from the 1950s. They wear cotton drill khaki jackets, black ties, brown trousers and highly polished black shoes. Over their shoulders they wear a 'Sam Brown' brown leather belt. The younger women are dressed in uniforms of green and

---

5 The Zionist Christian Church (ZCC) in South Africa has three to four million members across Southern Africa and is based in the lowveld town of Moria. Up to 2 million people converge on Moria each year during the mass pilgrimages at Easter. Healing is understood to be one of its primary strengths. The healing theology of the church traces it origins from John Alexander Dowie (1847-1907), a Scottish faith healer who founded and built his influential Christian Catholic Apostolic Church in Zion, Illinois, in the US. He established a 'holy city' of Zion after having been a pastor in Australia. Missions from this church were sent to the old Transvaal Republic (Zuid Afrikaansche Republiek) as early as 1895, and the church became established in the region over the next decade and a half. The ZCC eventually emerged from this Apostolic and Pentecostal background to become the region's dominant healing church.

yellow. The men in the choir are seated on a row of plastic chairs behind a 'high table' and are dressed in dark suits. All of their clothes are homemade. They only drink tea that is grown and marketed by the Church and have brought several sheep and a cow for slaughter, paid for by the chief and from ZCC-owned farms. They are a costly lot to host but are skilled in the art of protection from evil and, by doing so, protect others. The chief's belief in their belief makes them worth the price.

Chief Kenneth complains that he has had to 'pop out' several more goats and a cow as well. He has had to 'pop out' money for maize meal and other foods, even though the group is very strict about food taboos and what it can and cannot eat and drink. And then there are the contributions to the church to give thanks for its blessing. They stay for three days and have to be accommodated. Chief Kenneth is not a member of the church and is sceptical about the effectiveness of the blessing but he does not want to leave such important protection to chance. While it will involve some effort, the Traditional Authority and the chief himself will make a fair amount of money renting out spaces for people to sell food and drinks, homemade and commercial beer, and traditional and craft items. It is a local village fair with traditional dancing. Girls in traditional attire that leaves their breasts bare and men with bare chests and big bellies dance solemnly in loincloths of monkey and duiker skins. Cattle are slaughtered and people feast and get drunk. It is a fine time, and a high event that marks the emerging new traditionalism in South Africa.

The *ummemo* is the traditional Swazi chief's labour levy and village event. This is the occasion when the members of the community are meant to congregate after having rendered service to the chief. In this case, the community of Emjindini Tribal Trust is made up of families that have received grants of land from the chief. In fact, the participating audience is much larger and the legally mandated Tribal Trust is only a small section of a farm that was granted to some members of this community as part of a land redistribution and restitution process. The *ummemo*, however, is an important element of the re-traditionalization of the landscape and society in this increasingly densely settled rural area to the west of Barberton.

The re-traditionalization of land and landscape and of cultural life in parts of rural South Africa, exemplified by the *ummemo*, is an important reference point in the shifting grounds of traditional healing. It opens up space for traditional healers to dig wild herbs in the bush and to dance and drum in public. It does not, however, serve to give them wider public acceptance or more paying clientele but it allows them to be more publicly visible in the mix of healing options, despite obvious conflict. The protection rituals that the Christian ZCC has done are designed, for instance, to protect their members and clients (such as Chief Kenneth) from the bad influence of sorcerers, including some who are called *sangomas* or traditional healers. But Chief Kenneth seeks healing and protective services from both the ZCC and other healers. Many traditional healers are also members of churches such as the ZCC, and many of the healing/protective rituals that are conducted by the ZCC are very similar to those of the traditional *sangoma*. Thus, tradition and re-traditionalization in this context do not imply a *return* to a coherent or logically consistent culture. Rather, by re-valuing some elements of it, it further complicates an already complex cultural environment.

A few weeks later, I found myself shopping for my own traditional attire that I will wear for the first time at this year's *ummemo*. Sandile, my friend, needs another missing item from his traditional clothing. A woman in the community, who has just been nominated for the Traditional Music Award of South Africa, makes this item and offers to sell them to us. A month ago she had urged me to send as many cell phone messages to the competition as I could possibly afford, to vote for her. She had done well with her voice, CD sales and cell phone campaign, and was due to leave that afternoon for Durban where the awards would be announced, so we had to rush over to see her collection of traditional gear that she makes and sells as part of her business of tradition. Sandile was not impressed with the fluorescent green beads that she thought he would like. He took the garish set of beads but decided he also needed to shop around for something more traditional. (Later he bought a bandolier of pink ones.) Adding her voice to the rising chorus that wanted to see me in traditional attire that year, she loaned me a set of front and back aprons of vervet monkey skin, telling me that I would have to buy them if I wanted to use them again.

By believing in tradition and acting according to its precepts, we manifest its growing power, a power that traditional healers also make use of. Monkey-skin aprons and fluorescent orange-beaded bandoliers are worn over bare chests by big-bellied men using the latest digital cameras to document their participation in the chief's cultural revival. Similarly, protective bracelets of skin from sacrificial goats decorate the wrists of illegal young miners who use cell phones and lithium batteries to plan and prolong their raids on gold mines, feeding global markets from this out-of-the-way spot.

Tradition in the global market and the work of healing

Healing, tradition and traditional healing also do other work. On the way to her house, we pass four churches in less than a kilometre between the Chief's house and hers. We also pass two young men in the blue overalls that have been universally adopted by labourers throughout South Africa. They are wearing fresh strips of goat skin on their wrists and ankles. One of them is carrying plastic knee guards under one arm, while the other sports a massive gold chain around his neck. They are almost certainly illegal miners, young men who enter commercial mines and work old or disused stopes in gold mines in the surrounding hills. It is a major source of income for large numbers of young men in the area. Despite looking like ordinary labourers, they have clearly struck gold. The goat skins on their wrists are from goats slaughtered by traditional healers to protect them in the mines or to make them invisible to the guards as they enter them.

The economy of healing and other economic activities are linked in surprising ways. Most of the beads and paraphernalia that are used by traditional healers come from Indian-owned shops. Many of the items that local healers require come from the Indian Ocean, such as cowrie and other seashells, while the fabrics come from India, Mozambique and Swaziland. The practices of healers link the local economy to a regional and transnational economy, and the gold trade, protected by healers, links it to global markets. Several years earlier I had been in one of these Indian-owned shops. The husband of one of the *sangomas* that I was working with worked there as an assistant and had told me about it. I was inquiring then about the price of various items of the *sangoma's* kit, including the beads, shells, the items in the divination kit and clothes. When we were walking back then, a sermon was playing in English on the sound system.

This shop in the Barberton Indian quarter sells traditional regalia and requirements for rituals and religious groups. It has uniforms for the Zionists, for Swazi traditionalists, for other Christian groups and for *sangomas*. The Muslim owner of the shop, M, came to Barberton 30 years ago with his father who was a trader. M has been running the shop for many years and speaks fluent Swazi and is deeply versed in Swazi culture. When we entered the shop, we heard a Muslim cleric on the radio delivering a sermon in English and quoting frequent passages from the Quran in Arabic. The message of the sermon was, in essence, 'The Jews and the Christians will steal your faith. You must be constantly vigilant because they will do you wrong. You can be kind to them and treat them as if they were friends, but they have only one intention, and that is to undermine Islam and to destroy it.' When we entered the shop M was suspicious of us. As I explained my intention, he began to give us the prices of the items but seemed to want us to leave as soon as possible even though there was no one else there. The reason was the radio. The imam giving the radio sermon went on to consider whether it was the duty or merely an option for Muslims to kill Jews. Eventually, the sermon came to an end and we all relaxed. While the ordinary news was being read, M was much more willing to take time to chat.

Powerful international religious and ritual discourses meet and blend in this little corner shop that sells what might appear to be a mix of oddments in the old style of Southern African rural shops. The material particulars of rituals and powers to heal in Islam, Christianity and African traditional medicine are arrayed here under the glass counter and on the walls, sourced from all over the world. The market for healing has a distinct interface with global markets.

I was still unnerved by this experience when we walked into the shop again a few years later to buy traditional Swazi gear for the Chief's *ummemo*. This time the sound system was silent. When we arrived, M was telling a shop assistant that he must put price labels on tubes of rose-scented incense 'like the Germans'. 'You must do this with PRECISION! The way Germans do it, with precision,' he says to the bemused assistant. Looking up, he greets my Black companion, Sandile, in SiSwat, '*Sawubona, unjane*?', '*Yebo, sikhona*', then turns to me and asks 'Are you German?'. I say 'no', and he tries 'French? Canadian?'. I thought I should opt for one of the above but kept him guessing. Sandile, still not satisfied with the pink beads he had already bought in the Tribal Authority area, asked to see the beaded bandoliers that are part of the Swazi traditional attire. While looking for the item, the shopkeeper asked me, 'What's your surname?' He was determined to peg me down. 'Thornton,' I said. 'Oh, English.' 'No,' I said. Turning to ask Sandile his *isibongo*, he quickly placed my friend among Barberton's Black elite of landowners, businessmen and politicians. As I was examining the *mahiya*, traditional cloths that are part of the attire, he began to proselytize. 'You know, when we go on the *hajj* … you know the rituals of the *hajj*?'. 'Yes,' I said. 'On the *hajj*, we wear only an upper and a lower cloth, like the Swazis, like the Africans.' I did not contradict his bold generalization. 'Only ours are all white … only white. Very pure.' He went on to explain that men wear only the white cloths and, dropping his voice for emphasis, added, 'they don't wear underwear! They are all natural!' He looked at me to gage my reaction; I remained blank. 'Of course, the women are fully dressed,' he explained in case I felt ill at ease over this revelation. Since we were buying traditional attire, he began to develop his theory that the Africans must have adopted their own traditional attire from the Arabs because 'Arabs, during the *hajj*' wear only a top and bottom cloth wrap. This meant, he concluded, that 'the Arabs are much more ancient. They came first!' Religious differences could not have been starker and yet his business was built entirely around his trade in pagan goods and materials for religious observances of all kinds (except his own).

Sandile was watching me with one eyebrow raised. Turning to our friendly shopkeeper, I told him that I did not agree with him. 'How much is that cloth?' I asked, pointing to the most traditional of the trade cloths on display along a wire that stretched across the shop near the ceiling. I chose one and paid, heading for home as the first heavy rain of the summer hit and washed the dust on the roads down the gutters in a red torrent.

Competition in the market for healing

The traditional healers in Barberton are not traditional and simply deficient bio-medical doctors nor, on the other hand, necessarily possessed of ancient African wisdom and indigenous knowledge. In most respects they are not particularly traditional and are often not concerned with healing medical conditions as such. They compete intensely with one another and with a wide range of other religious, bio-medical, quasi-technical (healing technologies such as weight-loss machines), New Age, traditional Chinese medicine and many other healing systems and methods. When they use herbs in healing, it is rarely for their bio-medical or pharmacological properties, supposed or potential. Instead, herbs are used to smoke the whole body in smoke baths or are burnt and rubbed into the skin or into cuts in the skin, used in enemas, emetics and in (steam)baths or as packets of magical substances or charms. These substances index the healing power of the bush, nature and the uninhabited wild that is devoid of witches. The term *muti* can be translated as 'medicine' or 'charm' but also as 'bush'.

One such application is the use of *muti* in crime, especially theft. The house that serves as my research base in Barberton was recently burgled.[6] I had just arrived, and had unpacked my computer, camera gear, notes and bag. Before going to bed, I had been working on my laptop on the table in the lounge, leaving the computer and camera visible from the window. I did not wake as the thief bent the burglar bars away from the window, crawled through the gap and took the computer and camera. The next morning when I told the story to local friends, one immediately nodded his head and said, 'I'm sure what tipped you off was the smell.' 'What smell?' I asked. 'The thieves use a kind of *muti* to make sure that you don't wake up. It's made from the hair of hyenas, snake fat and other parts of animals. If they burn it by the window, you will not wake up and they can do what they like,' he told me. He believed this to be true: the market for belief leaves no one unaffected, even beyond the immediate market for healing.

In fact, I had not smelled anything and there was no evidence of burning by the window or anywhere else, but most people believed that I had slept through

6 The burglary occurred on Sunday 15 November 2009. The house is in a secure gated residential area, with a steel palisade fence surrounding it. This was not the first time. The house had also been burgled in February 2009 when they had tunnelled under the fence. After that, an electric fence was put around the area on the outside and on top of the steel palisade fence. The electric fence, however, did not go over the tops of the columns at the entrance. The tops of the columns had spikes on them, and when we examined the perimeter the morning after the burglary there was blood at the bottom and outside of the area. I followed the blood trail for a few metres into the bush, and then thought better of it. The trail led to an informal settlement known to be inhabited by illegal gold miners, many of whom were armed.

the burglary because a magic sleeping potion had been used. In fact, the thief had injured himself and I had followed the blood trail into the bush towards the squatter camp nearby. I tracked him only far enough to convince myself that the theft had been merely opportunistic; others strongly believed that magic had been used.

Since theft of all kinds – together with other kinds of crime – is a significant part of the economy in most South African towns, including Barberton, it is clear that thieves do pay significant amounts of money for magic of this sort. Although not a matter of healing, it contributes to the income of quite a few *tangoma*, *emagedla* and *emanyanga* (pl. types of healers and herbalists) and helps to sustain other healing activities. The large majority of initiated healers do not practice magic of this sort since to do so risks losing the powers bequeathed to them by the ancestors (*emadloti*). The role of the healer, as these cases show, is complex and multifaceted. The role they play and the contribution that they make – positive or negative – to the overall flow of money, goods and services, however, is impossible to assign a value to and is unpredictable and ambiguous.

In economic terms, the price of elasticity is near zero since prices to do not respond to supply, demand, assessed efficiency or the effectiveness of the product. In effect, the price of healing is the cost of membership in a community, be this a church, a network of knowledgeable people who can refer one to an effective healer of the traditional sort or any other. The effectiveness of any and all of these is not a foregone conclusion and some combination of them generally depends on what one believes, and belief is elastic. It changes to accommodate the need for healing.

Belief, the placebo effect and the market for healing

How, then, do South Africans in this diverse market of healing options make decisions on what to buy? I argue in the rest of this chapter that the choice of healing options has less to do with objective factors of disease or even perceived illness, and more to do with beliefs about what works. When even biomedical therapies have, in practice, only a slightly better chance of working, choices are made on the basis of what people *believe* will work.

But, more than this, the quality of belief is held to influence the quality of the cure. This may be understood as a complex placebo effect but it is more than this. Belief, like (rational) thought, allows us to assess our relationship to the world and to evaluate internal and external states. While rational or economic judgements allow us to evaluate evidence and reach conclusions based on an idea of cause and effect, belief permits us to evaluate moral states of being and to underpin knowledge and action with a sense of righteous certainty.

The centrality of belief in this market is manifested in two ways. First, it is widely believed that no therapy is entirely effective unless one *believes* that it will be effective, just as a witch has no power over those who do not believe in witches. Second, people also believe that every therapy has a reason why it is chosen that is not necessarily rational. Ancestors guide someone to a traditional healer, for instance. This is said whether or not the therapy s/he receives is effective. Similarly, someone who believes that they are healed by crystals understands this in terms of larger systems of belief about the mystical power of nature. One who attends a doctor's surgery has similarly decided to believe that this will be effective. Evidence of effectiveness after the fact is less important than prior belief, since belief in the cure as it happens augments its effectiveness.

It is belief, therefore, that makes therapies work, and belief – one could call it faith except for the fact that this term has strong Christian connotations – that provides structure for the market. For instance, it is widely believed that witches are never White. Black people often say, when asked, that witchcraft does not work on Whites. Whites, on the other hand, are often not entirely certain that witchcraft does not work on them, and fear it, even as they tell Black people that it can have no effect on them 'because we don't believe in it'. Whites, however, are often strong believers in many other kinds of spiritual influence, including witches, but most confine their beliefs to issues of Christian spiritualism and its dark twin, Satanism. On learning that I study witches, many White people in Barberton have asked me specifically whether I can tell them if witchcraft can affect them. Their question implies a belief that witchcraft is an objective fact and only its sphere of influence is in question. They are comforted by a kind of hopeful relativism.

Implicit in these systems of belief is more than belief as a state of mind, or an emotional commitment to a worldview or culture. Each system of belief has a set of practices and boundaries. The communities of belief divide the demand for therapy into different markets. More than the belief that sustains them, these practices are believed to be efficacious in a number of ways: as therapy, as (passive) healing and comfort, or possibly also as (active) sorcery, protection or defence from dangerous spiritual influences and aggression from others. Since they are opportunistic, shaped to the occasion and deployed for specific reasons, these practices range from active therapies for medical and psychological (spiritual) complaints or passive comfort and protection, to active aggression.

These therapies cost money to buy and often require additional equipment (even if this is just a bottle of beer, thread or cloth). There are markets for African *muti*, for pharmaceuticals, for recreational drugs, for foreign African *muti* (especially from Malawi or Mozambique), for animal and human body parts, for traditional African, Christian, Muslim or Hindu amulets and clothing, and many other items of spiritual-occult practice. And, as in any segmented market where boundaries limit knowledge in the market and thus the efficiency of the market (in the terms of the economist), there is ample opportunity for arbitrage and insider trading, fraud, schemes, gaming, double dealing and, of course, for just plain dealing across the borders of belief communities, and within them.

The nature of belief – why people believe one thing or another about unseen, non-empirical yet influential spiritual entities, including witches, ancestors, spirits, energies, aura, demons, fairies and many other sorts of non-material entities with power – is less important in the everyday economy of believing and healing than the limits, qualities and even quantities of belief in types of therapy or occult influences and the powers that enable them. The notion that only Christians can practice Satanism, for instance, or that African witchcraft cannot directly affect White people, places limits on the effectiveness of these practices. These limits are the boundaries of belief that structure the market.

In placing limits on their effectiveness, this places limits on the market for these practices. Not everyone can simply purchase healing that will work for them since there is another condition that must be met if it is to be effective: it must be believed and to be believed it must be part of a system of belief. Beliefs and therapies, thus, are goods in a complex market where utility is judged on the ability to make suffering more bearable, illness more meaningful, and healing more believable.

I am not alone in finding this incoherence and diversity puzzling. Carol Legg, writing a remarkable medical-ethnographic account of aphasia in a largely Black but polyglot suburb of Cape Town notes that:

> (T)here is no evidence of a discrete cultural account of aphasia (due to stroke) but rather a wide variation in causal notions that included biomedical causes, social and behavioural determinants, transgression of social rules, and the influences of supernatural powers such as witches and ancestors. … (T)raditional, biomedical and religious cures … were obscured by a burgeoning and not always ethical open market offering miracle cures. Uncertainty prevailed. (Legg 2010: 230-231)
>
> People were uncertain about the trajectory of stroke and aphasia, abut the possibility of treatment and about the integrity of healers and healthcare workers. People were also uncertain about their own alignments in this setting where Christianity, indigenous culture, biomedicine and western thought wrestle for hegemony. (*Ibid.*: 238)

Legg was writing about a suburb or township located in a very different part of South Africa. 2000 km away, but similar problems exist for both the local participant and the observer or analyst. Diversity, doubt and uncertainty prevail.

Not all therapies are effective in all cases and some are completely ineffective in all cases. Despite this, each therapy, however improbable, still manages to secure some part of the overall market. People may be spreading their bets but few have sufficient resources to gamble in the market for healing, and there are strong emotional and social limits placed on the degree of risk one can take with one's illness by betting on the wrong therapy for the condition, or the right therapy for the wrong condition.

Choice in the market for belief

All plural medical systems pose questions: (i) what counts as healing? (or how would I know that I am healed?), and (ii) what would I need to believe in order to believe that I am healed? It is therefore a search for a set of beliefs that would constitute valid conditions for healing to take place and to be assessed. In other words, healing is not merely conditional on biological or physiological states of the organism but on states of belief that provide sufficient cognitive and emotional conditions to believe that healing is possible, and to assess the outcomes.

It is thus inadequate to talk about the social causes of disease and illness here, as for instance in Kleinman (1978), Comaroff (1981), Lindenbaum & Lock (1993) sand Farmer (2006), since it is not the causes that are important but the conditions under which both an illness and a therapy may be assessed: the illness as amenable to therapy and the therapy as appropriate to the illness. In this plural medical system in which various practices and sets of healing cultures compete with each other, it must be possible for the patient to evaluate which sets of healing practices and beliefs give a reasonable chance of achieving health. There are also many types of illness and disease, some of which resolve themselves (by healing spontaneously), some of which proceed to morbidity and death, and some which come and go (like malarial fevers, TB coughs or AIDS symptoms) or maintain themselves at moderate, survivable levels of illness over long periods of time. People need a way of evaluating the effect of different therapies over time, in spite of remission, relapse and chronic illness.

This is a second-order question about the cultures that constitute medical pluralism in Southern Africa. A first-order question is 'How do I become healed?'. In systems where there is only one answer to this question, the first-order question is all that is necessary. Having asked it, people will go to the doctor or the healer and ask to be healed.

However, in a plural medical system there are many options for those who seek healing or who simply wish to preserve their health. Choosing the appropriate or right option or set of options requires an evaluation of the options available since in most cases there is no single 'right option'. Most people select a set of possible healing strategies, and multiple options may well be deployed at once. This is not just a question of how to be healed and what one believes, but of how to evaluate the premises of the healing system. To do this, the patient must ask what would count as 'being healed'. In a well-resourced, technical facility in which many of the measurement questions have been asked and answered, this is not an everyday problem for the patient, though it vexes scientists and philosophers of science. For the patient, s/he is healed when certain specific conditions, the knowledge of which is generally shared by healer and patient alike, are met. Did the fever go down to normal? Was the person's blood pressure corrected or blood sugar levels adjusted or the heart repaired?

Many of the illnesses that afflict people in South Africa are complex, of long duration and of uncertain symptomology. High blood pressure, diabetes, TB, diarrhoea, dehydration, malnutrition, HIV/AIDS and malaria manifest themselves in many ways and symptoms come and go. Others such as 'nerves' (generalized anxiety, depression), undiagnosed STDs and other common viral infections are often vague and hard to diagnose. Many of these are poorly treated in the Southern African medical system and some are simply untreatable given the technologies and resources available, while others, such as HIV and TB, often involve co-infection and drug resistance. When and if they are treated, a long treatment regime is involved with many opportunities for failure. Thus, the question of what would constitute 'being healed' is one that most people are forced to ask. It is frequently far from obvious.

There is also a continuum of states of health that might be judged as being 'healthy', 'relatively healthy' or 'healthy enough'. Illnesses and disease range from tolerable to intolerable and from something you can live with to something you die from. For instance, 'People *Living* with HIV/AIDS' (PLWA) is a formalized category of people with a recognized disease who may or may not be ill.

Part of this evaluative process involves an assessment of what kind of cure it is. A spiritual cure might mean that one is at least at ease with one's impending death and ready to die. Thus, healing in an environment of such medical pluralism involves more than the diagnostic categories of healing itself, but also a philosophy of types of healing. Implicit in this, of course, is a set of cultural categories of disease and illness but also a set of cultural categories of what constitutes the absence or cure of one or other of these categories of illness. This is, essentially, a set of positive (ontological, existential) cultural categories and their negations.

Each patient has to ask not only 'what kind of illness is it?' (the diagnostic question) but also 'how can I be healed' (a question about the choice of method) and 'what will I be healed of?' (the categorical question of what – body, blood, spirit or soul – will be healed) and also 'what must I believe in order to answer these questions?'. Thus, the question resolves to what is, at its core, a question of the sort that a cultural anthropologist asks. What is the context in which belief X makes sense, that is, how can we construct a cultural explanation for belief X? In the context of healing, this amounts to the question of what one 'must believe' in order to make a therapy work.

While this might seem strange, even farfetched, there is a constant conversation going on about who believes what, and with what consequences. When the newspapers print a story about a funeral business's worker who has sold the fresh hand and breast of a White woman to a healer or *sangoma* in Green Valley in the lowveld, everyone asks the question about belief. 'Why do these people believe that this will give them power?' is a typical question. People of every race, colour, class and occupation ask this question. Similarly, if one hears about a miraculous cure for AIDS at a Christian Church or how Mohammed, a healer from 'Africa' (South African's locution for anyone who is African but not South African), has healed a man in his 'surgery' in Barberton's main street, most people that feel inclined to discuss such things eventually come to the question of belief: What should one believe for such a cure to work. Virtually everyone I have known in a dozen years of fieldwork in this town does indeed discuss such issues of belief and healing. It is also true that no one seems to

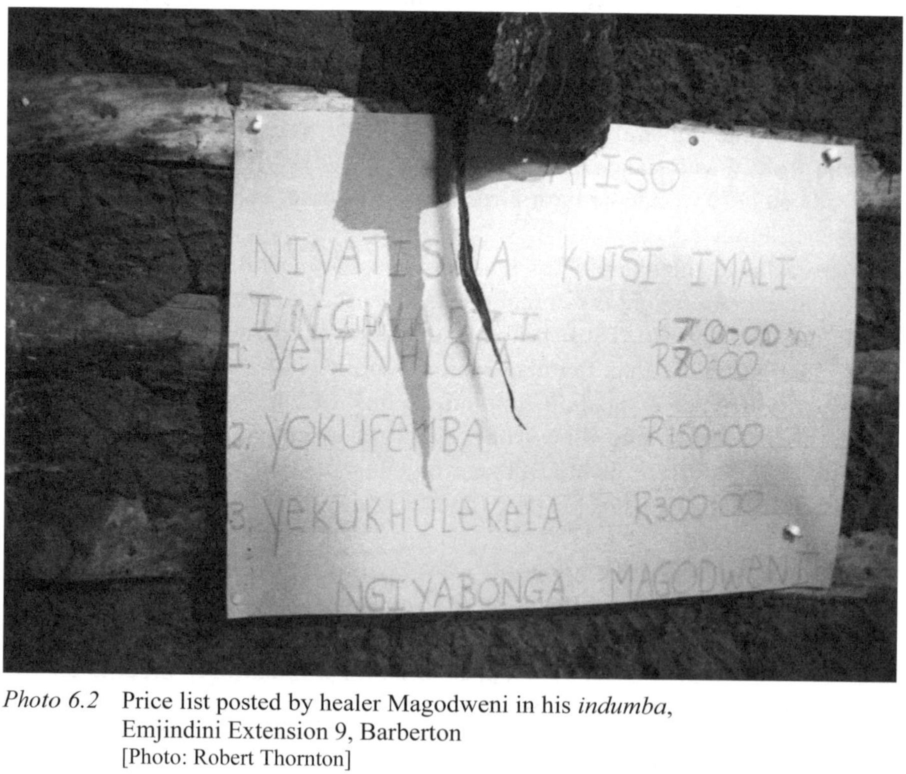
KUTSI IMALI
2. YOKUFE
R150-00
3. YEKUKHULEKELA
R300-00
NGIYABONGA

Photo 6.2 Price list posted by healer Magodweni in his *indumba*, Emjindini Extension 9, Barberton
[Photo: Robert Thornton]

question the fundamental premise that appropriate beliefs can cure certain illnesses and that belief can be acquired and dropped as necessary. What they seem to want to know is not whether belief X is valid or not, testable or not or true, but rather what is required for a belief to be effective. In this case, the strength of the belief that a cure or therapy will work is held to be an integral part of the power of the therapy and its strength.

Since value for money (or healing efficacy per investment of time, belief *and* money) is relatively indeterminate, prices are inelastic. Prices, in other words, do not vary with respect to the effectiveness of the therapy. Most therapies cost about the same, whether bio-medical, quasi-medical, traditional or other. Belief, however, does vary. A failed cure by Christian faith healers will cause a person to leave the church. In effect they cut their losses as they abandon the investment that they have put into the church. This is also true for traditional healing, New Age healing or other forms of quasi-medical and bio-medical healing.

The search for therapy is, therefore, less a search for the most efficient cure or a maximization of utility, as economists would expect, but is itself a diagnostic practice that judges which healing systems work and whether, and how much, to invest in them. What one 'believes' in this case has a pragmatic effect. It is not a market for simply things-with-a-price. Healing may be priced, as an insurer prices risk, but its price is – as with complex financial market derivatives and risk pricing – essentially arbitrary and risky in itself.

Not all healing works. According to one traditional healer, 'Some healers these days are just in it for the singing and dancing' (Mahlasela, Ext 13, Tingulubeni). Belief, then, allows some people to assume, independently of any evidence, that it is true, that is that it will work for them, as long as they continue to believe.

Conclusion

For an economist, the notion of elasticity typically refers to the responsiveness of price to demand, and vice versa. If price changes little with respect to changes in demand, then price is said to be inelastic; if it changes in response to changing demand, then price is said to be elastic. In a well-functioning market, price, supply and demand should change in step with each other, ideally in a one-to-one relationship. Economists can pretend to deal with ideal markets; anthropologists cannot. These ideal conditions are rarely met in real markets, and certainly not in the market for healing. The supply of healers is relatively fixed as new practitioners come into the market infrequently and most stay in it for long periods of time. Their supply and pricing has little relationship with the real burdens of disease, illness and misfortune. To a degree, prices for traditional healers are set by tradition and by communal consensus but they are mainly determined by what medical doctors charge, and South African law and insurance companies set this fee. Herbal medications often cost similar amounts to pharmaceuticals since these are usually subsidized by government. Prices have little elasticity in response to the market either with respect to supply or demand. Demand itself is often artificially low due to the fact that many people refuse to acknowledge illness, especially AIDS or TB, among other misfortunes such as trauma from drunken domestic fights, violence due to witchcraft accusations, jealousy and loans. The market for healing exists but is not an economy governed by price.

In addition, there is a very low level of specific knowledge about what various healers might offer, despite a generally well-informed public for healing. While in a more developed setting, bio-medical practitioners often have a significantly better success rate than other types of healers, in a small marginal town such as Barberton this is not always the case. Thus, no one assumes that bio-medical healers are necessarily going to be better or that they will offer better service or achieve higher cure rates. Many people have little knowledge of the validity, efficiency or theoretical basis any of the methods of healing might have. The patients' system of beliefs about what any form of healing might offer is therefore an important, if not the most important, element in the healing process. This is not to say that all methods of healing are equally good or are equally likely to succeed. They are not, objectively speaking. However, patients/clients often do not know this and the success rate of various healers – bio-medical doctors and clinic staff included – is judged by rumour, popular culture, the media (especially local radio and newspaper media that reflect local conceptions and beliefs most faithfully) and personal experience.

Belief, therefore, is frequently the most elastic factor in the local economy of healing. Beliefs change and adjust in response to changing ideas about what types of therapy work and what is available. Since the belief that a therapy will be effective is held to be one of the most important factors affecting its actual effectiveness, there is a market for belief. The market for belief operates as rumours, in self-advertising, through church efforts to recruit followers with offers of healing, prayer and protection from evil, the recruitment of traditional healers through dreams and affliction, and public health messages directed through the public media in favour of bio-medical therapies.

Ordinarily, the role of belief in medicine is held to relate to the placebo effect. The placebo (Latin: I please) effect refers to the fact that if a patient believes a medication might or should be effective, it will have some effect despite the fact that there is no active ingredient, or anything, that will have any measurable physiological, chemical or medicinal effect on the body. The placebo effect is the measure of the effect of belief on healing. In testing the real (chemical or physiological effect) of a medication, randomized controlled trials test the effect of the medication against the effect of the placebo. The effect of the drug under test is, then, the amount of healing that can be accomplished over and above what can be achieved by belief alone. Any surplus of effect caused by the medication or other intervention is held to be the real, measurable effect of the intervention.

But what if nothing works? What if all interventions are equal and they are all more or less due to faith and belief? If medicine is only as effective as the placebo, then placebos may be held to be as effective as the medication, and the net effect of healing is due to belief, its symbolic efficacy. Belief, in this case, may achieve what an economic rationality would fail to do. With limited exceptions, this appears to be the case in Barberton. The market for healing is a market for belief.

References

Amanzio, M, L.L. Corazzini, L. Vase & F. Benedetti (2009), A systematic review of adverse events in placebo groups of anti-migraine clinical trials. *Pain* 146(3): 261-369.

Anderson, A.H. (1999), The Lekanyanes and prophecy in the Zion Christian Church. *Journal of Religion in Africa* 29(3): 285-312.

Anderson, A.H. (2001), *African reformation: African initiated Christianity in the 20th century*. Trenton, NJ: Africa World Press.

Comaroff, J. (1981), Healing and cultural transformation: The Tswana of Southern Africa. *Social Science and Medicine* 15(3): xx.

Fafchamps, M. (2004), *Market institutions and Sub-Saharan Africa: Theory and evidence*. Cambridge, MA: Massachusetts Institute of Technology Press.

Farmer, P. (2006), *AIDS & accusation: Haiti and the geography of blame*. Berkeley, CA: University of California Press.

Finniss, D.G, T.J. Kaptchuk, F. Miller & F. Benedetti (2010), Biological, clinical and ethical advances of placebo effects. *The Lancet* 375(9715): 686-695.

Geertz, C. (1973), *The interpretation of culture: Selected essays*. New York: Basic Books.

Green, E.C., R. Thornton & Y. Sliep (2003), *Traditional healers and the bio-medical health system in South Africa*. Washington, DC/Johannesburg: Medical Care Development International (MCDI) & the Margaret Sanger Center International, South Africa.

Kleinman, A. (1978), Concepts and a model for comparison of medical systems as cultural systems. In: C. Leslie (ed.), *Theoretical foundations for the comparative study of medical systems*. Special edition of *Social Science and Medicine* 12: 88-93.

Legg, C. (2010), An ethnography of adults living with aphasia in Khayelitsha. PhD Thesis, University of the Witwatersrand.

Lindenbaum, S. & M. Lock, eds (1993), *Knowledge, power and practice: The anthropology of medicine and everyday life*. Berkeley, CA: University of California Press.

Thornton, R. (2009), The transmission of knowledge in South African traditional healing. In: T. Marchand & K. Kress, eds, *Knowledge in practice: Expertise and the transmission of knowledge*. Special issue of *Africa* 79(1): 17-34.
Waldram, J.B. (2000), The efficacy of traditional medicine: Current theoretical and methodological issues. *Medical Anthropology Quarterly* 14(4): 603-625.
Wittgenstein, L. (1952), *Philosophical investigations. Edited by G.E.M Anscombe & R. Rees and translated by G.E.M. Anscombe*. Oxford: Basil Blackwell.
Wood, K. & H. Lambert (2008), Coded talk, scripted omissions: The micropolitics of AIDS talk in an affected community in South Africa. *Medical Anthropology Quarterly* 22(3): 213-233.

7

Medicinal knowledge and healing practices among the Kapsiki/Higi of northern Cameroon and northeastern Nigeria

Walter E.A. van Beek

Kapsiki medicine is an example of traditional healing that is opening up to cosmopolitan systems of healing. Blacksmiths have always been the masters of health in Kapsiki society, with healing as one of their many specializations. The new healers do not depend on lineage but have chosen to become healers and are constructing their own pharmacopeia. Not only are they addressing new diseases, such as HIV/AIDS, they are also using modern means of communication technology, in particular the mobile phone, for a clientele that transcends community borders. However, their medicines are still rooted in the traditional definitions of healing herbs, with a central place for two plant species and an insistence on the plant specimen, in which specific properties are assigned to individual plants. This chapter is based on research spanning four decades and contains the medicine lists of a blacksmith grandfather and his grandson, throwing light on the dynamics of the transfer of medicinal information. The content of private and secret information appears not to be transmitted at all, and instead it is the ways of constructing knowledge that are being passed on. Comparing this insight with other studies on 'secrets', it is argued that private knowledge is being reinvented by each generation, unlike the more general, public knowledge whose content is indeed being transmitted.

Introduction

Healing in Africa has become an extremely complex field over the last few decades, with local traditional practices, cosmopolitan medicine and a host of interventions interacting and creating a maze of health options that people have to navigate. Previous generations in Africa lived with a bipolar system with traditional healing coexisting alongside more cosmopolitan methods although this often resulted in an uneasy truce characterized by fuzzy boundary markers but a definite hierarchical relationship. Over time, many expected to see a decline in traditional medication in favour of Western treatment; after all, the scientific approach of the North would surely usurp local practices. [1] But this has not happened. Cosmopolitan medicine is evidently not on the wane but neither are alternative forms, be they 'traditional' or 'esoteric'. Medicinal treatment has more than ever before become a market with stalls of different size and texture, with a competing and cross-cutting supply of care givers, a market in which the prestige and authority of the North have not been translated into a hegemonic position. Not only did healing systems from other continents arrive in Africa, such as Indian expert systems, but African healers also engaged in hybridization processes of healing practices, while more traditional forms remained on the market too.

This chapter focuses on the transformation, marketization and commoditization of one African medicinal system. New medical knowledge seems to exhibit both the rearranging of old elements into new wholes (*bricolage*) and the creation of new knowledge in an increasingly competitive, diverging and commercializing field. When navigating such turbulent waters, healers and patients have to continuously take their bearings, reapplying as well as reinventing their relevant knowledge in the new situations they face.

The first part of this chapter describes some new players in the field, a new kind of healer who has roots deep in local culture who is constructing new knowledge in the interface with Western medicine through creative applications and combinations of his own. In this, he also uses new forms of organization and technology, in local, regional as well as even national markets. The second part concentrates on the patient's navigation options, showing the increasing dependency there is on specialists as illnesses persist. Turning to the blacksmith, the traditional healer-diviner in Kapsiki society, the structure of traditional medicinal knowledge is sketched, showing the dominance of just two plant species. Finally, the various sectors of medicinal knowledge show diverse processes of transmission and non-transmission. Curiously, traditional experts' medicinal knowledge appears not to be transmitted at all, and the relevant knowledge has to be reinvented by each generation, exactly the kind of creativity we see among the new healers.

---

1 See Last (1986).

Map 7.1 Cameroon, showing research location

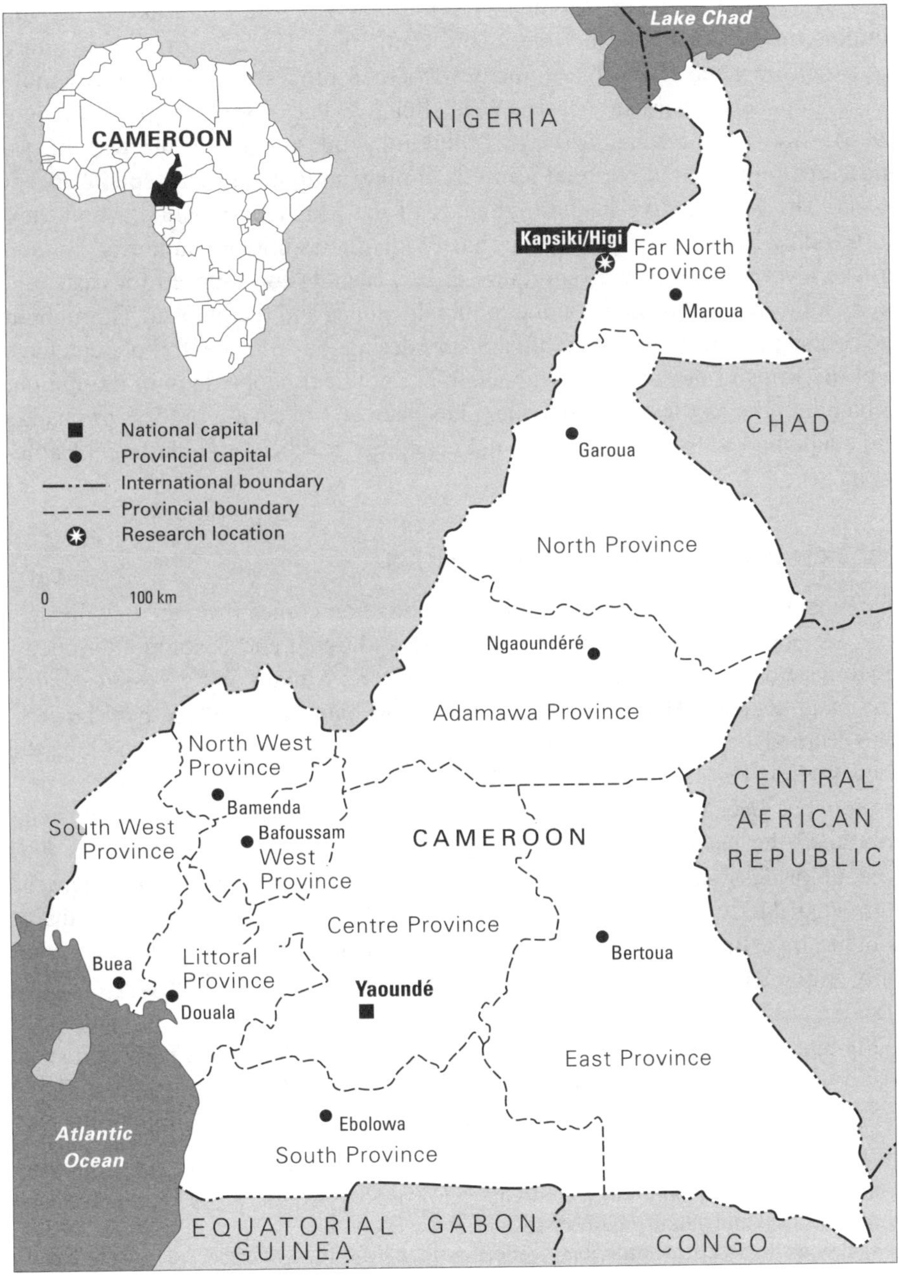

I take my example here from one specific culture, that of the Kapsiki/Higi[2] who live in the Mandara Mountains some 300 km south of Lake Chad and straddle the border between Nigeria and Cameroon. The data from this culture have their own specificity but in many ways their processes of healing resemble those found elsewhere in Africa (Winkelman & Peek 2004; Reynolds-Whyte 1996). Anyway, the Kapsiki[3] way of thinking about healing, health and illness, and cures represents a regional array of similar notions and concepts (Vincent 1991). The Kapsiki live in the highlands of the Mandara Mountains and their thirty-odd villages are quite autarchic, with no traditional authority beyond village level. They cultivate sorghum, millet, peanuts and tobacco for cash, and raise cattle, goats and sheep on the mountain slopes and the plateau. Throughout the course of history, the steep hillsides bordering the small central plateau have kept the Kapsiki out of touch with the main political happenings in the region; although in the last few decades, there has been an increasing process of change and adaptation to the new political and economic realities of Nigeria and Cameroon.

The new healer and the medical market

The most important dynamic in Kapsiki medication comes from the new healers who are operating in the space between the traditional and cosmopolitan medicinal systems. Two examples are presented here: a male and a female healer. The male healer is Haman Tizhè, an important man among these new healers[4] who learned his craft in Michika, the regional centre of the Higi part of the Kapsik-Higi. He chose to be a healer not because he was born into the profession but because of his personal history. Making the most of a difficult childhood, he used his stay among 'foreigners' to adopt and construct a new type of profession. From Michika, he ventured out into the bush where he cultivated the acquaintance of the healers in the area, usually blacksmiths or hunters. Investing time, money and energy in these relationships, he was gradually introduced to the secrets of Kapsiki medicine over a wider area. And he

2 My research into the Kapsiki of Cameroon and Higi of Nigeria has been carried out in various fieldwork periods from 1972/73 onwards and data have been gathered on return visits every four or five years ever since. The last visit was in January 2010. The work has been financed by WOTRO (Dutch Foundation for the Advancement of Tropical Research), Utrecht University, the African Studies Centre Leiden, the Hollandsche Maatschappij der Wetenschappen, the KNAW (the Royal Dutch Academy of Sciences) and Tilburg University.

3 The Kapsiki live in Cameroon, while the people on the Nigerian side of the border are usually called Higi. The term Kapsiki is used in this chapter unless a distinction needs to be made between the two groups.

4 For more details of his life story, see van Beek (2006).

watched wild animals feed, an important clue for many healers. He still spends a lot of time in the bush with old hunters and healers but also meets them in Sokoto, Aba and Gaitan in Nigeria and in Niger. And he has even communicated with *grand marabouts* from Mali when he was in Sokoto. One needs to travel a lot as a healer, so Haman was frequently away, though more so in the past than today: now that he is established, people come to him.

Haman has developed a new array of medications, mainly in the form of new medicines but also in ways of diagnosis and of administering the medication. More than in traditional settings and more than the blacksmiths, he addresses new problems in people's daily encounters: how to pass exams, how to achieve success at work or how to get revenge on one's enemies, using the word *voyance* (knowing the future) as well as 'blindage', which involves making one's enemies socially 'blind'. Traditionally, *voyance* came through in divination with a crab (van Beek 2010) but Haman does not perform divination himself, he just offers a diagnosis, basing his assessment on the client's somatic complaints and treats a wide array of ailments. He defines most as somatic, thus in contrast to the more divination-oriented ways of healing of the blacksmiths, the traditional healers, who first delve into their patients' social histories. But he claims, 'Not all new problems are somatic, however. For example, to have good luck in your car, you have to take some chameleon eggs and then you will not have any accidents and people will see you coming.'

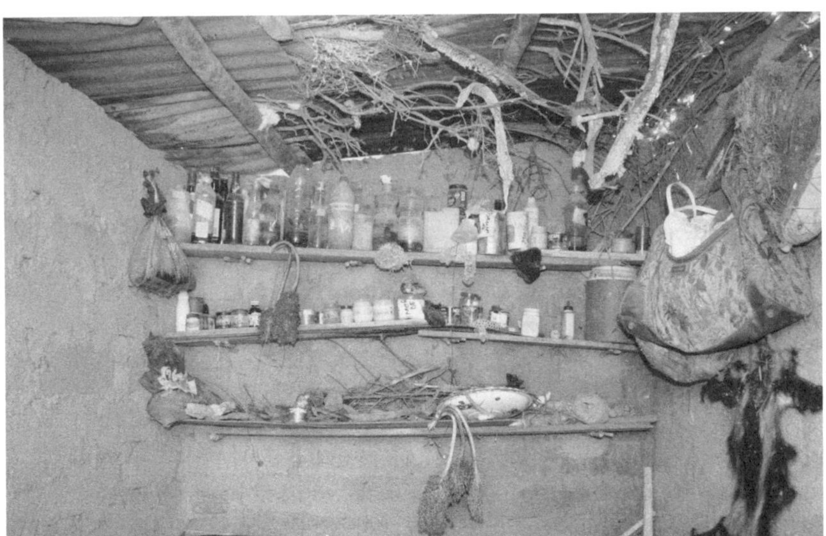

Photo 7.1 Part of Haman Tizhè's medicine cabinet
[Photo: Walter van Beek]

Evidently, as a new healer, he has had to turn his attention to HIV/AIDS and claims to be able to cure it, but only in the initial HIV stage. If a client tests positive, he gives him/her *calmage* (a traditional homologue to antiretroviral treatment) and treats the patient for three months. S/he is then retested and, if negative, has to continue both treatments and go for another test, preferably at a different hospital. He insists that with HIV/AIDS, healers have to cooperate with the local hospitals and dispensaries, and considers any healer a 'charlatan' if he refuses to send a patient to be tested for HIV at the hospital and to get antiretroviral medication.

Haman has developed what he calls a *passe-partout*, a general medication with a broad base, a composite medication made of five plants that has to be taken within five minutes of each other. This is especially useful for treatments by phone and at a distance, which is another important new development. When a new patient calls Haman on the phone, he asks what the ailment is, where it hurts and whether there are other problems. He also has to check what people have recently eaten and whether women are menstruating, as this precludes certain products. If the patient has no diarrhoea, he sends him/her his *passe-partout* and waits for its arrival before indicating in a subsequent call which product has to be taken first and what the waiting time between products should be. The patient has to call back within four hours and if the problem is abating a little, he instructs the patient what to take for the rest of the week before calling back six days later. If the medicine appears to have had no effect, another product is tried but this evidently takes time. He is now also using this *passe-partout* with patients at home where feedback is quicker. Such a *passe-partout* is not an easy thing to come by and he is proud to have it in his collection. But like everything in medicine, one has to exert oneself to get it or develop it. In his words, 'only a real healer who has genuinely "suffered" has such a *passe-partout*'.

Despite his proliferation of medication, the general principles of Kapsiki medication still hold, also for Haman. As we will see, one particular genus, Crinum (an onion) is the basic resource in the Kapsiki pharmacopoeia, with Cissus quadrangulatus (*hanggedle*) as a minor player. In both cases it is not the species but the individual specimen that is crucial: each individual onion has its own particular curative powers. However, in his hands, not only a specific Crinum or Cissus specimen is important: they always have to be mixed with other herbs, roots, barks, with concoctions of various compositions, and stored in plastic bottles, cups and other paraphernalia from the western system. Though many of his basic medicines include well-known folk medicines, these too are treated, mixed and made unrecognizable in his prescriptions.

Haman has not only built up an expanded pharmacopoeia but also an extensive network. A growing number of Kapsiki have migrated to the cities in the south, like Douala and Yaounde, the national capital, often forming *tontine*-like associations of *Ressortissants de Kapsiki* in those cities, and these people offer a natural clientele for the new healer. Haman is actively seeking clients and advertizes by word of mouth within this group and beyond. This means that he has to perform his diagnosis, prescribe medication and complete all the financial transactions at a distance by phone.

The new technology is part of a process of the commoditization of medication. A new patient has to pay his fees by transferring money by phone. In Cameroon, as in most African countries, money can be transferred by phone either as air time or as a real money tranfer to be cashed in at a telephone booth or with local entrepreneur, thus avoiding the high transaction costs and long handling time of official banks. After he has received the money, Haman sends the products to the PO Box indicated, with each package bearing a different number. When the patient has received the parcel, they call him and have to convince him that they are the patient in question. He asks again about their ailments and checks whether they are the same. He then tells the patient what the numbers stand for and how to use the various products – in what order, at what time, with what drink or food – and explains at some length the way they have to take the medicine. They have to repeat it back to him during the same phone call, and should not write the information down but remember it and not tell anyone else the details. Once healed, they are expected to phone him; and if they do not, he checks up on them by calling them about every two weeks. When they seem to be totally better, he sends no bill but asks them to 'send whatever Allah has provided them with' via Western Union, Moneygram or MTA transfer. But just what they can afford as, in his words, a patient should not become poor because of medical treatment. This is how he has built up a wide circle of patients in southern Cameroon and even in Norway and Paris. All are African and form an extension of the circle of clients for whom he needs a wide range of medications. All of them bring in more clients and remuneration. How much he earns in fees is hard to gauge but traditional medicine is neither free nor very cheap, and the same holds for Haman. He gives the impression that his prices are compatible with those at a dispensary, which after all is his 'relevant other'. This would put the first cost of treatment in the range of FCFA 500 to FCFA 1,500 (€ 0.75 to € 2.20), with the second payment varying according to the severity of the case and the patient's financial position. For local clients, payment in kind is also possible and for many is an attractive option.

Haman calls himself a *tradi-praticien*, (traditional healer) has initiated the *Association pour les tradi-praticiens de Mayo Tsanaga*, realized its membership of the national umbrella organization of traditional healers in Cameroon, and also received recognition from the *Organisation Internationale pour la Santé en Afrique* (OISA). This has not yet led to a standardization of practices or pricing as Haman still dominates the organization and is able to set his own agenda. He himself is positive about this organizational development, more positive than some of his colleagues. A nurse commented that the organization is probably beneficial to Haman. Yet, the organization is a sideline for Haman. Transcending the ethnic border, he has also built up a practice in Mokolo, the regional capital of the *préfecture*. He divides his week between the two places – three days a week in Mokolo and four in Mogode – and spends market day at his residence in Mogode which is across the road from the dispensary. His house in Mokolo is just around the corner from the hospital. The choice of locations indicates his desire for respectability from and cooperation with the Western medical system. The local staff at the Mogode dispensary are less impressed and, when talking about traditional healing (including Haman), complain about the delay in 'real' treatment these healers cause. 'People start with traditional healing and then appear at our door too late' is a frequent complaint among cosmopolitan health workers.

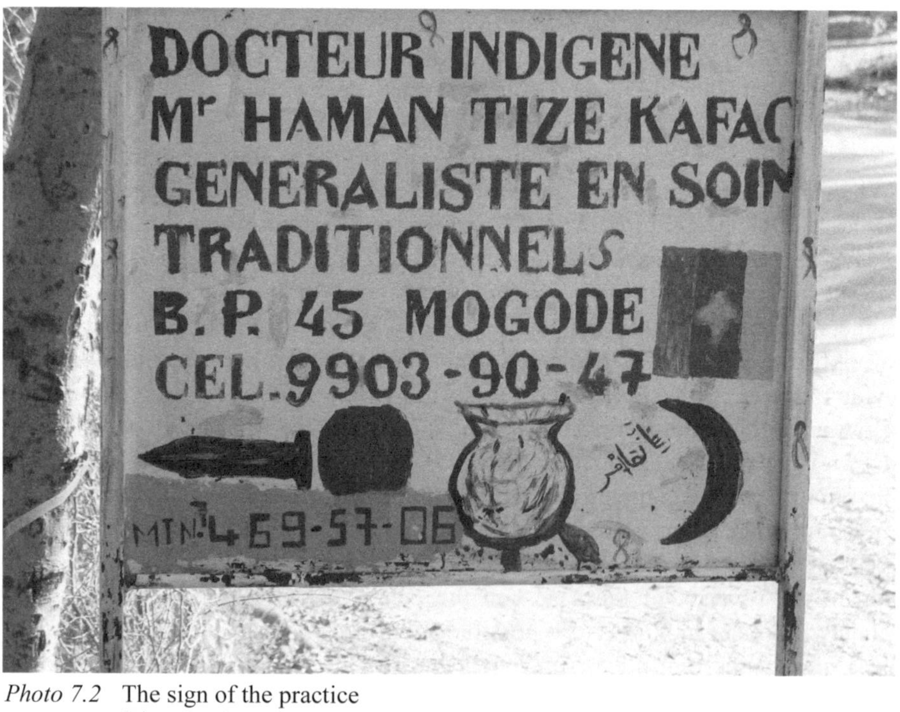

Photo 7.2 The sign of the practice
[Photo: Walter van Beek]

This new healing market does not only offer opportunities for men: new healers can be either men or women. In the past, smiths had a virtual monopoly on healing, with women specializing in children's problems, bloodletting and extracting foreign objects from patients' bodies. Today's female healers are non-smiths and have a wider array of expertise. For my female example I chose Masi Kantsu, who performs divination (with cowries), is *sage femme* and has her own array of medicine. She can deliver the medications as shown in Table 7.1.

Table 7.1 List of medications of Masi Kantsa, female healer and non-smith

Crinum specimen	Other plant species
Beshèngu (against sorcery)	Stomach ache (root)
Poison	Child birth
Gutuli (spirits)	Pregnancy
Protection (+ root + perfume)	
Success at market	

Masi claims to have been initiated into healing by spirits from the bush when she was about fifteen. Her parents are not healers, nor is she of smith descent and for her, being a healer was something completely new. However, she felt she did not have a choice once the spirit (*gutuli*) in the bush offered her instruction. She had to take it. What the spirit actually did was to activate what was already inside her: the whole array of medication was dormant in her brain, she says. But with the help of the spirit she can now discern what the matter is with a patient, and prescribe the appropriate medication. Masi Kwantsu has some issues with Haman, who she knows well, as they live in the same ward. As for the healers' association, she declares never having seen anything of the government money that should have been distributed among local healers through the association.[5] Nor has she seen any other returns from the contributions she had to pay. So she opted out.

What she exemplifies, with Haman, is the marginalization of traditional means of anamnesis (divination). The new healers tend not to rely on external mechanisms of diagnosis but follow a different strategy, inspiration first and then 'treat-and-see'. In fact, most of African cosmopolitan medication is done exactly the same way. As tropical diseases allow little time for lab research and the necessary lab services are not easily available or overly reliable, patients are routinely given a cocktail of medicines against the most probable diseases be-

5 The money never existed in fact, as the Cameroonian government is not in the habit of handing out cash to healers.

fore a full diagnosis is finally made. 'Treat-and-see' is the overall approach to African medication. As Haman's *passe-partout* has shown, diagnosis is made on the basis of self-description by the patient and by phone (!) using general observation, common sense and intuition. African somatic medication does not solve the puzzle (exactly what causes the ailment) but addresses the problem directly (someone is ill and has to get better), so the obvious way is, indeed, to treat and see.

Healing is increasingly becoming an open profession, and part of its appeal is in the remuneration it offers. People generally complain that being ill has become more expensive than ever, as hospitals and native healers have both upped their prices. In fact, healing was never very cheap to start with. Treatment with whatever medicine was also quite costly in the past and usually paid for in kind (chickens or an occasional goat) and only exceptionally as a monetary transaction. It is partly the monetization, thus the commoditization, that gives the impression of rising costs, and partly the expansion of healers' medicinal repertoires. And of course new illnesses are appearing, and so too are new healers.

These new types of healers are operating by expanding the existing market for healing and by creating a new one. Haman and Masi Kwantsu are a new type of medical entrepreneur, moving into the relative vacuum between traditional and cosmopolitan medicine where there is considerable room for manoeuvre due to weak national health institutions. The ideal of a harmonious blending or at least parallel cooperation with traditional systems and Western medicine is still a long way from being realized. And it may not even be possible at all in view of the contrasting epistemologies from which they operate. So, the market model fits the data much better, reflecting the fact that Kapsiki healing too has become part of a wider world, with an array of healing practices in tune with the more complex ramifications of modern society.

Navigating health in Kapsiki society

Any market is set in a cognitive system, in this case one of notions and values about health and healing, so the healing market and medicinal knowledge reflect the core aspects of Kapsiki culture. For the Kapsiki, health is not taken for granted, and is never a matter of fact. Health is not the absence of affliction but rather a fragile and temporary balance between personhood and external threats, a precarious equilibrium in human relations as well as a moment of absence of major external problems. Staying healthy implies a constant activity, as the body is always under siege in some way. This view of the human body also shows in the Kapsiki view of the compound, the larger body (van Beek 2007), as in the protection against evil (van Beek 1994). Evil influences are warded off by the wall of the compound, which can protect against witches, 'night stalkers' (*kelèngu*) and flying evil, so the man-high stone compound wall is the focus of major ritual protection. This is the first line of defence. The second is the skin; with its magical protection aiming at prohibiting intrusion by foreign objects, by making the skin ritually tough and impenetrable by iron objects, fleas loaded with 'evil stuff' and other possible misfortune (van Beek 1994). Like the greater body of the extended family, where harmony and good relations demand continuous work, keeping the body healthy requires constant exertion, while some temporal holes in the fortification are inevitable, as in any siege. This implies that medication serves as both a repository of cultural forms and as a creative space of invention where the old ways are being reinvented, amplified and adapted to new circumstances. This is elaborated on in the final section. Here the focus is on the way patients are orientating themselves to these new forms of marketized healthcare.

The first diagnosis in cases of illness is made at home: 'Is this illness common and will the patient get better without treatment?' The first response is 'wait and see'. 'Normal' diseases do not demand divination or specialist attention but if the affliction needs attention, the response starts from a pool of cultural knowledge about common illnesses and their treatment, the domain of folk medicine. And as most problems do go away without intervention, this often suffices.

Common knowledge about medication tends to focus mainly on plants. During my research, I collected 622 plant specimens,[6] which comprised an estimated 40% of the total Kapsiki botanic system,[7] and established their practical, medicinal or religious uses. Of the 622 randomly collected plants, 84 were medicinal (12.7%). Of these, about half were used for human somatic ailments, nearly 20% for animals (including hunting) and a third were of a more religious nature. Characteristically, the particular plants exhibit external characteristics that resemble the symptoms of the illness – e.g. a pocked calabash is used for smallpox – with 'fever' (usually meaning malaria for the Kapsiki) and diarrhoea being mentioned most often and, after that, ulcers (including oral infections) and skin problems. Leaves and roots are often pounded, boiled and applied as a paste, while tree bark usually involves using the *materia medica*. Some typical examples are:

---

[6] I greatly appreciate the help of Dr A. Leeuwenberg from Wageningen Agricultural University with collecting and determining the plants.

[7] This estimate comes from comparing two samples: the actual plants collected and an independent collection of plant names.

- *wumbela kaja*, Kotschya schweinfurthii (Taub.) Dewit et Duriga is used to treat diarrhoea and intestinal worms. The roots and/or bark are pounded, cooked and the infusion is drunk.
- *rhwè mezeke*, Haumaniastrum galeopsofilium, (Bak) Duvign. et Planch is used against itching. A paste of ground leaves is applied to the itchy spot.
- *manda kwadeva*, Plumbago zeylanica L. medicine is hung around the neck of a child to prevent stomach ache and inflammation of joints.
- *lerhwu*, Nauclea latifolia, L. is a well-known medicine that is used to treat hepatitis (but not the only one, see below)

Examples of the more magical-religious medicines are given below. In principle, the Kapsiki do not make a distinction between somatic and non-somatic medicines: they are all known as *rhwè* (medicine). After the wait-and-see period, the first line of medication is usually home treatment. Fever, itching, diarrhoea and constipation (the latter is hugely feared in large parts of Africa) are all treated with self-medication or folk medicine. As the main focus is on the symptoms, the illness is in fact defined as the symptom.

One peculiar element in the Kapsiki's pharmacopoeia is that they tend to link not only a plant species but even a specimen to one affliction, as mentioned

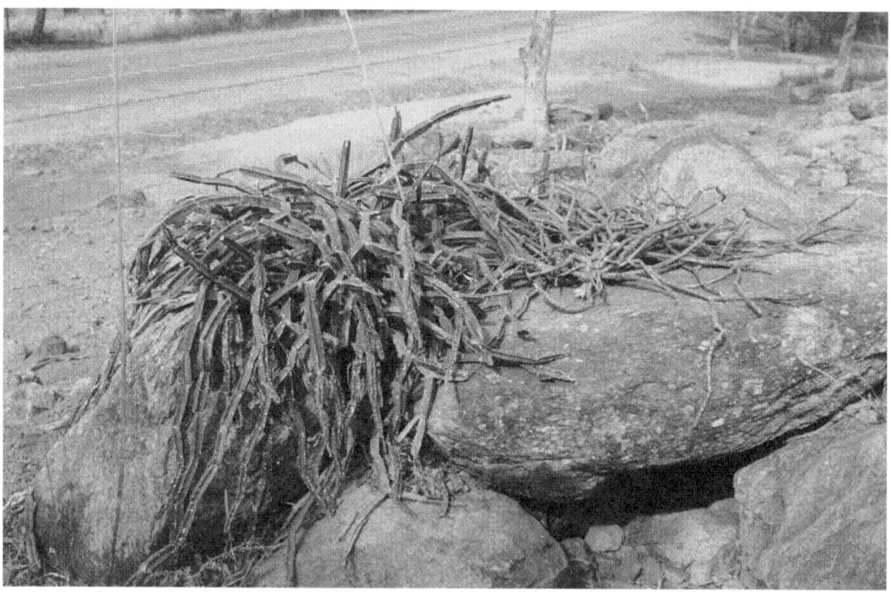

Photo 7.3 Cissus quandrangularis along the roadside
[Photo: Walter van Beek]

above. The most important medicines come from two plant species: *Crinum*[8] and *Cissus quandrangularis*.[9]

Cissus (*hanggedle* in Kapsiki) has a wide symbolic meaning but Crinum (*hwèbè* in Kapsiki) is the most important species medicinally. In principle, any of these native onion variants and often individual specimens of *hwèbè* offer medication against a specific affliction: each *Crinum* plant has its own illness to heal. Well-known illnesses, like 'fever', have more than one medicine. For example, four plants are used to fight malaria, though the *Crinum* medicine is deemed the strongest. Often the specific aim of the onion depends on its surface characteristics: a *Crinum* against smallpox is usually an onion with brown spots on its leaves. This homology between symptom and medicine is normal in Africa (Reynolds-Whyte 1996: 234) and medicine for *damara* (smallpox) has to be drunk from a calabash with *kwetlekwe damara*. As in many parts of Africa, smallpox is still considered a threat, even if it has been eradicated medically. But we are in specialist territory now. For other medicinal plants than the two mentioned, the relationship is between a specific illness and a specific species. Knowledge about medicines against scabies, intestinal parasites and hepatitis are quite widely known. The following example shows that symptom homology is often part of the medication, plus the central medicine that bears no symbolic association, illustrating the fact that the Kapsiki make no distinction between somatic and religious medicine.

> In case of hepatitis, take the bark of the *ndeweva vèra* (Ziziphus mauritiana) and boil it with lemon and acacia leaves for two hours. Two calabashes have to be filled with the bitter potion. The patient should drink from one in the morning and from the second in the afternoon for four days. They will then recover without further medication. (A prescription from Kweji Hake, a non-smith healer).

In this first line of health defence, it is the individual who is in charge, who tries to apply his/her own knowledge and searches for additional information on plants among kinsmen and friends, trying to navigate the pool of knowledge in the village. However, if the illness perseveres or seems unfamiliar, there are two ways of accruing more knowledge. The question is first to what domain the affliction belongs, to one treated at the dispensary or not. In the Kapsiki area, the first dispensary came with the Roman Catholic mission at Sir in the late 1960s, and others followed later, such as the one in Mogode. So these data on traditional medicine are set in a context of the availability of Western medication, usually at the level of nurses. Infected wounds, fever (malaria), diarrhoea and vomiting among children are first treated by self-medication but

---

8 The Crinum species we collected were all sterile.

9 The latter is widely used as a ritual, symbolic and medicinal plant in the whole Mandara area.

people quickly turn to the dispensary if there is one nearby. For most, this involves a journey, an overnight stay and thus some expense, which is the major parameter of therapy choice elsewhere in Africa as well (Janzen 1994). There is a hospital in Mokolo, some 60 km from most Kapsiki villages but again transport is never easy. Here we follow the health navigation within afflictions that are defined as being beyond ta dispensary's scope. The new healers define their expertise as overlapping or complementing cosmopolitan medicne but the more traditional healers, who are often blacksmiths, make a more rigid distinction between ' dispensary illnesses' and the ailments they themselves can address.

Some ailments that are deemed beyond the reach of a dispensary are stubborn and do not disappear quickly. The patient then has to choose between two pathways: looking for a more comprehensive diagnosis, a real historical anamnesis, or consulting a specialist healer within Kapsiki society. The first pathway is divination to acquire deeper knowledge of what is behind the somatic symptoms, which demands a personal history of the patient's relations.[10] The Kapsiki know various ways of divination – with a crab, stones, cowries or even with a tweaking bird (van Beek forthcoming) – and they all arrive at conclusions that define the illness as non-somatic but relational.[11] Then a series of smaller or larger sacrifices and offerings is prescribed to redress the problem. In effect, the curative aspects in divination are precisely in bringing interpersonal problems out into the open and acting on them.[12] Here I restrict myself to the second pathway, namely the transition from folk medicine to expert treatment.

Traditional healers and the market for medicine

Most medications stem from blacksmiths (*rerhè*), who form a separate category in Kapsiki society. This group, endogamous and clearly distinguished, has a lower but ambivalent status. In the eyes of non-smiths (*melimu*), blacksmiths are dirty (van Beek 1992), dangerous and full of mischief, but they know about occult matters, divination, magic and medicine. While considered the 'children of the village', they are also dangerous and, not being fully adult, are also unpredictable. Above all, they are the intermediaries between the ordinary people and the supernatural world. For a smith, his expertise in healing and the revenues accruing from it balance out his lower social status and the gentle disdain that other Kapsiki treat him with.

This combination of lower status and medicinal knowledge makes it possible for the patient to separate the expertise of the specialist and the knowledge of the technician and provides him leeway in navigating healing. As the social

10 For an in-depth treatment of this question, see Winkelman & Peek (2004).

11 Cf. Erdtsieck (2003) and van Dijk, Reis & Spierenburg (2000).

12 For an analysis of the internal dynamics of divination systems, see Jansen (2009).

superior of the specialist, the client or patient can cherish his/her independence from the specialist and feel free to reinterpret the lack of confirmation along the fault lines of society: 'Of course, the smith has said so because he is a smith (*rerhè*), not because it is the truth'. If predictions pan out, the technique produces the right knowledge and the belief is justified, but if they do not materialize, the smith is as irresponsible as any smith, and is out for his own gain.

The smith's low status may serve him well in harmonizing his role as healer with that of a fellow villager but it does hamper his entry into the new healing market to some extent. This low status is not only relevant within Kapsiki society but also translates into a network of lower-ranked individuals outside the group's area. Smiths are not the first to take advantage of the new opportunities and markets but are followers rather than leaders. On the other hand, they are trying to consolidate their position as healers within the community, addressing new afflictions and personal problems. So in a way, they are at a disadvantage from having taken an early lead.

Some afflictions that persist have a clear somatic aspect and demand a smith's specialist knowledge. It is not a deeper insight into relations but a different kind of knowledge that is needed, with more information about pharmacopeia, especially about combinations of medicines. Though a patient may attempt to navigate a higher level of knowledge once this pathway of healing has been chosen, his navigational freedom eventually becomes less. The first decision is about which specialist to consult, which blacksmith or other healer. Every traditional healer has a limited set of medicines, meaning too that s/he can cure a limited number of illnesses. So the 'therapy group' (Janzen 1994) decides which healer in their personal network could address these particular symptoms. Starting in their immediate vicinity, they contact one they trust and wait to see if he appears capable of diagnosing and treating the affliction. Though each healer has a limited array of medicines, they tend to first assess whether the illness falls within their competence. Only if treatment fails do they refer the patient to more specialized healers. Actually, most healers are quite clear about what they are able to treat and most of their medicines are related to general symptoms like 'malaria' (fever) or diarrhoea.

Some gender divisions prevail: female smiths specialize in medicines for children and in removing foreign objects from a patient's body (*kwantedewushi*: 'digging out things'). The Kapsiki have their own version of this almost-global technique and some ailments are interpreted as foreign elements that have entered the body, often through sorcery. Though few ailments are interpreted this way in Kapsiki aetiology, some are, especially with children.

Kwada,[13] a female smith, was treating a young boy for such an affliction: he was thin and had a swollen abdomen so her diagnosis was 'little frogs' (*kwankwèrèkwè*: the name is onomatopoeic) that had entered his body via his feet and had amassed in his stomach. So she had to take them out. With the boy kneeling before her and a large bowl of water between her feet, she rubbed his stomach vigorously with some special leaves (also called *kwanteÞewhus*hi, as well as *mezevezeve*[14]) and suddenly showed him – and me! – a little frog. She put the frog in the bowl, seemed to pound it with a stick, and rubbed again. Over the course of an hour she 'extracted' some twenty frogs from his stomach. Afterwards, she gently reproached me. When I had first contacted her, she sensed my doubts but now 'I had seen it with my own eyes'. Yes, I indeed had seen it, and had even taken pictures. In fact, I had wrestled with the Western idea that I should take the boy to the hospital. I did not, in the end. The boy had treatment for two weeks and got better.

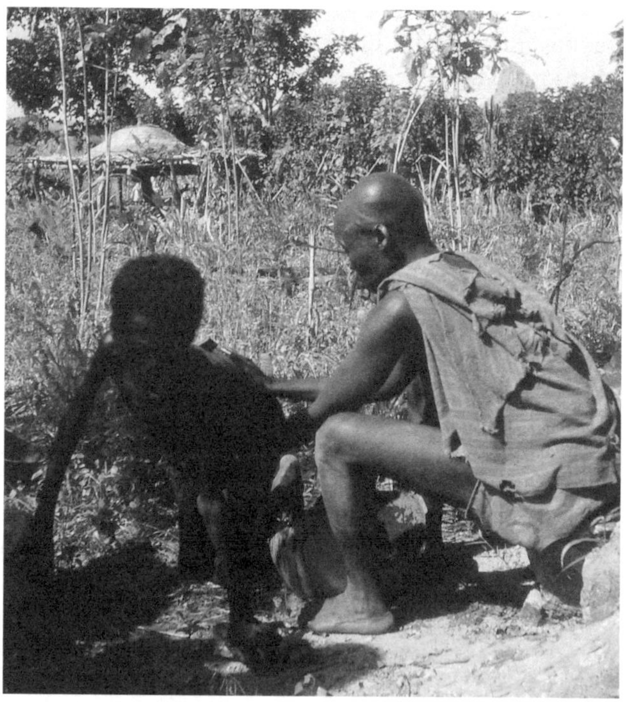

Photo 7.4 Kwada 'extracting frogs' from the boy's stomach [Photo: Walter van Beek]

13 The names of all concerned have been changed.

14 Probably Indigofera dendroides Jacq., (Papillionaceae) and Cassyta filiformis L., (Lauraceae).

As an example of a specialist treatment, the treatment of spirit possession may serve, an affliction the Kapsiki define as an illness and not as direct communication with the spirit world. As with persistent somatic afflictions, the treatment becomes much more complicated and demands the expert knowledge of a true specialist:

> At six in the morning, the healer cuts some leaves of *peha gutuli*, a wild aloe species, at noon some *zewe gutuli* (a wild grass) and at sunset some black groundnuts. He mixes this in the dark and rubs the mixture over his hands until they stink. While rubbing, he explains the medicine and the aim of the operation, who is ill and what should happen. The possessed perceives the healer coming from afar, 'even through walls', and tries to escape. His kinsmen have to tie him up. Then the healer rubs his hands over the forehead, nose, mouth and eyes of the patient who falls asleep. The healer carves two incisions on the patient's forehead with his knife, two on each shoulder, each hand and foot, and finally rubs a special Crinum (*hwèbè gutuli*) into the wounds. The next day the patient is better.

In this case, the navigation by the patient is restricted and his 'therapy group' – in this case his family – does the navigation for him. One reason for the restricted options for the patient and his group is the notion of secrecy in the form of private expert information. The healer has specific non-shared knowledge at three levels at his disposal. The first depends on the insistence on the specimen level in Crinum and Cissus (*hwèbè* and *hanggedle*): everybody knows these plants are medicinal but only the specialist knows which particular disease each of the individual plants serve. Some surface features of the plant may offer a hint but never more than that. What is kept secret is the exact nature of each individual plant plus the words that should be spoken. Non-healers have one or two onions for general purposes but specialists have many different specific ones and only they know the purpose of each.

Another level of specialist knowledge resides in additional knowledge about the common stock of medicinal plants. Basing themselves on the general knowledge, they 'just know better':

> In the case of the *lerhwu* (medicine against hepatitis), a healer confided that this could also serve for another problem: Anyone who has drunk poison and could not vomit should drink a potion of crushed *lerhwu* roots in order to induce vomiting after five days. Or, for the *mezeke* mentioned above, the same healer stated that this would be better if used with *nyi cènè* (mahogany oil) and ochre.

The third level is the array of different plants and mixes of medicinal plants that are the most efficacious, and here each healer has his specific prescription. This somatic way of healing not only has more complex prescriptions but also separates the patient from the specialist. No longer are they kinsmen or village members, and no longer has the patient any idea what the medication is made of. This has to do with secrecy, as the real specialists are extremely secretive about their knowledge, but also with the danger inherent in healing, not only for the patient but also for the healer. A serious illness is a force in itself, and healing means that the illness has to go elsewhere. To paraphrase Mary Douglas: 'Illness is evil out of place'. Just as in Kapsiki sacrifices, evil is chased from the compound to the potential detriment of neighbours.[15] Healing one patient implies risk for a bystander and, above all, for the specialist. So this level of knowledge can become dangerous and one has to attain the status of healer first before venturing into such a hazardous field. During treatment, the healer communicates with the illness itself, addressing it as a person. Some illnesses, especially smallpox, are considered a personage, dangerous and wild yet approachable, but only by someone who has the complete knowledge. A serious illness is somebody else, dangerous and erratic but with a distinct identity, someone the healer has to 'know'. So the real specialist keeps his distance from his patients.

A final reason for distance is the performance character of some of the healing, especially treatment dealing with the most persistent kind. This is crucial in many Central African afflictions (Janzen 1994; Reynolds-Whyte 1996) but, even for the privacy-oriented Kapsiki, a performance can be an additional means in the healing process.

> For a tenacious case of possession, Miyi, the most famous of all blacksmith healers in the region, is called. When he arrives, the neighbours flock to the hut where the patient, Tizhè, is sitting on the floor tied with ropes and screaming incomprehensibly. Miyi has Tizhè's head shaven and makes some room around the patient. From his leather document case, he selects a few small packages of medicine and burns some in front of and behind the patient. He circles the smoking stuff around the patient's head, enveloping Tizhé in a cloud of smoke. Other mixtures of medicine are lighted all around his body, medicine is smeared on his nose and mouth, and by now Tizhè has become calm. His kinsmen and neighbours, by now quite a crowd, look on in awe at the proceedings; even those who are healers themselves cannot guess what Miyi used for this session. Meanwhile, Miyi works quickly, efficiently and with determination, allowing the crowd full view of the proceedings. After half an hour, the patient is asleep and everybody is convinced that Tizhè is healed. Not Miyi, though, not the healer. He leaves some follow-up medication with the family, warning them that the affliction may return.
>
> Miyi's very professional performance made a huge impression and even though Tizhè suffered a relapse later, public admiration was not eroded. In fact, the return of the 'possession', which Miyi had feared, meant that the diagnosis had to be changed. It was not the *gutuli* (bush spirits) but a Fulbe marabout that was the cause of the problem. So Miyi advised writing a letter to the marabout of a nearby Fulbe pastoral group to ask him to heal Tizhè. And so Tizhè got rid of his 'possession' in the end.

[15] See van Beek (1994).

Trust and insecurity, or uncertainty, operate together in the healing process. Insecurity and uncertainty are fundamental aspects of life and trust *in* the specialist – which is greater than the trust *of* the specialist – can make any insecurity bearable. And a good performance helps too, including a show of certainty from the healer. Combined with the notion of the body as a fortress under siege, a show of confidence can have a peculiar result. People take medicines that give them a limited certainty of healing but the healing is nevertheless considered to be immediate. The medicine works instantly and is deemed to instantly repair the hole in the body's defence. No further medication is thus needed. When taking antibiotics, patients tend not to complete the five-day cure and after the first injection they consider their body healed. After being bitten by a poisonous snake, a famous healer and a personal friend of mine just had the first injection at the dispensary and then sold the rest. He died a week later.

In some *rhwè* applications that are not specifically aimed at healing, performance becomes a purpose in itself. Socially inferior blacksmiths in particular may boast their prowess in the field of *rhwè*. When a blacksmith is buried, for instance, they whole group flaunts its *rhwè*, in the public dance with the corpse. No non-smith will dare to mix with them, afraid of the power of the publicly displayed 'medicine'. Even beyond the ritual context, some specialisst may boast their prowess, at least verbally.

> A healer once told that he took his 'stuff' to the market in the next village during the dry season. When he sat down with his vials and stick, leaves suddenly appeared on the empty branches of the tree. Everybody was scared, he told us, running to and fro, shouting and pointing. The women were afraid to bring him beer and had to be forced to do so. When he stood up, all the leaves disappeared. The people in the village gave him money and chickens and implored him not to come back.

Performance separates the specialist from his patient and from the audience, and makes a rigid distinction between knowledge and ignorance. Language becomes less important, knowledge about the variety of medications for the treatment all the more so.

Not only does the specialist put a distance between himself and the 'case' but the patient does so too, for several reasons. First, healing, as we have seen, involves certain risks. Not only has the affliction to move elsewhere, the Kapsiki hold that any intervention in the normal course of life has inherent danger. Each attempt to change things with *rhwè* runs risks and costs money, and if one relies on these means, one has to be prepared to deal with all the side effects. A little knowledge and a partial application are dangerous. The following is a complex example of such a chain of side effects:

> Marriage is one of the focal points of Kapsiki society. Women tend to leave a marriage easily and quickly, and men are constantly trying to induce women to stay with them. Medicine, of course, is available. A complicated prescription[16] involves hiding several plants and objects in the small pillow a woman uses to carry things on her head. Then she will follow the man to his compound but the side effect is that she will not stay long. Another *rhwè* has to guarantee her stay, binding her to the house. But then the other women will be jealous. This problem can be helped but then she will be infertile. Again, medicine is at hand but any children, when they grow up, will not want to leave the compound. A daughter would turn down any suitors unless another *rhwè* sets her free. A son will look for a woman only after another small ritual. And then he has to marry a girl first, but not a runaway bride, as they are more available.

One wonders about the timeline in this long series of medication. In theory, this would tie a client to the healer for a generation, which would mean they would both have to stay in one place and alive, which is reminiscent of the treatment received and given. This is asking a lot of fate and memory, so much so in fact that in all probability the complete package of this kind of medicine is seldom actually given. So the prescription, though given to me in all privacy by an old healer who was a good friend, has to be more discourse than practice, a discourse that establishes the healer as a full-blown specialist and the client as a dependent. The purpose of such a discourse is to establish authority and, in the end, to attract clients for different treatments.

Anyway, the prescription shows that there is a notion of a natural course of events and of the risks of intervention in it, and that non-specialists should stay out of this realm. The sheer complexity of the medication sequences and the risks involved induce the patient, in fact any non-specialist, to profess ignorance. To win trust, the patient has to construct his own ignorance; to let the specialist be an authoritative guide in the dark maze of medication so that some trust can be salvaged despite the fundamental insecurity. Thus, all parties – the specialist, the patient and the therapy support group of kinsmen – are interested in the 'creation of ignorance' (Hobart 1993). The unequal division of expertise is productive in the healing process and, as such, is a more or less conscious choice on the part of the patient. Also among the Kapsiki, healers are the worst patients.

Transmission and invention of medicinal knowledge: Elements for a medical market

How is medical knowledge actually transmitted? In principle, smiths state that this is done between kinsmen, usually father and son, or father and grandson,

[16] For a more detailed description, see van Beek (forthcoming: Chapter 7).

with the mother's brother often playing an important role as well. Some elements are clearly transmitted between kinsmen and kinswomen, the most obvious being treatments that are mainly technical. One instance is bloodletting, which is indeed transmitted from mother to daughter, among blacksmiths.

More cognitive elements are less clearly transmitted. Young smiths always claim that their (grand) fathers have told them everything. However, talking with the older generation, I got the impression that they were reticent about imparting their knowledge and judging the youngsters too immature for the accumulated knowledge. Recent research indicates that the process of preparing one's son or grandson for the arena of healing might be even more complicated and that there is hardly any transmission of actual knowledge. This sounds strange in the field of traditional medicine, as it seriously questions the very notion of tradition. My thesis here on the transmission of specialist knowledge is that the content of medicinal plants or means is not transmitted. Instead, it is reconstructed by each generation. What is transmitted is the way to construct this knowledge, the pathways and how to find out what plant does what and what mixtures are effective. My data here are longitudinal as I was able to collect the medicinal lists of different generations within the same family due to

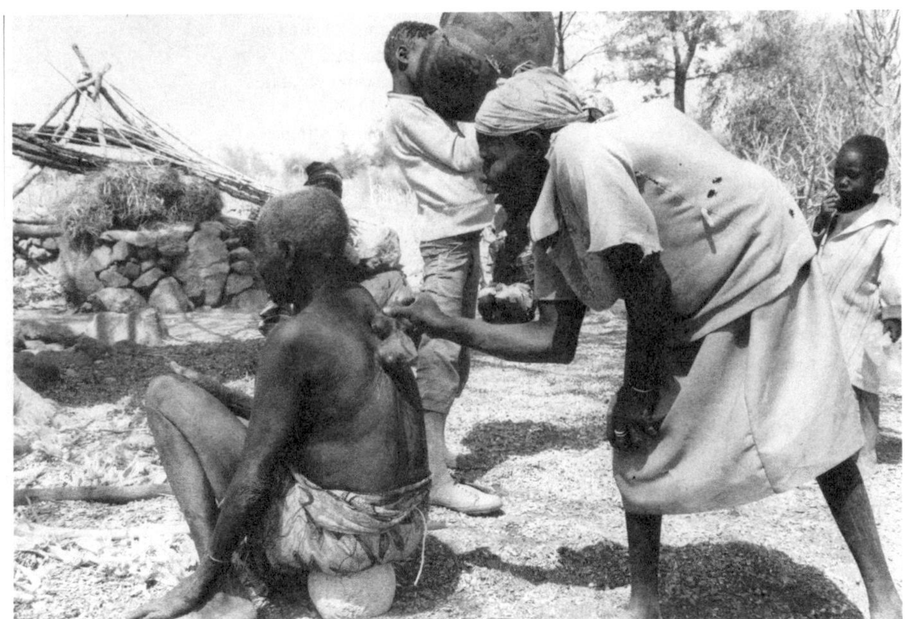

Photo 7.5 Bloodletting by a smith woman
[Photo: Walter van Beek]

my long involvement with the Kapsiki. Tables 7.2 and 7.3 list the medicines of the chief smith in 1973 and his grandson's list in 2008.

The notion is that knowledge in a traditional society is handed down through the generations, and that private knowledge of medicine should 'run in the family'. After all, that is what tradition is about: handing over the accumulated wisdom of the past from the ancestors to the present. But that is not at all what these lists show as they hardly match.

To be the same, two medicines should have identical goals and come from the same plant, so they would at least be in the same column. Some medicines do appear to be the same, i.e. against sorcery (*beshèngu*), for a too rapid successive pregnancy, i.e. a pregnancy immediately following a birth without menstruation in between (*matini* in Kapsiki, a pregnancy with no prior menstruation), and against worms/intestinal parasites. The medicine against curses (*bedlam*) is on both but in clearly different ways. All other medicines are different. So of the 26 medicines Gwarda had, his grandson only inherited possibly two – 'possibly' because even if both used Crinum against sorcery, it is dubious

Table 7.2 Chief Smith Gwarda's medicine list, 1973

Crinum specimen	Cissus specimen	Other plant species	Other means
Beshèngu	Witches	Stomach ache (child)	
Sekwa (guilt magic)	Epidemic	Snake bite	
Childbirth		Intestinal parasites	
Too rapid pregnancy		Senility	
Headache		Scorpion sting	
Stomach ache		Cold	
Travelling abroad		Foot infection	
Threshing sorghum		Hepatitis	
Prevention of revenge magic			
Against poison			
Against *bedla*, curse			
Leprosy			
Lack of breast nilk			
Toothache			
Wounds			
Smallpox			

Table 7.3 Medicine list of Gwarda's grandson, Maitre Kwada, 2008

Crinum specimen	Cissus specimen	Other plant species	Other means
Beshèngu		Worms (tree bark)	*Gutuli* (stone)
Adultery (wife)		Bilharzias (mix)	Miscarriage (2)
Too rapid pregnancy		Against curse	Weight loss of child (lizard)

whether they will be the same specimens; in fact, viewing the age of individual plants, this is highly improbable. Crinum specimens do not last very long, and bulbs seldom flower. Most are found in the bush, dug up and planted at home, so transmission of a lasting line of Crinum medicines is very unlikely.

Gwarda's list is much longer but he was older at the time and a long-established chief smith who people depended on for treatment. The question is whether this partial transmission of knowledge is the rule or an exception, or whether it can be seen as a sign of erosion of the smith's function as a medicine man. For the latter, the list can be compared with that of Dzule, a smith of the same generation (Table 7.4).

Table 7.4 Dzule's medicine list, 2008

Crinum specimen	Cissus specimen	Other plant species
Beshèngu	Witches	Arthritis
Poison		How to steal unnoticed
Epidemic		Headache
Chickenpox (+ other plant)		Childbirth
Snake bite		Miscarriage
		Gutuli spirits

Dzule's list seems to overlap most with Gwarda's, even if he is neither his descendant nor close kin, but similar ailments are treated with different means, like epidemics, snake bites, headaches, poisoning and childbirth. Everyone has medicine to combat sorcery (*beshèngu*) though the actual medicines may well differ. However the younger generation also has the means to fight bush spirits (*gutuli*) which Gwarda does not have. Protection against sorcery has always be a subject of discussion but the notion of dangerous bush spirits is quite recent and is probably an influence of Christianity. Formerly, *gutuli* were more or less equated with God (*shala*) but Christianization turned them into small, black demons (van Beek 2007), so protective medicine is called for. The same was seen in the case of Masi, the new female healer, whose list of medication looks similar to the ones cited here. As Dzule is from the generation between Gwarda and Maître Kwada, the common elements with Gwarda might well stem from a larger overlap in definition of what the greatest threat to health is.

Drawing conclusions from these lists is not easy but some trends run parallel to processes already mentioned in Kapsiki ethnomedicine. The first is that of secrecy, keeping relevant information very close to one's chest, even regarding kinsmen. Healers stress the fact that getting the information involves suffering, and sometimes money, but always their own research and trying out hunches. What is important, our new healer Haman explained, is to look carefully at what wild animals eat and, in particular, what they spurn. Then one takes that plant and shows it to someone who knows, and one produces new medicinal knowledge. Another issue is the medicine the smiths in question are still looking for. Each has a short list of medicines they hope to find. For Dzule, this was the medicine for flying, but he knew nobody who had one.[17]

These tales and the lists suggest that specialist knowledge is not transmitted but reinvented by each generation. This kind of secret knowledge is thus produced, not reproduced. Traditional expert systems seem to have little history and what is traditional about them is the process of constructing the knowledge, more than the knowledge content itself. So for private knowledge, tradition has no content, only method. It should be remembered that even if the list shows medication against the same affliction, the medicine itself might well be different, a different Crinum specimen for instance. What is traditional is the fact that Maitre Kwada explicitly states that 'all his medicines came from Gwarda'; although in actual fact, they did not but his grandfather did teach him how to construct the knowledge. This is what tradition often amounts to: not the transmission of knowledge but the way to reinvent knowledge. The notion of tradition itself serves as an invocation of authority: invoking the past gives credence and weight to one's construction of knowledge, so this use of tradition is more an *argumentum ad autoritatem*, a way to load one's knowledge with authority than its actual direct transmission.[18]

Conclusion

It is the mechanism of constructing knowledge in medicinal knowledge that seems to be the stable factor. Expert (traditional) knowledge in itself is not transmitted and it is only ways to acquire such information that are handed over. One important reason for this is secrecy and the wish to keep one's knowledge to oneself, a tendency that fits well with Kapsiki culture, but is in fact much more general. Bellman (1984) revealed how, anthropologically, secrets can be semantically empty, especially collective secrets. For instance, initiation secrets are often public knowledge that one is not allowed to talk about, so instruction

[17] Except, of course, the *nasara* (white people).

[18] A similar observation is made by Thornton (2009: 29) about South African *sangomas*, the 'traditional healers' who are not very traditional, certainly not in the content of their knowledge or their transmission of knowledge. A more fundamental critique on the relationship of tradition and truth is offered by Boyer (1990: 79 ff.) who treats the discourse on tradition as 'customized speech', which may lack meaning because it is never intended to have any meaning other than the ritualization of knowledge.

during initiation teaches initiates what they already know and can now talk about amongst themselves.

> For instance, at the end of their initiation, Kapsiki initiates (*gwela*) are shown the traces of the old habitats in the mountain area and are told the story of the history of the village. They already know this tale but have never been told it at the 'proper' spot. The discourse is context-dependent. Among the Dogon, the great secret is that masks are normal men who have dressed themselves as a 'mask'. At least *vis-à-vis* the women this is considered a secret, but of course no Dogon woman is ever fooled as they know exactly who is dancing with what mask, and how well their sons are performing. The discourse on masks, however, is male territory. And when the bull roarer is whirled at a Dogon funeral, it is the voice of the 'big mask' (*èmna na*) for the women and the small boys. Young boys will soon learn that they are next in line to whirl the device, but should never tell their women how it is done.

So secrecy, like tradition, is mainly a discourse and it is often about discourses. These public secrets serve to define authority, structure intra-group relations and construct borders with the outside.

The social dynamics of private secrets, however, are quite different. Whereas public secrets are easily transmitted and even get special attention in cultural transmissions such as initiation, private ones are not. Throughout Africa, expert knowledge on healing is highly personal, the content secret and ways of application secluded from prying eyes. It is this very secrecy that precludes transmission. One reason for this secrecy is in the construction of this kind of knowledge itself as it demands the direct involvement of the healer with his *materia medica*, a personal link that is often expressed in terms of suffering. Expert knowledge is thus private by definition. The same holds for the application of this same knowledge in healing practices, though not all healers need to have suffered from the diseases they address themselves (the phenomenon of the 'wounded healer') but a healer does have to build up a personal acquaintance with the affliction somehow. The Kapsiki definition of some illnesses in terms of supernatural entities does necessitate such a personalized approach.

So the non-transmission of knowledge content points the way to how experts should gain knowledge. This also implies that knowledge, though highly adaptive, is not cumulative and that knowledge is not subject to the selective pressures of application and transmission and no longer carries the traditional guarantee of time-tested methods, as they have neither the time nor the mechanism to be part of any serious trial. Of course, specialists will glean whether their *rhwè* works but the absence of interpersonal testable anamnesis precludes much of the testing. And anyway both the complex mix of medicine and the treat-and-see methods of healing make an evaluation of specific medicines very difficult. Indigenous knowledge systems often focus on specialists and their reclusive information but my data point the other way. If any integration between Western and indigenous medication is to be reached, it should not be with specialists' information, but with general folk medicine, with the kind of information that is shared and transmitted and thus is open for testing over the generations. The generalized cultural information on medicinal plants and practices seems a better partner to such an enterprise than the indigenous specialists who establish much of their authority on secrets that are elusive and ephemeral.

Finally, the market. Medicinal knowledge is power as well as money. Clearly these kinds of private secrets are also encouraged by the very market forces that we started out with. Healing in Africa, as in the case of the Kapsiki, has always been a lucrative business in terms of remuneration and prestige, and the coming of Western medication and the appearance of new healers have increased both the prestige and the money. The new healers, just like the old ones, are protecting their monopoly, not through certification (which is the Western way) but by the individualization of knowledge. In fact, most of the information I collected on blacksmiths' medicine lists was given to me in the last month of my first field stay. Not only did this demand considerable trust before they consented to do so but they also delayed doing so until a time when I could not be of any competition to them. I was leaving so their knowledge could be shared without me being able to assist another healer in the village.

Medicine tends to be a closed shop, and not only in Africa. In the past Kapsiki blacksmiths guarded their healing monopoly very carefully and dominated divination and the making of poison (for arrows) and magic. They also had an absolute monopoly on funerals, which was embedded in their complete control of all metal work. The fact that their endogamous group was ranked lower than non-smiths is surprising, but works well in healing.[19] The phenomenon of the blacksmith healer and general specialist is not unique to the Kapsiki,[20] as similar patterns can be found throughout West Africa. The dynamics of the smiths' dominance are clear as well. The medicinal market is opening up, with non-smiths breaking in and taking over the area between Western and traditional forms of medicine, creating new ways of addressing health problems. They use new technologies and modern forms of organization yet remain rooted in their local cultures by translating the new challenges of life and the navigational hazards into existing interpretative frameworks. And even more crucially, they are using the same mechanisms of knowledge production as their blacksmith predecessors. The old professionals are making way for new professionals,[21] but some of the structures of the medical field still remain.

19 Author's own fieldwork.
20 See Schmitz-Cliever (1979) for an overview.

References

Bellman, B.L. (1984), *The language of secrecy: Symbols & metaphors in Poro ritual.* New Brunswick, NJ: Rutgers University Press.

Boyer, P. (1990), *Tradition as truth and communication. A cognitive description of traditional discourse.* Cambridge: Cambridge University Press.

Erdtsieck, J. (2003), *In the spirit of Uganga: Inspired healing and leadership in Tanzania.* Amsterdam: AGIDS.

Hobart, M., ed., (1993), *An anthropological critique of development; The growth of ignorance*, pp. 44-60, London: Routledge.

Jansen, J.A.M.M. (2009), Framing divination: A Mande divination expert and the occult economy. *Africa* 79(1): 110-127.

Janzen, J. (1994), The drums of affliction: Real phenomenon or scholarly chimera? In: T. Blakely, W.E.A. van Beek & D.L. Thomson, eds, *African religion: Experience and expression*, pp. 165-190. London: James Currey.

Last, M. (1986), *The professionalisation of African medicine.* Manchester: IAI & Manchester University Press.

Reynolds Whyte, S. (1996), *Questioning misfortune. The pragmatics of uncertainty in eastern Uganda.* Cambridge: Cambridge University Press.

Schmitz-Cliever, G. (1979), *Schmiede in Westafrika. Ihre soziale Stellung in traditionellen Gesellschaften.* Munich: Klaus Renner.

Thornton, R. (2009), The transmission of knowledge in South African traditional healing. *Africa* 79(1): 17-34.

van Beek, W.E.A. (1992), The dirty smith; smell as a social frontier among the Kapsiki/Higi of north Cameroon and north-eastern Nigeria. *Africa* 2(1): 38-58.

van Beek, W.E.A. (1994), The innocent sorcerer; coping with evil in two African societies, Kapsiki and Dogon. In: T. Blakely, W.E.A. van Beek & D.L. Thomson (eds), *African religion: Experience and expression*, pp. 196-228. London: James Currey.

van Beek, W.E.A. (2006),'Een slaaf voor een kalebas'. De stuiptrekkingen van de slavenjachten in Adamawa (Noordoost Nigeria & Noord-Kameroen), In: K. Koonings, ed., *Antropologie en Afro-Amerika als passie en professie. Opstellen aangeboden aan Wim Hoogbergen*, , pp. 73-121. Maastricht: Shaker.

van Beek, W.E.A. (2007), Agency in Kapsiki religion: A comparative approach. In: M. de Bruijn, R. van Dijk & J-B. Gewald, eds, *Strength beyond structure. Social and historical trajectories of agency in Africa*, pp. 114-143. Leiden: Brill.

van Beek, W.E.A. (2010), Crab divination among the Kapsiki of north Cameroon. In: P. Peek & W.E.A. van Beek, eds, *Reviewing reality dynamics of African divination.* In press.

van Beek, W.E.A. (forthcoming), *The Kapsiki blacksmith.* Bloomington: Indiana University Press.

van Dijk, R., R. Reijs & M. Spierenburg, eds, (2000), *The quest for fruition through Ngoma: Political aspects of healing in Southern Africa.* London: Currey.

Vincent, J-F. (1991), *Princes montagnards du Nord-Cameroun. Les Mofou-Diamaré et le pouvoir politique.* Paris: Harmattan.

[21] On professionalization, see Last (1986).

Winkelman, M. & Ph. Peek, eds, (2004), *Divination and healing. Potent vision*. Tucson: University of Arizona Press.

8

The commodification of misery: Markets for healing, markets for sickness

Nadine Beckmann

The opening up of the healthcare sector to privatisation in Zanzibar has led to a process of marketization that captures both biomedical and non-biomedical forms of healing. The emerging market for health has created opportunities for some but is increasingly closing off routes for treatment for those who cannot afford the rising costs. This shift in focus from healthcare provision to profit-making, it is argued, promotes emotional distancing and the disintegration of care relationships that used to be structured by moral responsibilities. The transgressive processes of commodification have become particularly visible in the global 'fight against HIV/AIDS', where an industry is emerging in which the very state of 'being sick' can become a commodity. Feeding donors' demands for participation in a rights-based agenda of 'making the voices of the afflicted heard', HIV-positive people are joining the bottom rung of the AIDS industry. This commodification of people's misery in the form of treatment testimonies and illness narratives is the epitome of marketization in a world in which an infected body assumes a market value and suffering becomes a way of surviving.

Introduction

The last decades have seen the large-scale ideological and financial promotion of biomedical rationality and an increasing shift in responsibility for health and well-being onto the individual. In Zanzibar, as elsewhere, neoliberal reform packages have pushed for the state's withdrawal from the provision of healthcare and other social services and the introduction of privatization and cost-sharing models, and a relatively new consumerist and entrepreneurial dimension in the provision of healthcare (Parkin 2006: 713). These trends have led to an increasing need for cash in the quest for well-being and care and have created the opportunity for some to make considerable profits. This raises new questions around commodification and the creation of markets in areas that used to be structured by moral responsibilities and kinship relations rather than economic opportunity and profit.

HIV/AIDS has highlighted an increasing dehumanization of affect, emotion and care, as has been shown in a number of studies investigating how social support networks break down under the burden of the disease. The stigma related to HIV/AIDS is one reason for the disintegration of care relationships and emotional distancing; and the high cost involved in caring for a chronically ill person – or several, as often more than one family member is infected – is another. I argue that this breakdown of social and emotional support is indicative of a broader process of commodification that is emerging in other areas of treatment and care-giving too. It includes hospital wards and clinics where quality care is often only provided on the payment of cash, as well as non-biomedical practitioners who have started to view their services as a marketable commodity. These emerging markets for health and well-being are resulting in increased competition among a range of different healing practices and practitioners, and to progressively less access to treatment options for patients who lack financial resources.

Commodification processes are particularly visible surrounding HIV/AIDS, which has become a lucrative business. With vast amounts of money having been invested in the 'fight against HIV/AIDS', an industry has emerged that is providing new market opportunities for a range of actors from the global to the local. Simultaneously, it painfully illustrates the constraints faced by the poor and marginalized who see that donors are often more interested in physical, countable lives ('our investment in antiretrovirals/information and education/condom distribution saved x number of lives last year') than in livelihoods, and in 'AIDS victims' rather than persons who need to survive both physically and socially.

In this industry, the very state of 'being sick' can become a commodity and a source of income. Afflicted with a deadly disease, faced with the loss of jobs, friends and support networks, many of my HIV-positive research participants had nothing but their sick bodies as a resource. Feeding donors' demands for PLHA (People Living with HIV/AIDS) participation in a rights-based agenda of 'making the voices of the afflicted heard', they are joining the bottom rung of the AIDS industry, using their sick bodies and PLHA identities as a 'commodity of last resort' (Scheper-Hughes 2002: 2). In such contexts, commodification becomes highly transgressive and can pose serious risks.

This chapter follows the processes of commodification of well-being and misery in Zanzibar that are particularly apparent in the management of HIV/AIDS. It starts with a discussion of the general deterioration and privatization of Zanzibar's health services, and the ensuing emergence of a market for health and well-being that goes beyond biomedical services and increasingly includes 'traditional' healing, thus shifting the focus from healthcare provision to profit-making. The devastating impact of these processes on the provision of care for impoverished HIV-positive people, whose support networks often crumble under the emotional and financial cost of the infection, is then explored. The final sections analyze their efforts to build alternative social networks by joining PLHA support groups and highlight the precarious nature of their participation in the AIDS industry, which frequently exacerbates their already vulnerable situation. The commodification of people's misery in the form of treatment testimonies and illness narratives is the epitome of marketization in a world in which an infected body assumes a market value and suffering becomes a means of survival. The chapter concludes with an analysis of the strategies HIV-positive people use to negotiate a fragile balance between global discourses on openness and disclosure and living with a highly stigmatizing infection.

The findings presented here are based on twenty-two months of ethnographic fieldwork on living with HIV/AIDS in Zanzibar that was undertaken in 2004-2005 and during several follow-up visits in 2007 and 2008. Using mainly participant observation, I lived with a local family and worked closely with a group of HIV-positive people who had formed a support group, the Zanzibar Association for People living with HIV/AIDS (ZAPHA+). I spent my days in the ZAPHA+ office, accompanied ZAPHA+ members as well as my friends and my host family on visits to hospitals, healers and midwives, visited people in their homes, took part in AIDS- and health-related education sessions, policy planning and monitoring meetings by a range of NGOs and development organizations, and participated in daily life on the islands.

Emerging markets for health in Zanzibar

Zanzibar is a small island archipelago off the Tanzanian coast with a predominantly Muslim population. Formerly an important trading post, it has a long history of trade and migration across the Indian Ocean. Zanzibar's golden days of economic success are long gone and the economic situation today is extremely fragile. A legacy of extensive plantation agriculture, the socialist policy of isolation and self-reliance from 1964 to the mid-1980s and the neo-

Map 8.1 Zanzibar

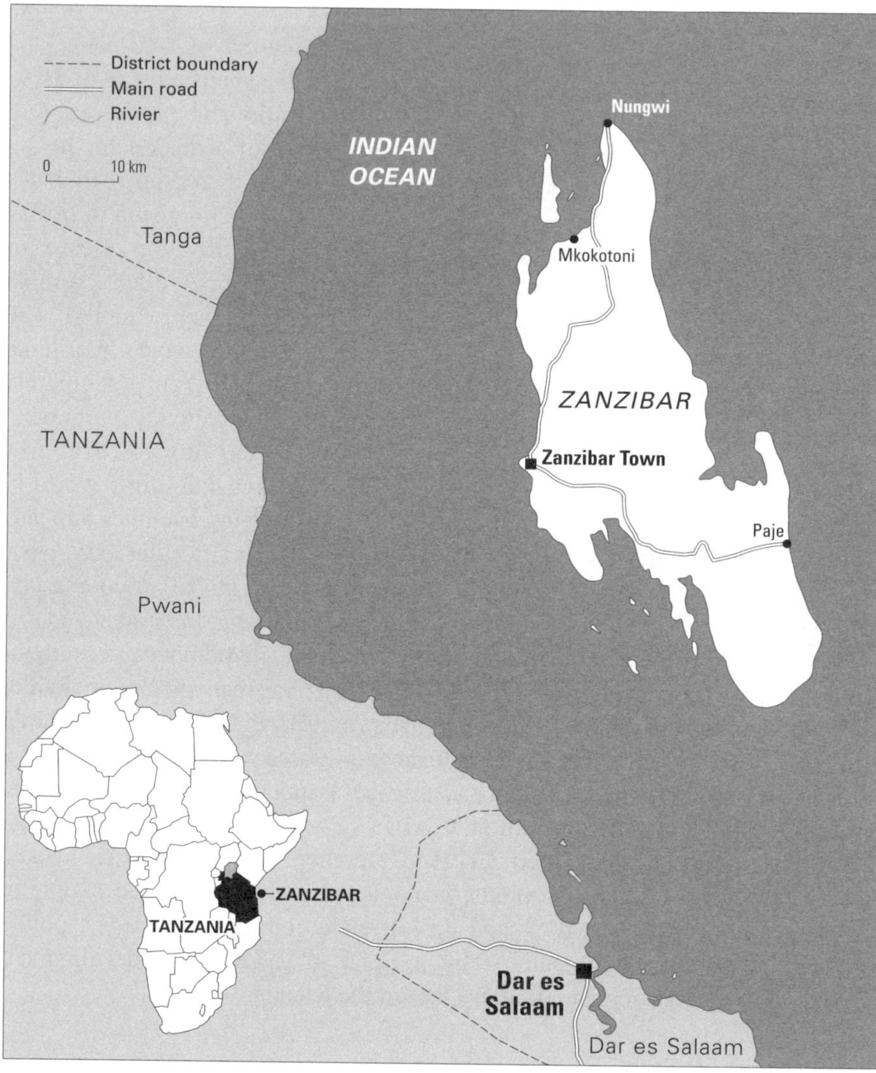

liberal reforms of the late 1980s/early 1990s with their thriving corruption and recurrent political turmoil have created an environment of instability and economic fragility combined with a profound lack of state-sponsored social-security services.

After the 1964 revolution, the new socialist government heavily promoted biomedicine in Zanzibar and proclaimed a commitment to free and universal biomedical healthcare. At the same time, practitioners of non-biomedical diagnostic and healing techniques[1] were regarded as backward and their methods as being based on 'superstition' and thus not fit for a socialist society. As a consequence, many were forced to flee the islands (Parkin 2006: 698). However, the commitment to provide free healthcare for all proved impossible to fulfil, and these policies ushered in an era in which neither biomedical nor traditional treatments were easily accessible. The biomedical health system – formerly in much better shape in Zanzibar than on the mainland – started to deteriorate in 1970 when the government banned private medical practices. Subsequently, patients had to wait for treatment at government hospitals and clinics for days or go to Dar es Salaam for treatment (Martin 1978: 60).

After two decades of economic and political isolation, the socialist experiment was abolished, resulting in a de facto return to capitalism and political liberation in the mid-1980s, which has enabled the return of private practitioners, pharmacies and small hospitals. Traditional Muslim Zanzibari healers have also started to practise more openly again (Parkin 2006: 699).

The neoliberal move towards the privatization of public services in the past two decades has included the health sector, and cost-sharing models for public health facilities have been introduced. Patients now have to pay a hospital admission fee, buy many of the drugs they are prescribed themselves,[2] and cover the costs of surgery and other procedures,[3] often on top of the bribes they had to offer in many of their encounters with the health system before. While medicines and services were often simply not available[4] in socialist times, the increase of private-sector health provision on the islands has meant that the problem has shifted from *availability* to *accessibility*: better-quality healthcare is in reach although most struggle – and fail – to afford it. The two accounts that

---

1 These are often labelled as 'traditional' healing. While some of the practices indeed go back to long-standing local aetiologies and therapies, new practices are constantly being developed and imported. Zanzibar, with its long history of migration and cosmopolitanism, is prone to the import and mixing of new approaches, and healers are often sought precisely because their origins are outside the islands.

2 While officially the under-fives, pregnant women, the disabled and HIV/AIDS patients are exempt from the health fee, my HIV-positive research participants complained that this rule only seemed to apply when they sought treatment at the HIV clinic. When referred to another department, fees were usually incurred.

3 Roughly Tsh 70,000 to Tsh 100,000 for routine surgery, such as a cesarean section in 2007. (The exchange rate was US$ 1 = Tsh 1,457 on 22 June 2010.) In middle-class private hospitals in Dar es Salaam, these cost between Tsh 1.5m and Tsh 2.5m in 2010 (*Daily News* 2010).

4 This is true for the majority of the population but excludes the elite who had access to preferential treatment and a VIP ward in the hospital with private rooms and better service. These VIP rooms are available for those who can afford the extra charges.

follow show the precarious position people are faced with should they need medical care. The first captures the situation in a ward in Mnazi Mmoja, the islands' referral hospital.

In August 2008, my long-term informant and friend Zakia[5] was hospitalized with final-stage AIDS. Apart from 18 occupied beds, the ward was empty and lacked mosquito nets, sheets and pillows; and everything was very dirty. Zakia's parents mobilized all their resources to buy the intravenous fluids and medicines that the doctor had prescribed to prepare Zakia's weak body for the start of antiretroviral treatment. Yet after six days in hospital, her IV drips were still sitting on her bedside table and her dressings had not been changed and were yellow with pus.[6] The only diagnosis she had received was 'stomach problems'. In the mornings, a nurse came in to sweep the floor but did not clean the tables or wash the patients. Even when asked for help, many of the nurses did not react but became angry and mean. None of the people visiting Zakia – family and fellow activists from ZAPHA+ – were able to get the nurse to fix the drip, and they could not afford to pay her to 'ease' the service. Zakia's friend came in every day to care for her, take her to the toilet, and wash and feed her. The woman in the next bed, also suffering from AIDS, had nobody to look after her. A family member came once a day to bring a plate of food but nobody took the time to feed her. Too weak to eat herself and abandoned by her personal networks, she was left on her own.

The poor quality of services in Zanzibar's public health facilities is not only due to a constant scarcity of basic equipment and drugs and a severe shortage of clinicians but also to what seems to be increasing indifference among staff towards their patients. Several of the older nurses complained that trainee nurses often joined the programme not because they liked the profession but because they had connections with the authorities. In addition, Structural Adjustment Programmes have led to rapidly decreasing salaries for public-sector employees (Dilger 2010: 103), who generally need to have several jobs to make a living. The opportunities offered in the private healthcare sector mean that increasingly doctors are starting their own private practices to which they devote much of their time and energy, reducing their hours at the public hospital

---

5 All the informants' names have been changed, except for those who are openly HIV-positive and have assumed publicly visible roles in ZAPHA+.

6 Hygiene standards were generally extremely poor, which resulted in widespread bacterial co-infections in patients. According to the Health Information Bulletin 2008, the third-highest cause of death in Mnazi Mmoja Referral Hospital and Bububu Military Hospital (the hospitals with the highest mortality rates on the islands) was septicaemia (blood poisoning), which accounted for 7% of all deaths (MoHSW 2009: 45). This could point to shortcomings in hygiene and poor surgical management in these hospitals.

to the bare minimum. Nurses equally try to supplement or replace their meagre public-sector incomes, for example with work in foreign health development projects. The impact of such trends on the provision of care in emergency situations is highlighted in the following account from the same hospital.

A woman from a village on the east coast who was obviously in pain was rushed by ambulance to the maternity ward. This was the first time I had ever seen the hospital ambulance in operation. She had been in labour for almost three days, her relatives said, but the birth was not proceeding. She was admitted to the ward but shortly afterwards the doctor came out and told them that she needed an urgent caesarean section and that they should find Tsh 70,000 to cover the operation. The relatives rushed off to mobilize the money and I heard other people talking about another woman who had been in hospital since the day before waiting for a C-section, but her family could not pay for it.

This delaying strategy was obviously dangerous for both the mother's and the baby's health. While the woman did receive the surgery some hours later, the doctors put recovering the costs before their patients' welfare and showed little concern for their suffering. This is not an exceptional case and similar situations arise all over the country. For example, the death of a woman in the maternity ward made the headlines in Dar es Salaam in 2008,[7] and in 2010 a newspaper report warned women of being talked into unnecessary caesareans by 'selfish doctors' who value personal gains over patients' lives (*Daily News* 2010).

As a result of so many negative experiences with the public healthcare system, trust in biomedicine is not pervasive. In fact, many of my informants were afraid of visiting the hospital and were terrified of having to be admitted. 'The only way you get out of the hospital is wrapped in a cloth [i.e. dead]', I was often told, and people always took care not to touch anything when visiting a patient for fear of catching 'bugs' (*wadudu*). While the large majority are forced to cope with what they can afford, the small mobile elite turns to one of the better-equipped but expensive private clinics that have sprung up on the islands, pointing towards an increasingly 'class-based' differentiation of healthcare provision (Parkin 2006: 699).

The privatization of healthcare delivery has, in turn, led to the creation of a market for health in which practitioners of non-biomedical healing, too, have started to view their services as a marketable commodity, resulting in increased competition among a range of different healing practices and practitioners.

---

7 The incident is reported to have taken place in June 2008 in Mwananyamala Hospital in Dar es Salaam, which has been at the centre of scandals involving the intimidation of pregnant women to the extent that some mothers and/or their newborn babies have died during delivery. A probe team exonerated the hospital in the former case (*Daily News* 2009).

Many of my informants claimed that the once-common herbalists, massage therapists, and spirit and Qur'anic healers who offer their services as a charitable act and pious deed have become very rare. Indeed, Zanzibar's Traditional and Alternative Medicine Policy (2008: 6) calls for the regulation of local traditional healing and proposes developing 'appropriate and profitable marketing, pricing and post-harvesting systems so that it can match with world market trends'.

The need for cash to access hospital-based and non-biomedical treatment has reached such an extent that deaths and severe complications caused by medical negligence due to the patient's inability to pay have become common occurrences, and accounts of traditional healers detaining patients until they can pay their fees and threatening them with witchcraft attacks should they escape have posed a real concern for many of my research participants.

The treatment of AIDS (and the promise of a cure) has become a particularly lucrative business, fuelled by the rise of the AIDS industry that emerged out of globally concerted efforts to fight the pandemic. HIV-positive people in Zanzibar are very aware of the influence of economic considerations on their health and their dependence on donor support for the antiretroviral treatments that keep them alive. The stigmatizing nature of HIV/AIDS, the debilitating symptoms of the disease and the high costs of biomedical treatment make it an especially attractive market for treatments.

While my informants praised the introduction of free antiretroviral treatment in 2005, a cure (*kupona kabisa*) was what they were really hoping for. Consequently, many had already tried out one or several treatments that promised to eradicate the virus completely, and news about new, allegedly successful medicine against AIDS frequently arrived. People went home to their villages to find their own healers and bought medicines from all over the country, from places as far away as Kagera (where the Tanzanian epidemic started and people were thus assumed to have experience with its treatment), Dubai and Saudi Arabia. Herbal concoctions (*dawa za miti shamba*), the composition of which would come to the healer in a dream or with the help of spirits, and fumigations (*fukizo*: incense burning), often in combination with Qur'anic supplication (*dua*), were administered and supported through prayer and abstinence, following the way of the scriptures. Some of these cures were developed by longstanding healers, others traded by entrepreneurial self-pronounced healers, and some were even sold in backrooms by biomedical doctors who then observed their clinical effects on patients. While genuine attempts to relieve suffering undoubtedly are a motivation, healers also seem to be doing good business,[8] to the extent that in 2004 advertisements that claimed to offer a cure for AIDS were made illegal. However, this did not stop constant demands for new therapies and treatments for opportunistic infections.

How do people cope with the high costs of severe and long-term illness in an increasingly monetized environment where most diagnostic and treatment routes require cash payments? Here the availability of a functioning social-support network becomes all the more important. Building up and maintaining extensive networks of support helps to spread everyday risks and uncertainties. However these networks often crumble under the stigmatizing and costly burden of HIV/AIDS.

Disintegrating networks of social support

There is common consensus among Zanzibaris that the extended family serves as the prime network of support. Nothing is considered as important as family relations, and a strong emphasis is placed on harmony within the family. Wealth does not necessarily need to be shared equally among family members, and in a community deeply involved in trade it is acknowledged that some people make more profit than others. In situations of need, however, it is compulsory to help. In addition to family obligations, neighbours (*majirani*) in Zanzibar also act as an important support system: living together creates relationships of responsibility, and community cohesion is generally strong. Neighbours play a central role in providing support for larger occasions such as weddings and funerals, and are supposed to recognize when a person needs help. Some of my informants reported that their neighbours occasionally gave them food or money when they were desperate, or gave their children a meal to relieve them of the stress of feeding their family.[9] Work also creates relationships and feelings of responsibility. Colleagues support each other, and employers often help in case of sickness by contributing to the cost of medication and hospital visits, or they might even send the sick person on paid leave.

Together, the social network of family, neighbours, friends, colleagues and employers thus works as an insurance system in which moral debts are created for which a return can be claimed afterwards. But members of the social

8 Payments usually ranged from Tsh 150,000 to Tsh 500,000, which is a lot of money but not unaffordable. Many of my informants had mobilized their social networks to raise it.

9 Some long-standing community members (usually not recent immigrants) who do not have family even received constant support from their neighbours, as was the case of Mariam, an old widow with no children, who was fed and dressed on a daily basis by all the neighbours on her street.

network do not only extend economic support; the emotional support they give by enquiring about a sick person's health, by visiting and generally by showing that they care is often regarded as important as material aid. Nevertheless, long-term illness puts enormous strain on a social network and with rising costs it is often impossible to provide comprehensive and enduring care.

Moreover, situations occur in which disputes about family members' liabilities arise, and support is denied or kept to an absolute minimum. These conflicts tend to take place in cases where the person in need is thought to have brought an emergency situation upon themselves through immoral behaviour, e.g. through drug or alcohol abuse, or through sexual promiscuity. All these behaviours are closely associated with HIV/AIDS, which is predominantly explained in Zanzibar as divine punishment. Local mosque communities do not play a major role in caring for the sick, and the moral interpretation of AIDS on the islands frequently leads to further ostracism from the community and exacerbates rather than helps the situation. Stigma, blame and financial costs come together and result in the disintegration of social support networks: it is plainly easier to justify high treatment expenses for a family member who is deemed an 'innocent victim'. Recently, however, attempts in the Muslim community have been directed at redefining the 'AIDS-as-punishment' message into one of 'AIDS-as-a-trial-from-God', focusing on Muslim principles of compassion and caring for the sick rather than condemning or blaming them (Beckmann 2009). Ashura's story offers insight into the self-sacrificing care that is extended by some family members, but tensions that arise even within the nuclear family demonstrate the fragility of the relationships of care that can easily break down from one day to the next leaving the patient to their own fate.

In 2005, Ashura, a 30-year-old mother of a small son, was terminally ill with AIDS. She had been hospitalized for four months with diarrhoea, severe nausea and serious dehydration. During this time, her mother had been with her: she slept at the hospital, went to work during the day, then home to wash Ashura's clothes and prepare food for her, and came back to the hospital to care for her daughter. Three weeks after Ashura started to take antiretrovirals, a ZAPHA+ member took her to the hospital for a chest X-ray. Her mother had broken her foot and was hospitalized. Now Ashura did not have anybody to care for her, and there was no money for food. The family lived in a very basic *makuti* (coconut-palm leaves) thatched house in Kwahani in the Ng'ambo area of Zanzibar Town. They were having lunch when I visited some days later, a plate of plain rice with a small handful of spinach to share between everybody. Ashura's mother was sitting on the floor with outstretched legs, unable to walk. 'But we have a hospital appointment tomorrow, again,' she said, biting her lip. 'Last time Ashura just didn't want to go, she couldn't face making the journey down to the street to get a bus. But we had to pick up those drugs! So I had to get a taxi to come directly to the doorstep and pay the driver to take us to the hospital.' Ashura's sister, who also lived in the house, constantly scolded and blamed her for the infection and for bringing shame on the family. She had not made any effort to ensure that Ashura took her drugs while her mother was in hospital. She made it clear that she could barely tolerate her presence in the house and took care not to let her children get too close to their sick aunt. Weakened physically and mentally by the symptoms of AIDS, Ashura relied exclusively on her mother for her daily care, while the rest of her family network limited their care to ensuring she did not starve. Despite her antiretroviral treatment, Ashura died a year later in the summer of 2006.

Ashura's story highlights the vital importance – and volatility – of a functioning social-support network for survival in Zanzibar. If this breaks down, the consequences are usually deteriorating health and death. While HIV rates are comparatively low on the islands,[10] AIDS is perceived as a major threat. A person who is often sick or shows any of the symptoms associated with AIDS attracts rumours, neighbours and friends stop visiting, and people in the street point fingers. 'The worst thing about AIDS, the reason why we are so scared about it, is that if you have it, you won't have any friends', 29-year-old Hassan explained. The painful loss of part of or even one's entire social network is not only emotionally scarring, it is also physically dangerous. In the absence of state-sponsored social-security services, a social network is vital for physical survival. Indeed in most cases I encountered in Zanzibar, the disclosure of one's HIV status led to immediate abandonment or divorce, which hits women especially hard. Many HIV-positive women are left with several children and no, or only minimal, financial support. Many, therefore, hide their HIV status from their partner and family members. Once it becomes known that a person is HIV-positive, business often goes down: 'who would want to buy anything from a *mwenye UKIMWI* (a person with AIDS)?' Zainab, an HIV-positive woman in her mid-forties explained. One member of ZAPHA+, Zanzibar's only support group for those who are HIV-positive, reportedly died because nobody cared for her when she was sick and people threw stones at her and refused to sell her food. Such extreme cases of stigmatization occasionally occur in Zanzibar but usually families provide at least a minimum level of care, supplying food and help with daily household tasks, such as washing clothes and cleaning the house. But many of my informants deplore the lack of kindness and compassion, and report that they are scolded by family members and treated with contempt. The family might attend to (*kuhudumia*) but not actually care for (*kujali*)

[10] Officially, Zanzibar has one of the lowest rates of HIV infection in Sub-Saharan Africa. According to the only published survey, HIV prevalence was 0.6% in 2002 (ZAC 2003: 1).

the person. This points to the fact that caring for a sick person needs to be more than providing basic assistance – emotional support, expressed by showing empathy (*huruma*) and love (*upendo*), and a respectful way of interacting with the sick person (*kumheshimu*) are viewed as essential features of relationships with the surrounding social environment. Without these, several of my informants pointed out, life is not worth living, and suicide is sometimes considered.

Ashura's story also demonstrates the financial costs of caring for a sick person, which go well beyond hospital bills and charges for drugs, and include expenses for food, water and transport. Ashura's mother had never before taken a taxi, and the trip swallowed up a major part of the family's income, but empathy and love for her daughter led her to decide against cost-effective considerations. Ashura's sister considered it an unfair waste of precious resources on an undeserving, dying person. Such considerations about the efficient use of household resources are found in other parts of the region too. In northwestern Tanzania, for example, health staff often advise AIDS patients' relatives not to waste any more money on medical treatment (Dilger 2010: 107). While free ARVs have been available to all eligible patients since 2005, the constant need to treat opportunistic infections could not be met by the majority of my informants. Antifungal creams, Septrin, Cotrimoxazole, painkillers, TB and STD medication, vitamins and good-quality food all place considerable pressure on family budgets. Although these drugs were officially free for PLHA at the government hospital, they were often not available, or were only given subject to bribes. Infections were left untreated, courses of treatment not finished[11] or other forms of treatment were sought in an increasingly competitive market for health and well-being. So how do HIV-positive people cope with the loss or disintegration of social relations?

Purposeful relatedness: Entering the AIDS industry

An important part of coming to terms with the infection for most of my informants was the process of protecting their existing social network and building up new social relationships to replace those they had lost. One way of creating new support networks is to join a support group for HIV-positive people, such as ZAPHA+. As the only organization in Zanzibar that exclusively caters for and is run by HIV-positive people, it forms a self-governed self-help group for people living with HIV/AIDS. ZAPHA+ members provide mutual emotional comfort and reassurance, information about life with HIV/AIDS, and practical support through home-based care and help with household chores,

[11] This results in ever-increasing drug resistance. Multi-drug-resistant strands of TB, for example, ravage the continent and cost uncounted numbers of lives every year (cf. Farmer 2001).

food and drugs. New friendships develop and reciprocal responsibilities are established. Moreover, many joined in their search for a marriage partner, since rumour spread that this was the only place where HIV-positive people would find someone willing to marry them. Newly diagnosed single patients were often referred to ZAPHA+ by a concerned nurse for just this reason.

The extent to which these new social relationships can provide economic stability is relatively limited, however, since members largely come from the poorest sectors of society. But, importantly, membership of ZAPHA+ promises access to financial support through participation in the organization's income-generating activities, projects and events, and thus the AIDS industry, that rapidly growing economic sector that comprises doctors, donors, foreign experts, government officials, and those worst off, namely the sick.

The heavy involvement of donors in the field of HIV/AIDS (as, to a lesser extent, in other areas such as poverty reduction and women's empowerment), boosted by the design of the Millennium Development Goals and the establishment of several large funding instruments known as Global Health Initiatives in the twenty-first century, have led to the emergence of a global industry in which new career opportunities are arising. The value of this industry is enormous: global spending on HIV/AIDS totalled US$ 13.7 billion in 2008 (KFF 2009). Tanzanian government expenditure on HIV/AIDS for 2007/2008 was predicted to reach Tsh 568 billion, 'a staggering one third' of all aid flowing into the country and far beyond the 'best case' scenario of the 2007 National Multi-sectoral Strategic Framework's financial assessment (TACAIDS 2007: 8). A small part of this funding is dedicated directly to supporting the activities of HIV-positive people.

However, members' and donors' views on the best way to support those who are HIV-positive have diverged. While members hoped that being poor and HIV-positive would entitle them to a share of the vast amount of money dedicated to HIV/AIDS that was reportedly entering the country, donors generally opposed the idea of funding basic needs.[12] Relatively little support so far has come in the form of charity, and the needs that were most urgently felt and frequently vocalized were food and money to pay for rent, clothing and children's schooling. Deemed unsustainable, these were usually not met by donors, who do not intend to encourage the development of a permanent community of aid recipients (although that has been happening) but to 'build capacity' and 'empower' people to 'help themselves'. Income-generating activities and the provision of micro-loans to enable members to start their own small business are therefore central components of economic empowerment programmes.

[12] With the exception of acute emergency situations: money spent on saving lives is generally considered money well spent.

ZAPHA+ started to make soaps, AIDS-awareness ribbons, clothes and knitted baskets. Some more entrepreneurial individuals sell food and drink in the queues at HIV clinics or products that cater specifically to this new target group, such as soaps and creams against skin rashes and barks and herbs against upset stomachs and headaches, which are common side effects of antiretroviral treatment. Overall, however, these income-generating projects were unsuccessful in providing a living for members who frequently complained that they did not get any or only very little payment for their work. They instead saw it as a pastime and their contribution to the organization. This has created conflicts with foreign volunteers who have invested their time to find opportunities for income generation because they felt that members were not pursuing their jobs seriously, and accused them of being lazy and opportunistic.

At a training course for peer educators facilitated and financed by Medicos del Mundo (MDM), for example, ZAPHA+ members complained that they did not get enough money for attending the course as the allowance was lower than usual (Tsh 3000 per day and no meals). The MDM representative replied that the training would give them the opportunity to get paid work afterwards without them having to disclose their HIV status. The argument escalated, with MDM accusing the ZAPHA+ members of being lazy and self-centred, and ZAPHA+ members in turn reproaching MDM unkindness and negligence towards the needs of sick people. 'How can we concentrate all day if we don't even get anything to eat? Your nutritionists teach us that we have to eat quality food, and then you make us sit here without lunch until the evening!', a long-standing ZAPHA+ member angrily exclaimed.

While members who joined in search of substantial charity or business opportunities that would generate a viable income were mostly disappointed, they began to realize that their HIV-positive status could offer the opportunity of making a living from participating in the world of international development. Those who had been members of the organization for some time had certainly learned how to 'navigate the AIDS industry' (Boesten 2008). The importance of the role of people living with HIV/AIDS in the fight against the global pandemic, the perspective and the commitment they can bring to care and prevention was officially recognized in the promotion of the strategy for the Greater Involvement of People with AIDS (GIPA). This was formally adopted as a principle at the AIDS Summit in Paris in 1994, where 42 countries declared the Greater Involvement of People Living with HIV and AIDS to be critical to ethical and effective national responses to the epidemic (UNAIDS 2007). All major global players in the AIDS response have taken this on board. While the GIPA was criticized for being largely tokenistic and not providing any real opportunity for HIV-positive people to participate in decision-making processes, one result of the new strategy has been that ZAPHA+ members are now regularly invited to take part in stakeholder meetings, seminars and workshops on a whole range of subjects related to HIV/AIDS. These meetings grant a sitting allowance, usually upwards of Tsh 5,000 per day to every participant, and a hot meal is often provided too. As many ZAPHA+ members have no income at all and rely on support from family, friends, and neighbours, this has proved a real incentive for them to take part in meetings.

Project funds have additionally been sought from a wide range of national and international aid agencies and ZAPHA+ has been able to secure large amounts of funding from leading international organizations (e.g. the Steven Lewis Fund, the Clinton Foundation, USAID). ZAPHA+ has in fact served as a locomotive for other local HIV programmes, and donors – in line with GIPA principles – have been eager to fund projects that involved people living with HIV/AIDS, unlike local organizations.[13] This donor demand for HIV-positive people has turned their sick bodies into a potentially valuable resource, and members have quickly learned to adjust to the logic of international development, which requires an amount of suffering to justify intervention. They have become skilled at 'telling a good story' and whenever potential donors show up, one of the members 'presents her story' (*kutoa hadithi*), realizing that the more heart-breaking it is the better the chance of getting through to the donor. 'You have to make them cry,' Rahma was advised when preparing her speech for World AIDS Day, 'and don't forget to ask for what we want: more support, more respect, and treatment'. This ability to tell a good story, Nguyen (2005: 133) points out in his analysis of a local grassroots organization in Burkina Faso has become key to survival and the narratives of distress are used tactically, especially in contexts characterized by limited resources. Ironically, AIDS, the very thing that resulted in them losing their economic basis, has now become a major source of income for those who have managed to turn their HIV-positive status into a marketable commodity.

---

[13] There were over twenty local non-governmental organizations and several governmental institutions working specifically on HIV/AIDS in Zanzibar, but many have neither visited nor collaborated with ZAPHA+ in any way. While all the local HIV/AIDS NGOs were part of ZANGOC, a Zanzibari umbrella organization, there were few connections between them. For example, there is no formal referral system between the Zanzibari organization for AIDS orphans and ZAPHA+ (arguably a major 'producer' of AIDS orphans), and many ZAPHA+ members did not know that support was available for orphans. A striking example of the reluctance to work with ZAPHA+ was Zanzibar's First Lady and ZAPHA+'s patron, who organized a concert to raise money for HIV/AIDS but did not even inform ZAPHA+ about it. Several ZAPHA+ members have suggested that prejudice and the fear of contact with HIV-positive people are the reasons for the widespread unwillingness to let them participate, claiming that even Ministry of Health officials (who should know about HIV transmission) were afraid of shaking their hands.

ZAPHA+ members also understand the kinds of suffering that are particularly likely to attract funding: mothers and children, and orphans who have been abandoned by their families. Projects aimed at supporting these vulnerable sectors of the population are likely to receive support, as are projects geared at self-sufficiency, such as micro-loans and small-business development. The importance of juggling the catch phrases of the development industry has been recognized: all ZAPHA+ proposals boast development terminology and acronyms such as 'home-based care' (HBC), 'income-generating activities' (IGA) and 'poverty alleviation', 'capacity building', 'peer education' and 'peer counselling', to name but a few. Moreover, people have learned to fashion these projects to their own needs and circumvent donor agencies' conditions, a practice that has been observed in other parts of Sub-Saharan Africa too.[14] Instead of merely asking for food support, for example, ZAPHA+ applied for (and received) US$ 25,000 for a one-year nutrition project, where a 'nutrition committee' consisting of ZAPHA+ members prepared a meal for all members twice a week, using locally available, reasonably priced but nutritious ingredients. The recipes were to be collated in a cookbook for HIV-positive people in resource-limited settings. It is these kinds of projects – that can be applied to other geographical settings and are not predominantly directed at 'feeding' people – that, not surprisingly, are enthusiastically received by donors, although for the majority of members the important part of the project was being fed a hot meal twice a week. The large amounts of money flowing into the country for AIDS thus make acutely visible the areas that are *not* supported, such as pervasive food insecurity, unveiling neoliberal agendas of state reform that shift responsibility for basic services to the population. The fact that so much money seems to be available has given rise to heavy competition and damaging rumours: about the West already knowing of a cure for AIDS but withholding it from Africans for economic, political or racist reasons, or about HIV-positive people who are allegedly getting rich from these funds.

Indeed, many ZAPHA+ members are trying to live off the various training courses, meetings and workshops run by external agencies that supply an irregular but considerable income from which beneficiaries can live quite comfortably. The AIDS industry can thus offer new opportunities to the impoverished and marginalized. These include financial opportunities but also the potential to establish new identities and social status through acquiring leadership positions and gaining respect within ZAPHA+ and among stakeholders. Activism as part of ZAPHA+ means creating and maintaining links with national and international organizations, gaining access to governmental meetings and engaging with local, regional and national government authorities

[14] For a compelling account of a youth group in Burkina Faso, see Nguyen (2005).

– in short, establishing links with and gaining insights into institutions and processes that previously were entirely beyond the reach of most members. Participation in PLHA groups can thus be empowering and an opportunity to take agency: a form of self-marketing that can lead to self-reflection and self-construction as a 'person living with HIV/AIDS', and to 'producing and feeling' their identity as PLHA, similar to the processes of 'ethno-preneurialism' – the commodification of ethnicity and indigenous identity described by Comaroff & Comaroff (2009). Financially, participation in the AIDS industry can, for a few, lead to personal relationships with a wealthy Westerner who may provide substantial on-going support. This is the lottery ticket that many hope for, and a major incentive for investing time in participating in activities that do not always carry meaning or produce immediate benefits.

However, this is not a certain game. Some individuals manage to carve out a living by giving testimonies, participating in workshops and seminar, and working as home-based carers, peer counsellors or income-generators. But with growing numbers of members, many will never get the opportunity to enter the ranks of the AIDS industry. At the same time, these opportunities come at a cost as the disclosure of one's HIV status can pose risks, as the following case studies demonstrate.

Markets for sickness: The commodification of misery

On 1 December 2004 I joined some ZAPHA+ members at the Amani Stadium in Zanzibar, where the annual World AIDS Day was being celebrated. These celebrations culminated in the presentation of prizes by Zanzibar's President Amani Karume to organizations that had carried out outstanding work over the past year. While ZAPHA+ members felt honoured to receive a prize, it was difficult to find volunteers willing to accept the certificate in public. Only a handful of people on the islands were openly HIV-positive, mainly among ZAPHA+'s leadership. Most ordinary members preferred to keep their HIV status secret. Two members finally decided to 'go public' to show that they were not ashamed of being infected. One was Rahma, a 43-year-old single mother of four children. She had tested HIV-positive in 2000, having cared for her sister who suffered from AIDS for over a year. After her sister's death, she took in two of her sister's orphaned children and supported the remaining three. The other woman was Amina, a 30-year-old mother of one son. Both were divorced, had been members of ZAPHA+ for several years, and were outspoken and self-confident. Amina's family, and Rahma's employer and colleagues at the hospital, where she worked as a cleaner, knew of their HIV status and had been supportive. However, when Amina proudly accepted the certificate from

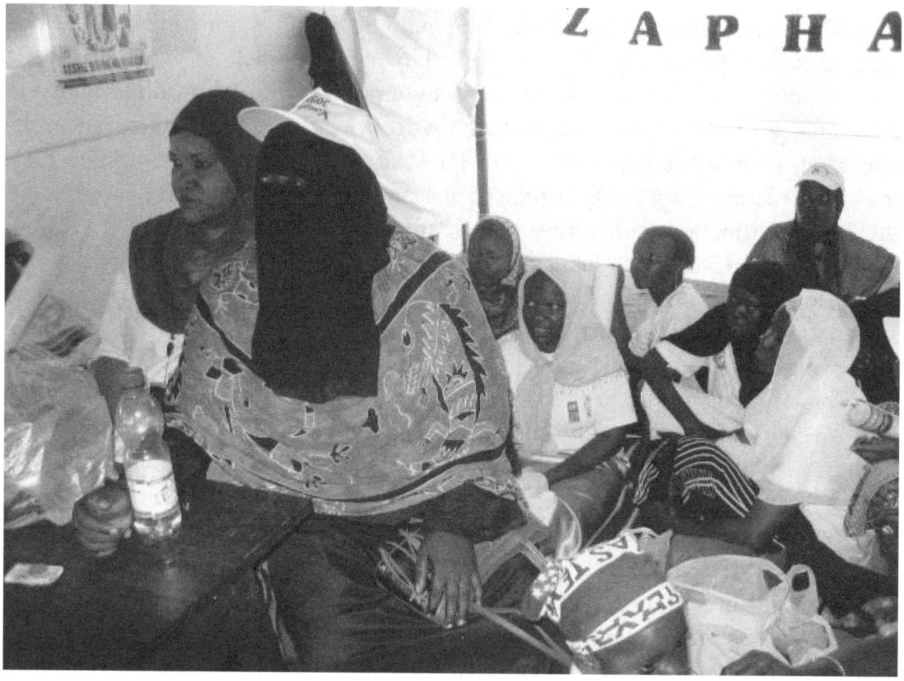

Photo 8.1 ZAPHA+ stall at the World AIDS Day celebrations 2004, Amani Stadium, Zanzibar: Showing solidarity without risking disclosure
[Photo: Nadine Beckmann]

the President, and when Rahma gave a passionate speech advocating the rights of HIV-positive people, the local TV station TVZ transmitted their public acts into the households of the Zanzibari people. The next day, Rahma was dismissed from her job and Amina was chased away by her family.

Both recounted how their families, friends and colleagues had not blamed them for their condition, but that the public disclosure of their HIV status was unacceptable to them. To have AIDS is *aibu* (shameful) and to admit it openly meant they had disqualified themselves from participation in the social world of 'normal', i.e. non-infected, people. As part of a social network, Rahma and Amina had disregarded the needs and feelings of their networks' other members. Disclosing their HIV/AIDS status in the workplace could scare off clients, especially in a hospital setting due to fears surrounding the infectiousness of the virus, and the family of an HIV-positive person is subject to stigmatization in the wider social environment too. Since AIDS is so closely associated with moral failure, HIV infection is seen to reflect on the person's upbringing and thus on his/her family. Implying that moral and specifically sexual norms must have been broken, it indicates a clear disregard of the rules of respect and obedience to one's parents and elders. A family who has a member who is known to be HIV-positive will become the centre of attention and gossip, and the family members' general *tabia* (character, behaviour) will be re-evaluated. Consequently, it may be more difficult to find appropriate marriage partners even for non-infected family members. A person's public disclosure of their HIV status thus has implications beyond the individual sufferer and affects the larger social network of which s/he is a part.

Openness and testimony, emphasized in the global discourse on AIDS as an important means of fighting stigma and coping with one's infection, for individuals like Amina and Rahma thus carry the danger of destroying what is left of their social support network, and harming those closest to them. Not many are willing to take such risks. To still benefit from the AIDS industry, members have devised strategies to minimize the dangers disclosure entails. Just as in their private lives, they disclosed their status step-by-step, carefully testing the waters and weighing up the risks before they trusted a person with such powerful and dangerous information. Many chose to engage in lower levels of disclosure, guarding the spaces in which they speak about living with the virus: they avoid public and broadcast events, but attend closed donor meetings and workshops where the possibility of running into a relative or neighbour is low. Others justified their presence at ZAPHA+ by claiming to do HIV charity work. Ahmed, a carpenter in his mid-thirties, for example, collected training and workshop certificates he had gained through his work within ZAPHA+ so that he could show them to his employer and colleagues should they ever wonder why he spent time with HIV-positive people. In fact, when the organization received a new door sign that suggested the group's association with HIV/AIDS, many members refused to come in for fear of stigmatization, and women started to wear face veils when entering, although the sign did not even mention that the organization was only for HIV-positive people.[15] These members' strategies about hiding their infection contradict the discourses on the value of openness and empowerment that form part of the donor script and that are promoted within ZAPHA+, despite the fact that many genuinely want to make a change.

Knowledge of and openness about one's HIV status, HIV policy planners assume, will reduce the stigma over time. '*Pima ufaidhike*' ('test for your own benefit') is what a T-shirt by the Tanzanian Commission for AIDS (TACAIDS) declares. Many however cannot afford to carry the burden of stigma and complain that donors do not really care about their daily struggles: 'What benefit do

[15] It reads: 'ZAPHA+. Place of friendly services for young people, on reproductive health, AIDS, teenage pregnancy and drugs'.

I get exactly?' Zaina, a poor, older member, asked bitterly. Maria, a former member of the Kigoma branch of Service, Health and Development of People Living Positively with HIV/AIDS (SHEDEPHA) received a place on an HIV-awareness seminar, and thus a daily allowance. In return, she was asked to tell her story and disclose her HIV status in a large hall in front of an audience of Kigoma citizens. 'I did it, I said openly in front of all these people that I was HIV-positive, and what do you think I got? Only Tsh 5,000. I took this risk while other PLHA leaders just sat there and said nothing and got all this money.' After this experience she told them she did not want to be a part of their group any longer. Although Maria subscribes to global scripts of openness and de-stigmatization, she was explicit about feeling exploited by donors' consumption of PLHA stories in the drive for increasing openness about HIV/AIDS, and the fact that they rarely ask what happens to people after disclosure. The lack of support mechanisms that buffer the impact of disclosing in a largely hostile environment, in combination with the extreme poverty of

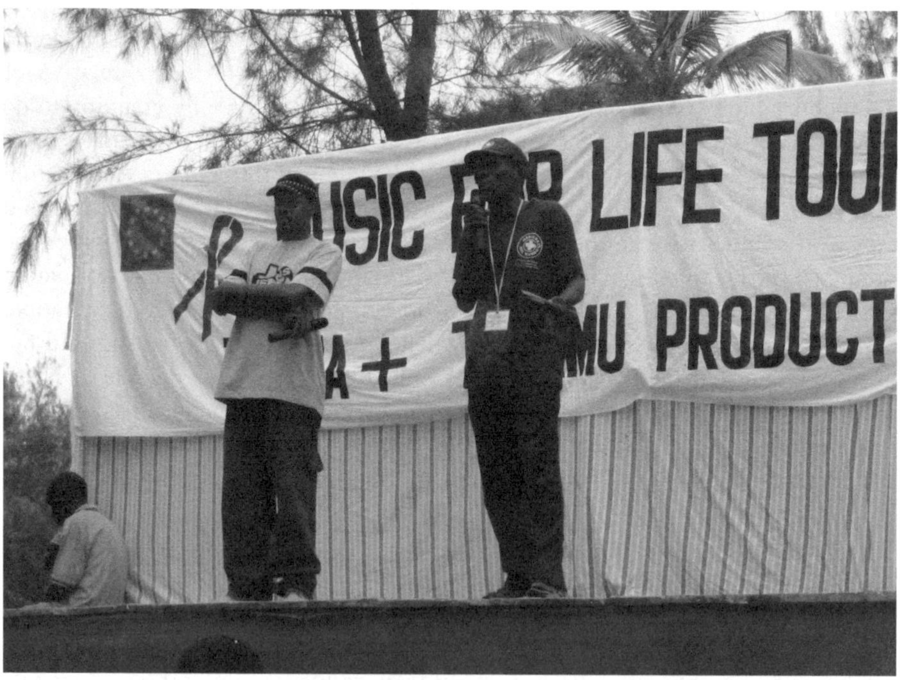

Photo 8.2 ZAPHA+ member and peer educator testifies on his life with HIV/AIDS in Zanzibar at Medicos del Mundo's HIV/AIDS awareness activity in Kiwengwa, 14.8.2005
[Photo: Nadine Beckmann]

many PLHA who are responding to the demands of a powerful industry that promises both life-saving medication and financial benefits, makes the commodification of sickness and misery highly transgressive, and the sick body a 'commodity of last resort' (Scheper-Hughes 2002: 2).

Their public acts resulted in Amina and Rahma losing central parts of their support networks, leaving Rahma to feed her children without an income, and Amina without a caring family or a place to live. Rahma started offering laundry services to get by, which is physically arduous and badly paid. She claimed she earned Tsh 10,000 to Tsh 12,000 per month from this job, not nearly enough to sustain a family. 'If I really stretch it,' she said, 'I need Tsh 25,000 per month to feed them all. I can't even think of the last time I ate meat; it must be at least three months ago. One kilo of meat is Tsh 2,000, you know, and a small piece of fish is Tsh 800. And to prepare fish you need tomatoes, onions, potatoes … I use *dagaa* (small dried fish), and in the morning I eat a cup of *uji* (porridge). Sometimes I boil water without tea leaves because I can't afford any.' She now relies on her income from the AIDS industry, micro-loans and income-generating projects, participation in meetings and education sessions and money from weekly Saturday 'therapy' meetings. This way she can accumulate Tsh 30,000 per month, but this sort of income is irregular. If there is no work within ZAPHA+, she makes soaps and sells them in the neighbourhood. Smiling proudly, she tells me that her neighbours say she takes care of her children better than most men. The neighbours also help out from time to time. 'I pray to God,' Rahma says, 'I ask Him to help me with the children and to find us something to eat. And sometimes I'm walking home and a neighbour says: "come on in!" and gives me beans, rice or Tsh 500. There were so many things I wanted to do, so many plans I had made. But now it is difficult because of the virus. Now I only want to live until my children are grown up.' Rahma has to deal with enormous stress. Her nineteen-year-old son is living with his friends: he left their home of his own accord in order to help her. One of her deceased sister's children is being abused and beaten by her aunt. 'When she ran away and begged me to let her stay here with me I said: "Endure (*stahimili*)! I don't have any space for you at home". But both children are supported by me. If I could afford it, I would want them all with me at home.' In such circumstances, public disclosure of her HIV status may be seen as a desperate attempt both to gain access to financial support and to redefine a highly stigmatized identity by emphasizing altruistic motives and moral responsibilities to care and protect. Its potential for empowerment and agency through self-marketing is limited by the constraints of the market, where capacity for sickness stories is limited in the face of increasing competition, and where financial value placed on narratives of suffering is too low to provide a sustainable livelihood for most PLHA.

At the same time, self-marketing as an AIDS sufferer and an ARV-supported survivor can contribute to crumbling social relationships by evoking the appearance of making money from their stigmatized condition. Amina managed to carve out a career for herself within ZAPHA+: she was elected the group's secretary, which provided a small monthly salary. More importantly, as secretary, a number of invitations from development organizations to participate or speak at meetings and seminars were addressed directly to her, and thus opened up opportunities for further income. Allowances paid for participating in such meetings usually range from Tsh 5,000 to Tsh 10,000 a day, and up to US$ 50 per day if the workshop is held outside Zanzibar. These are considerable amounts of income compared to the average salary on the islands.[16] However, spaces were limited and competition was high – ZAPHA+'s membership had grown to several hundred by the summer of 2007, due to an efficient referral system of newly tested HIV-positive people by ZAPHA+ members working as peer counsellors at HIV-testing sites in Zanzibar.

While for some members, like Amina, ZAPHA+ had replaced social networks that had disintegrated under the burden of the stigma of HIV, the newly built relationships were subject to conflict and tension too, many of which arise from the competition for scarce resources.[17] The fact that money seemed to flow to ZAPHA+ in amounts almost incomprehensible to many members, who come from the poorest sectors of society, was a major incentive for joining the group, which managed to secure several large grants worth thousands of US dollars. Apart from initial attendance expenses of Tsh 3,500 per person for the weekly 'therapy meetings'[18] (which soon declined when membership rose), most members saw very little of this money, which was invested in running an office, providing home-based care for sick members and income-generating activities. The fact that funds were too scarce – and not intended – to care for every member's needs was a constant source of tension and led to conflicts within the group. Difficult decisions had to be made: ZAPHA+'s leadership had to negotiate the demands of stakeholders who requested PLHA participation by *qualified* individuals who would follow and engage in discussions at meetings or reliably present their testimonials, with their members' demands. Spaces for attendance at meetings or workshops had traditionally been allocated by voting

---

16 Mean per capita annual income in Zanzibar was Tsh 198,907 in 2004/5 (Zanzibar Household Budget Survey 2004/5: 108).

17 There are other sources of tension too, including romantic and sexual affairs among members and resulting jealousy, and cases of abuse of power for sexual favours and privileges.

18 These meetings were intended as group therapy meetings, but organizational matters, upcoming events or projects were discussed, or the sessions were used to run education sessions on HIV/AIDS-related topics.

at the Saturday meetings. Spaces were assigned on the basis of need and level of involvement: active members and those who were in acute financial difficulties were usually particularly favoured so that they could benefit from the daily allowance and the food provided. As a result, members with no English skills or technical knowledge sat in important policy-planning and donor meetings and could neither represent ZAPHA+'s interests nor report back to their members.[19] The following example illuminates the difficult negotiations between ZAPHA+ and their stakeholder network.

Khadija had been pushing for a workshop place for months. She and other 'ordinary' members were angry at the leadership who she claimed used their privileged position as gatekeepers to limit opportunities for members to gain access to workshop spaces. Khadija was a long-term member of ZAPHA+ but had never been able to connect well with the other members. As a barmaid selling sex and alcohol and drinking regularly, she had been marginalized within the group, despite the organization's strong commitment not to stigmatize anybody. After she and various other members had caused some stir in a meeting with ZAPHA+'s main funder by openly accusing the leadership of siphoning off money, she was finally selected to tell her story at a teachers' workshop organized by the Peace Corps. When they came back in the afternoon, Tausi, an experienced public speaker who had accompanied her, was fuming: 'Khadija pulled out! First she made such a fuss and kept hassling us about getting a place at a workshop, and then she doesn't do her job! Charles [the Peace Corps trainer who recruited ZAPHA+ members for his workshops] was also angry and said he'd never work with ZAPHA+ again!'

Khadija's story demonstrates how ZAPHA+ members were very aware of their dependence on donors and the need to play by their rules, which include reliability in providing the services demanded, accountability and transparency in implementing projects, and demonstrating eagerness to provide voluntary or low-paid services in the 'fight against AIDS', to be fought in unity as HIV-positive people, side by side with the organizations that supported them. Some members had embraced the struggle to contain the epidemic and protect others from infection. For many, however, participation in the AIDS industry came out of the desperate quest for survival when there was no one else to turn to anymore. Yet donor dependency, the insufficient availability of funds and the diverging views of members and donors on appropriate ways to invest these funds have been a major hurdle to building the unity that is considered so

[19] The fact that high-level meetings were usually held in English, without translators, and that a level of technical knowledge beyond most members' ability was required for full participation demonstrates the lack of commitment among donors to involving PLHA in decision-making processes in a meaningful way.

important to make headway in the fight against AIDS. It instils tension and conflict among members, and thus directly opposes their efforts to build new social relationships that can be trusted in times of need. The uneven dispersal of funding generates mistrust, which can erupt in open conflict and threats, as in the case of Amina.

Amina had been at the ZAPHA+ office almost every day for years, and had worked hard to gain members' respect. In her position as secretary, accusations grew louder, however, about how she misused her position by taking up the invitations to send a ZAPHA+ member to meetings herself without giving members the chance to choose a suitable representative. When Amina died of AIDS in the summer of 2008, very few attended her funeral. I was struck by the division among formerly close ZAPHA+ members at the funeral: they formed two groups and sat on different mats, some feet apart. Some were crying but there were also whispers: that Amina had brought her demise upon herself; that she did not deserve better. Her friend later recounted: 'Some members are glad that she died, they were happy! They said she had taken money and didn't pass on letters (invitations), so that she always got to go to seminars. Some even wore *kangas* that read: *Umeuliza umepata* ('you got what you asked for!').' As assistant secretary, she became ZAPHA+'s new secretary, usually a highly desirable and prestigious position, but she only took the job reluctantly: 'I'm scared of being secretary. They said I should quit my other job and work for ZAPHA+ fulltime, but I won't do it. I'll get a fly stuck in my nose (*nitapewa nzi puani*) for nothing.'[20]

These conflicts have reached beyond ZAPHA+'s members and have included the wider society. The vast amounts of money circulating in the newly emerged industry around AIDS have led to accusations that ZAPHA+ members only pretend to be HIV-positive in order to make money. These accusations reflect the perceived injustice of investing so heavily in people who are largely thought to have brought their own suffering upon themselves, while neglecting the needs of the 'innocent' people who are also suffering from poverty and illness. Moreover, with antiretroviral treatment available on the islands now, HIV has become more invisible, and many PLHA look as healthy as everyone else. ZAPHA+ members must therefore constantly take care that they reconcile conflicting sick roles, as Zanzibari society defines an AIDS sufferer by physical symptoms and mistrusts claims to HIV-positive status by healthy-looking individuals. The donors' desired 'sick role' is tending to be that of the empowered survivor, healthy through antiretroviral treatment, and transformed in attitudes and behaviour through their interventions. The accusations show how the AIDS industry could damage the fragile position of PLHAs even more, adding another

[20] This alludes to her fears of being targeted by witchcraft attacks out of jealousy.

layer to HIV-related stigma by inserting an economic component in the already existing fear and hatred. They also demonstrate the extent to which monetization has become a focal point of referral, and how the fierce competition for scarce resources in an increasingly monetized environment serves to instil jealousy and suspicion and threatens to damage carefully rebuilt social relationships.

Conclusion

The rise of markets for health in the wake of neoliberal moves towards the privatization of healthcare has shifted the problems concerning health services in Zanzibar from availability to accessibility, and increasing the need for hard cash has limited poor people's access to healthcare and treatment options. This trend captures biomedical and non-biomedical sectors of healthcare alike. I argue that related to these trends towards marketization, privatization and individual responsibility is a decline in affect and emotion in the provision of care. The newly emerged AIDS industry shows these trends very clearly, opening up opportunities to make profits on a previously unknown scale. In this industry, the very state of 'being sick' can become a commodity, a source of income. Consequently, not only have healing practices and substances become commodified, the diseased body and its stories of suffering can also be turned into a commodity, something that can be marketed and serve as a potentially major source of income.

However while the AIDS industry has opened up new opportunities for the impoverished and marginalized, most do not enter into it lightly as they are fully aware of the dangers involved in the disclosure of their infection. Just like the commodified organs Scheper-Hughes (2002: 2) describes in her analysis of organ trafficking, which become 'an object of desire for one population and a commodity of last resort for "the other" and socially disadvantaged population', HIV-positive people in Zanzibar (and other poor and marginalized countries) are using their bodies, their stories of suffering and recovery, and their HIV-positive status as a last resort. The fact that they risk so much by taking this step is evident from the small number of people who dare to do so: only a handful of people in Zanzibar are open about being HIV-positive and are willing to speak in front of others about their infection. As long as openness and disclosure of one's HIV status result in the destruction of a person's social relationships and means of survival, and in the absence of real participation in decision-making and planning processes, it is difficult to see how PLHA participation in the AIDS industry can lead to their empowerment, as envisaged by many organizations working in the field. Under these circumstances, their gains rarely move beyond the short-term financial benefits offered in return for their testimony, and HIV-positive people become collaborators in their own exploitation, consenting to being reduced to a 'most miserable commodity' (*Ibid.*: 8).

Ironically, it is the more philanthropic, human-rights-based approach to HIV/AIDS intervention that places HIV-positive people as actors in this industry, calling for interventions to be based on principles of positive living, empowerment and partnership. Yet the donors' preference for saving lives, while neglecting the livelihoods and social persona of the saved, exemplifies the reduction of life to 'bare life' (Agamben 1998). This is becoming more and more apparent in neoliberal regimes of care. Anthropology has an important role to play in unveiling these processes that are found in the multiple layers of meaning produced at the intersection of local and global discourses and practices around the control of large-scale health threats. Analyzing strategies for the fight against AIDS through the lens of processes of commodification highlights the potentially transgressive nature of (undoubtedly well-meaning) approaches to de-stigmatization and empowerment and points to the contradictory forces at play in the realm of global health interventions.

References

Agamben, G. (1998), *Homo Sacer: Sovereign power and bare life*. Stanford: University of Stanford Press.

Beckmann, N. (2009), AIDS and the power of God: Narratives of decline and coping strategies in Zanzibar. In: F. Becker & P.W. Geissler, eds, *AIDS and religious practice in Africa*, pp. 119-154. Leiden: Brill.

Boesten, J. (2008), Navigating the AIDS industry. Paper presented at workshop entitled 'Poverty, Exclusion and Abjection,' University of Leeds. 12 November 2008.

Comaroff, J. & J. Comaroff (2009), *Ethnicity Inc.* Chicago: University of Chicago Press.

Daily News (2009), 'Team to probe dead infant switch'. 25 November. Accessed 15 January 2010: http://www.dailynews.co.tz/home/?n=5627

Daily News (2010), 'Mothers warned of surgical operations during delivery'. 4 July. Accessed 10 July: http://www.dailynews.co.tz/home/?n=11424&cat=home

Dilger, H.J. (2010), 'My relatives are running away from me!' Kinship and care in the wake of structural adjustment, privatisation and HIV/AIDS in Tanzania. In: H.J. Dilger & U. Luig, eds, *Morality, hope and grief: Anthropologies of AIDS in Africa*, pp. 102-126. Oxford: Berghahn.

Farmer, P. (2001), *Infections and inequalities: The modern plagues*. Berkeley: University of California Press.

KFF (Kaiser Family Foundation) (2009), Fact sheet: The global HIV/AIDS epidemic. Accessed 10 April 2010: http://www.kff.org/hivaids/upload/3030-14.pdf

Lock, M. & V.K. Nguyen (2010), *An anthropology of biomedicine*. Oxford: Wiley-Blackwell.

Martin, E. (1978), *Zanzibar: Tradition and revolution*. London: Hamilton.

MoHSW (Ministry of Health and Social Welfare Zanzibar) (2005), *Situation and response. Analysis of the health sector on the HIV/AIDS epidemic in Zanzibar*. Revolutionary Government of Zanzibar

MoHSW (Ministry of Health and Social Welfare Zanzibar) (2009), *Health information bulletin 2008*. Revolutionary Government of Zanzibar.

Nguyen, V.K. (2005), Antiretroviral globalism, biopolitics, and therapeutic citizenship. In: A. Ong & S.J. Collier, eds, *Global assemblages: Technology, politics, and ethics as anthropological problems,* pp. 124-144. Oxford: Blackwell Publishing.

Parkin, D. (2006), The commercialisation of biomedicine and the politics of flight in Zanzibar, Tanzania. *Journal of Ethnic and Migration Studies* 32(4): 697-714.

Parkin, D. (2007), In touch without touching: Islam and healing. In: R. Littlewood, ed., *On knowing and not knowing in the anthropology of medicine,* pp. 194-219. Walnut Creek: Left Coast Press.

Revolutionary Government of Zanzibar (2006), *Zanzibar household budget survey 2004/5*. Zanzibar: Office of Chief Government Statistician.

Revolutionary Government of Zanzibar (2008), *Zanzibar traditional and alternative medicine policy*. Zanzibar: MOHSW.

Robins, S. (2005), Rights passages from 'near death' to 'new life': AIDS activism and treatment testimonies in South Africa. IDS Working Paper No, 251. Brighton: University of Sussex, Institute of Development Studies.

Scheper-Hughes, N. (2002). Bodies for sale – whole or in parts. In: N. Scheper-Hughes & L. Wacquant, eds, *Commodifying bodies*, pp. 1-9. London: Sage Publications.

TACAIDS (2007), *Tanzania public expenditure review. Multisectoral review: HIV/AIDS*. Dar es Salaam: Ministry of Finance.

UNAIDS (2007), *The greater involvement of people living with HIV (GIPA)*. Policy brief. Accessed 10 February 2010 at: http://data.unaids.org/pub/Report/2007/JC1299-PolicyBrief-GIPA_en.pdf

ZAC (2003), *Report on situation and response analysis of HIV/AIDS in Zanzibar*. Zanzibar AIDS Commission.

9

Individual or shared responsibility: The financing of medical treatment in rural Ethiopian households

Marleen Dekker

Illness and health feature prominently in the debate on poverty and there is an extensive literature on vulnerability, risk-coping strategies and the relationship between risk and poverty. It mostly considers the household as the unit of analysis and decision-making and assumes all household members are equally protected when confronted with illness. Although some studies have documented that certain individuals, notably women, are less protected, the mechanisms underlying these outcomes are not well understood. Based on a survey in Ethiopia, this chapter discusses whose assets, savings and relationships are used to meet the costs of treatment. Despite the customary norm that the male head of household is responsible for healthcare expenditures and the wide range of intra-household arrangements, it was found that particularly polygamous women who become ill source money for treatment by themselves, using their own savings, selling assets or acquiring a loan or gift through their networks. Oromo women are an exception as their husbands finance their treatment. These findings suggest that risk-coping strategies are not applied equally between sick household members. With the increasing monetization of healthcare, this adds a differential level of vulnerability to health shocks.

Introduction

Health shocks feature prominently in the debate on poverty. In a context where both biomedical healthcare and traditional healing practices have become increasingly monetized, the costs of treatment can be high and absorb a very significant amount of a household's income (Xu *et al.* 2003; Wagstaff & Doorslaer 2003). If the availability of cash is limited, individuals and households depend on risk-coping strategies to finance access to healthcare and treatment, and may reduce spending on basic needs, sell (productive) assets or borrow money. Such strategies are expensive and may endanger a household's future economic status by depleting its finances through indebtedness and reducing its income-generating capacity by selling productive assets (Scheil-Adlung *et al.* 2006). This, in turn, increases the risk of ending up or being trapped in poverty. Bogale *et al.* (2005), Dercon *et al.* (2005) and Krishna *et al.* (2006) have all demonstrated how the costs of illness contribute significantly to the impoverishment of households in rural Ethiopia and Uganda respectively. If health shocks are salient to understanding poverty dynamics, then understanding the strategies people employ to cope with health shocks is also important for development policy and practice (Bhattamishra & Barret 2010).

Most of the literature on coping with risk considers the household as a unit of analysis and decision-making (Burger *et al.* 1998; Rosenzweig & Stark 1989; Dercon & de Weerdt 2006; Dekker 2004) and assumes unexpected health shocks can be fully insured against within the household. There is now empirical evidence documenting the unequal effects of unexpected health problems on different individuals within the same households (Duflo & Udry 2004) and previous work in Ethiopia has shown that women often bear the brunt when confronted with illness. By considering the nutritional status of individuals, Dercon & Krishnan (2000) showed that women in poor households in southern Ethiopia find it more difficult to recover after illness. And Dekker (2008) found that illness-related labour needs are often not cushioned in the household and can only be met through personal support networks of female relatives. In the absence of such networks, women struggle to respond to the labour needs associated with health shocks.

The above-mentioned studies suggest that individual household members are not always protected against the consequences of illness by other household members. They do not explain the mechanisms behind these outcomes, but note that the vulnerability of individuals within a household is critical in understanding household vulnerability more generally (Alwang, Siegel & Jorgenson 2001). This is especially relevant when access to healthcare becomes monetized and individuals and households have to navigate markets to find treatment. Based on the data set used by Dekker (2008), this chapter considers the extent to which household members can rely on the social, financial or buffer stock assets of fellow household members to gain access to treatment when they are ill. Such intra-household responses to healthcare expenditure are important in the Ethiopian context where costs for care and treatment are rising and treatment is increasingly tied to transactions in the healthcare market. Despite the customary norm that the male head of household is responsible for meeting healthcare costs, polygamous women who are ill often source money for treatment themselves. The extended family, friends and local organizations may provide informal insurance in terms of assistance but the women also use their savings or sell assets to finance treatment.

This chapter is organized as follows. The first section provides a brief description of the Ethiopian healthcare sector today. This is followed by a description of the data and the context of this study, including access to health facilities. The following section discusses the strategies used to finance treatment and provides more details about these strategies and whose savings, assets and relationships are used. These descriptives are then contextualized in some case studies before the factors that explain the differences in savings, assets and relationships are analyzed.

Illness and health in Ethiopia

The Ethiopian public healthcare sector is characterized by low coverage rates for modern healthcare, and the country scores low on health outcomes. The 2009 Human Development Report ranks Ethiopia 171st out of 182 countries on the Human Development Index. Life expectancy is 54.7 years and the country has a malnutrition rate among under-fives of 38% (UNDP 2009). Between 60% and 80% of the country's health problems are estimated to be caused by preventable infectious diseases and malnutrition. Despite the high rate of disease, health-service utilization remains low, particularly for clinical care. In the 2004 Ethiopian Welfare Monitoring Survey, less than half the respondents who reported having health problems had consulted modern health institutions or traditional healers for assistance. Consultation rates are lower in rural areas and among women (CSA 2004). The average distance to a person's nearest health facility was 7.7 km in 2000 (Federal Ministry of Health 2006). Healthcare utilization is hampered by shortages of personnel and medical equipment, high expenses, long waiting times, the unavailability of drugs, a lack of laboratory equipment for simple tests and the non-cooperative behaviour of staff (*Ibid.*).

The provision of health services in Ethiopia has long been dominated by the public sector and the number of facilities run by the Ministry of Health has expanded considerably in recent years. After the legalization of the private sector in the mid-1990s, the numbers of private (profit-making) facilities, retail pharmaceutical outlets, and NGO and faith-based providers have risen steadily, especially in the urban areas. The government has made the expansion of the private healthcare sector a clear policy objective but the institutional framework remains weak (Lindelow & Serneels 2006).

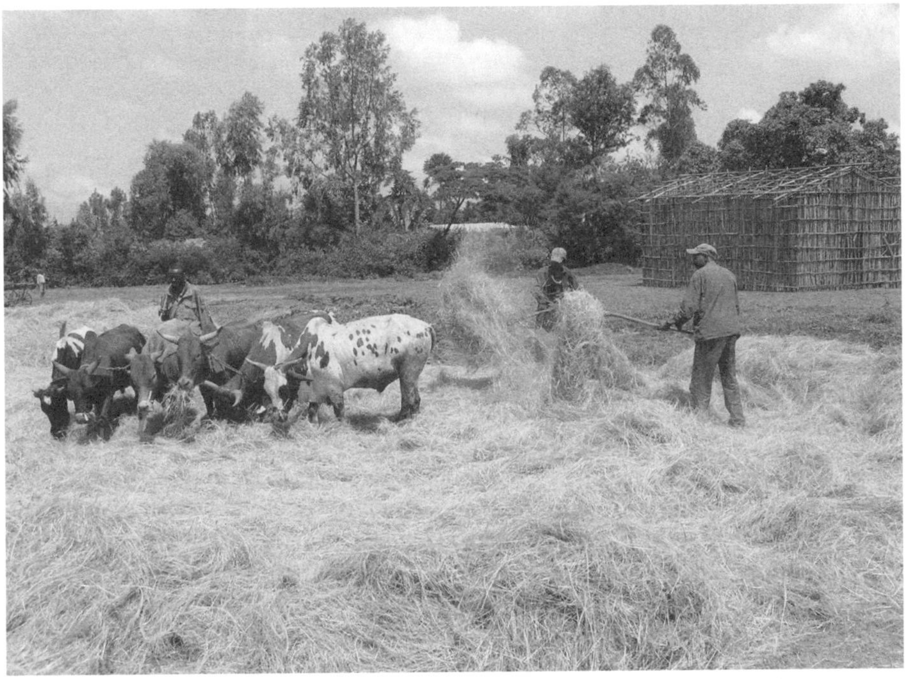

Photo 9.1 Farmers winnowing *teff* in Turufe Kecheme
[Photo: Marleen Dekker]

Since the early 1950s, cost recovery has been part of Ethiopia's public healthcare system. Nominal amounts are charged for outpatient registration, consultations, lab tests, routine diagnostic procedures and hospitalization costs. Higher fees are asked for prescription drugs and (inpatient) surgical procedures. When originally introduced, the fees covered a substantial part of the total costs of the services. However in the last five years, fees have become merely symbolic from a cost-recovery perspective but still pose a significant obstacle for those seeking care, especially the poor and those with limited access to cash.

Per capita spending on health in Ethiopia remains among the lowest in the world. Spending from domestic and external sources accounted for 49% of total spending on healthcare in Ethiopia in 2000. Private expenditures constitute 36%, while NGOs cover nearly 10% and private enterprises 5%. Private expenditure predominantly comes from out-of-pocket (OOP) expenditure (80%), which indicates that market transactions are important in the health sector (Tigandebage & Macintosch 2005). OOP expenditures on health account, on average, for approximately 1% of total household expenditure (50 Birr or US$

6) and are mainly for pharmaceutical products and transportation (World Bank 2005).

Data and the context of the study[1]

The data used in this chapter are from a survey conducted in the Ethiopian village of Turufe Kecheme (see Map 9.1). They are unique in the sense that all the households in the village were visited and the aim was to interview both the husband and the wife (or wives) in every household. A total of 357 households and 670 individuals were interviewed.[2] Given the cross section of the data, the results presented describe only a snap-shot in time. Reference to other research material on the village allows insights into additional on-going processes.[3]

Turufe Kecheme is one of three villages in a *kebele*[4] in Shashemene *wereda* in the Eastern Shewa Zone of Oromiya Region. It is situated in a relatively fertile area and has two rainy seasons that allow the cultivation of cereals (*tef*,[5] maize, millet and wheat) and vegetables (potatoes and onions) for own consumption and to sell at market. Many residents are actively engaged in trading and other non-agricultural activities to generate or supplement their incomes. The village has small shops with basic necessities and drinking houses that sell locally brewed spirits. Turufe Kecheme is well connected to local markets and government services by an all-weather road that connects the village to the main road between Addis Abeba and Kenya. Products can be sold at Kuyera market which is 2 km away or at the markets in Shashemene and Negele, which are slightly further away (Gezahegn *et al.* 2006).

Turufe Kecheme was set up in 1985 during the villigization programme when people who were living across the *kebele* territory were organized into compact villages to facilitate the provision of services. Although located in an

---

1 The Turufe Kecheme data set (TK data set) was collected between May 2005 and August 2005 in collaboration with the Department of Agricultural and Resource Economics, Debub University, Awassa. The funding for data collection by the Amsterdam Institute of International Development and the Netherlands Organization of Scientific Research (NWO) is gratefully acknowledged.

2 The data set and the village are described in more detail in Dekker (2008).

3 Turufe Kecheme is part of two long-term research projects involving the collection of qualitative and quantitative information as part of the Ethiopian Rural Household Survey (ERHS): http://www.csae.ox.ac.uk/datasets/Ethiopia-ERHS/ERHS-main.html and the Well-being in Developing project (WeD-Ethiopia): http://www.wed-ethiopia.org.

4 A *kebele* or municipality is the lowest administrative division in Ethiopia.

5 *Tef* or *teff* is a local grain.

Map 9.1 Ethiopia, showing research location

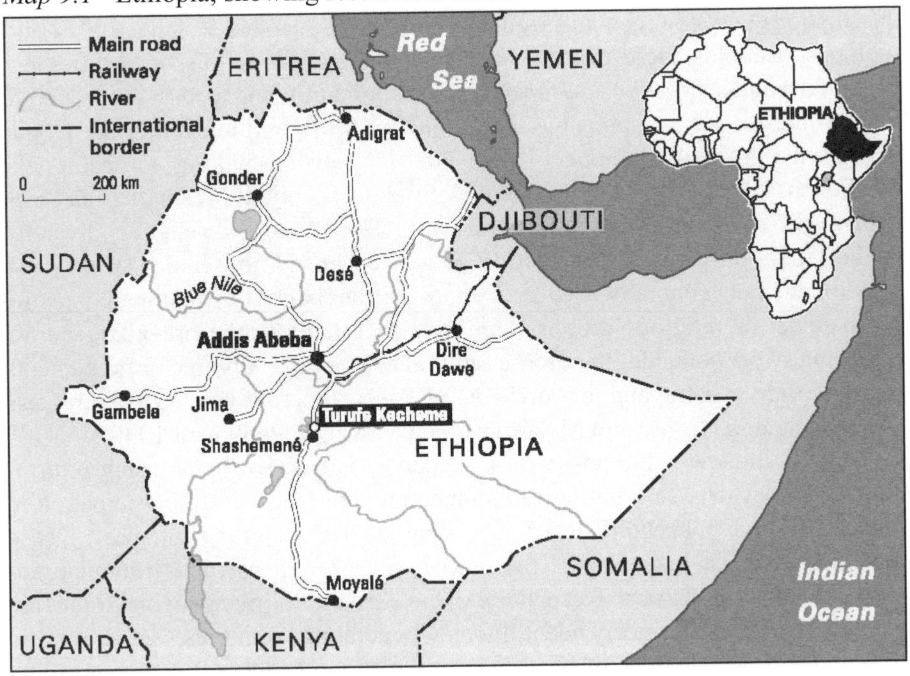

area originally inhabited by the Oromo, the rural areas surrounding Shashemene town are known for their history of migration (Gezahegn *et al.* 2006). This is reflected in the village's ethnic composition and religious diversity. Just over half of the respondents in the study were Oromo. Amhara, Tigrayan and Wolayita people formed relatively larger minorities, while the Kambata and Hadiya were considerably fewer in number. Gamo, Gurage, Sidama and Silte make up only a tiny fraction of the population. There are four religious denominations in the village: Islam, Orthodox Christianity and Kalehiwot (Protestant Church) have the largest followings, while a minority attend the Catholic Church. There are many local associations such as funeral and cattle associations (*iddir*, *tera*) or savings clubs (*equb*) but these are not organized along strictly ethnic or religious lines.

Most households consist of a married couple and their children and other extended (parents, siblings, grandchildren) or unrelated (servants) household members. In polygamous households (some 10% of couples), wives may live on separate residential plots or may live together on one plot. Approximately 15% of households are headed by a woman, (widows, divorcees or wives with husbands working elsewhere). Many studies have reported asymmetric power distributions between men and women in Ethiopia (Seebens & Sauer 2007), and within households there can be substantial differences in responsibilities between husbands and wives. Women are predominantly engaged in reproductive work while men are responsible for productive work and allocating the labour of household family members (Dito 2010). Decision-making regarding expenditures is generally left to men, with the exception of smaller incomes generated by women through off-farm work. The ethnic and religious diversity in the village influences the position of women in the household. Oromo and Muslim women generally live in a more patriarchal set-up compared to the other ethnic or religious groups. This may be related to the prevailing norms regarding work outside the house and marriage and divorce arrangements (higher bride wealth and no division of assets upon divorce) that are less common among Oromo and Muslim women (Bevan & Pankhurst 1996).

Box 9.1 illustrates the position of women in Turufe Kecheme using information from our data set relating to income-generating activities, participation in public life and household decision-making on risk-coping strategies.[6] These indicators suggest that, despite the patriarchical set-up of rural Ethiopian society, women in Turufe Kecheme do have room to manoeuvre: some are actively engaged in independent income-generating activities, some discuss development with leaders of local organizations and *kebele* officials but only a very small minority have any independent say in decisions on coping strategies.

Illness and health in Turufe Kecheme

Illnesses that are common in the village include tuberculosis, eye diseases and kidney problems in the dry season and malaria and colds in the rainy season (Gezahegn *et al.* 2006). There are also outbreaks of cholera, leprosy and tuberculosis. Given the difficulties in access to healthcare in Ethiopia reported in the previous section, it should be noted that Turufe Kecheme is not representative of the Ethiopian context as households have easy access to Shashemene General Hospital, which is only 2.5 km away. The facilities at this public hospital, which include a leprosy centre and an eye clinic, are not rated highly by the villagers and shortages of medicines are common. Those who can afford it prefer to go to private clinics in Shashemene town or Awassa for

---

6 This question was asked independently of the actual illness(es) experienced and coping strategies used and therefore does not necessarily relate to illnesses but to a broader range of decision-making.

Box 9.1 The position of women in Turufe Kecheme

One indicator concerning the position of women in the village relates to income-generating activities. Most economic activities undertaken there are joint (farming) activities with the husband and wife (and other household members) working in the family fields. Some 60% of the women reported alsobeing engaged in some other economic activity independently of their husband. These are usually non-farm activeities such as weaving, pottery, petty trade or brewing.

Another indicator of their position in society relates to their position in public life and the extent to which they participate in discussions about village issues. In the questionnaire, respondents were asked if they discussed issues related to their village with other members of their household, their neighbours, co-members of local organizations (such as *iddir* or *equb*), leaders of these organizations, the *kebele* leadership or people living outside the *kebele*. Not surprisingly, men were more likely to discuss issues related to the development of their *kebele* than women, and these differences are statistically significant at the 0.05 level. More than half of the women discussed issues related to the development of the *kebele* within their household and with neighbours or fellow members of one of the local organizations. 20% discussed community issues with people from outside the *kebele*. About 40% of the women also discussed these issues with the leaders of the local organization or with *kebele* officials (compared with 55% and 62% of the men respectively).

There were also questions about decision-making concerning risk-coping strategies within households and whether couples decided jointly on the type of coping strategies or whether one of the spouses made the decision. Just over half of the women reported using risk-coping strategies, such as selling assets or asking relatives or neighbours for help. In only a few cases (3-8%) did women decide on these strategies themselves, while in 34-40% of the cases the men decided independently. This was slightly different when working to earn additional income; 13% of the women reported that they decided on this independently, while 45% said that this was their husband's decision and 40% indicated that it was a joint decision.

serious illnesses. In addition, there is a Catholic mission with a health centre and a Seventh Day Adventist clinic within 6 km of the village (Pankhurst & Bevan 2007). There is a private doctor and pharmacy some 2 km from the village and respondents reported using self-medication and treatment too. The village has two traditional birth attendants and two health workers who were trained by the Ministry of Health and an NGO. These health workers do not give consultations but do provide condoms and assist in vaccination campaigns. The nearest ritual healer (*Kaleecha*) is two-hour walk away but there are traditional doctors who set bones and prescribe herbs in the *kebele* (Gezahegn *et al.* 2006).

This range of medical services can be put in a quantitative perspective by using data from the 1995 ERHS Survey (CSAE 2010). Here we specifically refer to the data collected in Turufe Kecheme. In 1995, households in Turufe Kecheme reported 70 cases of illness in the month prior to receiving the questionnaire. In more than 75% of these cases patients sought treatment for their illness, and those who did not reported that the illnesses were mild or could not be treated. Other patients forewent treatment because it was too expensive. Given the short distance to healthcare facilities, distance or transport costs did not feature among villagers' reasons for not seeking treatment in Turufe Kecheme. Most patients went to Shashemene General Hospital (64%), the nearest health centre (4%) or the nearest pharmacy (9.5%). Some 7.5% of patients visited a hospital or health centre further away, sometimes because they considered the nearest hospital or health centre to offer poor-quality service or facilities or because they wanted to visit a private or NGO facility. The remaining 15% visited traditional healers.

Data from the ERHS show an increase in expenditure on health and healing over the past two decades. The survey measured nominal expenditure on modern medical treatment, medicines, traditional medicines and healers separately. Comparing household expenditure over the four months prior to the survey of households in Turufe Kecheme shows an increase in average expenditure on biomedical care from Birr 9.5 in 1995 to Birr 33.7 in 2004. Costs for healing were Birr 1.5 in 1995 and Birr 3.4 in 2004 respectively. Not only did average expenditure increase but the range increased considerably too. In 1995 the maximum amount paid for biomedical care was Birr 285, while in 2004 the figure was Birr 740. For traditional healing and medicines, the maximum increased from Birr 143 Birr to Birr 370.[7]

According to custom, it is the head of the household, in most cases the husband, who is responsible for covering health costs (Gezahegn *et al.* 2006; Bevan & Pankhurst 1996; Ellis & Woldehanna 2005). Women in the village also mentioned that husbands take their wives to the clinic or hospital and buy fruit or slaughter a beast for her if she needs to regain her strength. *Iddirs* may provide loans to finance healthcare expenditure but these need to be repaid and failure to do so may lead to exclusion from a funeral association (Pankhurst & Bevan 2007). The poor and destitute can obtain free healthcare at public hospitals with government support. To access those free services, households need a letter from the local *kebele* office for which 'proof of need' has to be obtained from other members of the village (Dekker 2008). At a national level, some 5%

---

7 Similar trends were found for the other villages in the ERHS. Expenditure was comparable to the national average of Birr 50 in 2005 (World Bank 2005). The increases reported are higher than the level of inflation.

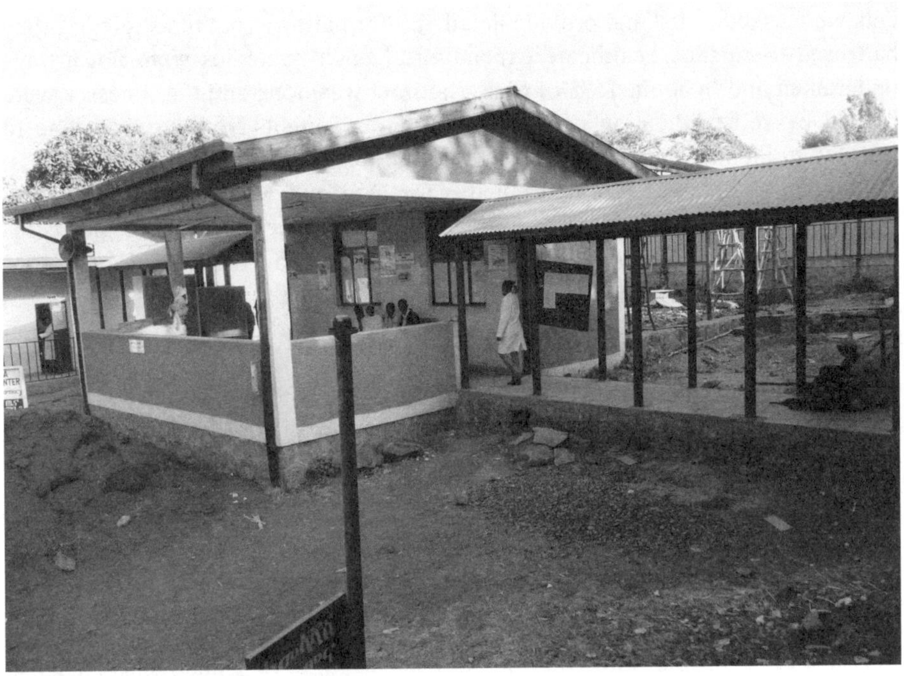

Photo 9.2 A clinic in rural Ethiopia
[Photo: Marleen Dekker]

of outpatients and 25-35% of inpatients have access to free services (Stierle *et al.* 1999).

As is customary, the male head of the household is responsible for healthcare expenditure and a distinction is made here between male-headed households and female-headed households. Those without a male head are likely to experience different dynamics and this distinction has thus to be considered in the analysis below.

Illnesses and financing treatment

In the individual questionnaires in 2005, respondents were asked about the incidences and severity of health shocks that had affected respondents, members of their household and family members over the previous twelve months. The question was worded in such a way that it solicited information on major illnesses only. These were referred to as illnesses that led to a reduction in asset holdings, income or consumption. The 670 individual respondents reported 374 illnesses among themselves, 320 illnesses among household members and 91 illnesses among family members. When such illnesses were reported, respondents were asked to list and provide detailed information about the strategies they had used to finance healthcare expenditure.[8] Such strategies were not always undertaken and in about 15% of cases, nothing was done and the illnesses were treated by self-medication or no treatment was sought. Nothing was done to respond to labour shortages or a reduction in income resulting from the illness. Taking no action was reported equally for men and women who fell ill but female-headed households more frequently reported having no strategies compared to male-headed households. Questions focused on risk-coping behaviour and did not look into the type, quantity or quality of the treatment sought.

Respondents who sought treatment indicated a wide range of strategies in response to the financial needs related to treatment, comprising both traditional and biomedical care and medicines.[9] Usually, one type of strategy was undertaken to deal with the health problem, while a small minority (6%) reported adopting more than one strategy to finance treatment. Table 9.1 shows that the majority of individuals reported having sold assets (39%), used savings (23%) or received informal assistance (20%) in response to the unexpected health problems they or their household/family members experienced. Free medical care or assistance from a local organization, such as an *iddir*, was reported only in 5% and 3% of the cases respectively. The proportion of recipients receiving free medical care is in line with the national average for outpatients. This also suggests that OOP expenditures were the village's main form of healthcare financing and that most healthcare transactions take place in markets (Tibandebage & Mackintosch 2004).

The sale of assets or assistance categories encompasses a range of activities. This refers predominantly to selling produce from expected harvests in advance (61%), and selling animals (21%) and domestic assets (16%). Occasionally equipment (2%) or a house or piece of land (2%) is sold. These items suggest asset sales can indeed be expensive coping strategies. Selling grain before it has been harvested and selling animals, equipment or land can easily endanger a household's food security or future economic productivity.

Assistance networks are primarily composed of links in the proximity of the village. Assistance mostly came from someone living in the village (69%). Some 15% reported assistance from someone living in Kuyera, the market village 2 km from Turufe Kecheme. Assistance was predominantly received from local organizations (*iddir*, *equb* or NGOs) and immediate relatives, while 20%

---

8 The information available on the nature of the symptoms was not sufficient to be included in the analysis.

9 The questionnaire did not address details on spending patterns (type of facility, medication, transport etc).

Table 9.1 Coping strategies to finance the treatment of ill household members (%)

Strategy	All households (N=626)	Male-headed households (N=529)	Female-headed households (N=97)
Savings	23	24	22
Sold assets	39	39	38
Informal assistance	20	22	13
Money lender	4	4	7
Increased work	4	3	5
Free medical care	4	4	8
Local organization	1	1	0
Other	4	4	6
Total	100	100	100

Source: Household Survey (2005)

reported assistance from friends. Assistance is clearly linked to indebtedness as most of the assistance was provided as a loan that was to be repaid without interest (48%) or with interest (23%). In 29% of cases, assistance was offered as a gift. In the majority of cases (84%), assistance was provided immediately when the need arose and came in response to a request by the respondent or another household member. Assistance did not come automatically but was usually requested: in 10% of cases it was offered to a household without them having to ask for it. The data also suggests that assistance is provided in reciprocal networks that span time: 88% of respondents indicated that they had received assistance from this person before, and in 82% of cases the respondent had provided assistance to this person as well.

The third and fourth columns in Table 9.1 show the strategies taken by male- and female-headed households respectively. Although the differences in percentages are small, they are statistically significant (Chi-squared test: 12.7 at 0.08 level). The use of savings, the sale of assets and informal assistance are dominant in the coping strategies for female-headed households but they are less prevalent than in male-headed households, especially with respect to informal assistance. Female-headed households more often reported receiving free medical care, borrowing money from a money lender, increasing the amount of work undertaken or using other strategies to access money to pay for treatment. This is what might be expected since female-headed households tend to be poorer.

Tables 9.2a and 9.2b illustrate the proportional breakdown of whose assets or savings and which relationships are used to finance healthcare expenses for the three dominant strategies, again for male- and female-headed households respectively.[10] For male-headed households (Table 9.2a), in all three types of strategies it is predominantly the head of household who uses his savings, sells his own or the household's assets and uses his social ties to obtain informal assistance. Although of lesser importance, the spouse is also active across the three categories, particularly when it comes to using her social ties to access informal assistance. Other household members, including adult children, are only partially involved. A different picture emerges for female-headed households (Table 9.2b). The heads are dominant when it comes to selling assets or informal assistance but when savings are used to finance treatment these are often the savings of other household members. Given the relatively small number of observations in these categories, conclusions from this comparison should only be drawn with care.

A more diverse picture emerges when the amount of money generated from these strategies is considered. Tables 9.3a and 9.3b present the average proceeds in Ethiopian Birr for each of the three strategies per type of household member, in male- and female-headed households respectively. Table 9.3a shows that the amount generated in male-headed households by drawing on cash savings is on

Table 9.2a Assets, savings and relations used to cope with illness-related costs in male-headed households (%)

Household member	Use of savings (N=106)	Sales of assets (N=168)	Informal assistance (N=100)
Head	77	79	61
Spouse	17	13	36
Other h'hold member	6	8	3
Total	100	100	100

Source: Household Survey (2005)

Table 9.2b Assets, savings and relations used to cope with illness-related costs in female-headed households (%)

Household member	Use of savings (N=19)	Sales of assets (N=32)	Informal assistance (N=10)
Head	37	88	80
Other h'hold member	63	12	20
Total	100	100	100

Source: Household Survey (2005)

10 Due to missing information on the identity of the person whose assets, savings and networks were used to finance treatment, the total numbers in these tables do not correspond to the total number reported in Table 9.1.

Table 9.3a Proceeds of strategies undertaken by household members (in Birr) in male-headed households

Household member	Use of savings	Sales of assets	Informal assistance
Head	66	140	94
Spouse	65	116	89
Other h'hold member	35	198	87
Total	66	150	97

Source: Household Survey (2005)

Table 9.3b Proceeds of strategies undertaken by household members (in Birr) in female-headed households

Household member	Use of savings	Sales of assets	Informal assistance
Head	37	142	711
Other h'hold member	230	440	103
Total	147	165	495

Source: Household Survey (2005)

average only Birr 66, while sales of assets and informal assistance via networks generate larger amounts. Across all three strategies, the amounts generated by the head of household are higher than those generated by their spouses, although the differences are not large. It is interesting to note that in male-headed households, other household members can make an important contribution. They are not frequently involved in strategies (Table 9.2a) but if the need arises, they can use valuable assets or access assistance through their networks to finance treatment. The distribution in female-headed households is more skewed and the amounts generated are higher. Although female-headed households use informal networks less frequently (Table 9.1), when heads do ask for assistance, they are able to secure large amounts of money. Other household members invest a lot of their savings or sell high-value assets to finance treatment for household or family members.

To address the division of responsibilities in more detail, the identity of the patient is considered in Tables 9.4a and 9.4b, which cross-tabulate the position of the patient in the household with the person who used his/her assets, savings or relationships to finance treatment for male- and female-headed households respectively. Table 9.4a shows that when the male head of household was sick, the large majority financed healthcare expenditures themselves, while some received finance from their spouses, (adult) children or other household members. For a small majority of the spouses (58%) who were ill, their husbands provided the money needed for treatment. There was, however, a substantial minority (39%) who financed their treatment themselves. Detailed information on the provider of informal assistance reveals that these women were to some extent assisted by their male blood relatives (father, uncles, brothers) but friends and local organizations provided assistance to a greater degree. The costs of treatment for other household members were predominantly catered for by the head of household or by themselves but they were also assisted by relatives outside the household.[11] In female-headed households, the ill head of the household predominantly financed her own treatment with help from her children and other household members. A similar but reverse picture emerges for other household members, who cater for themselves but are also assisted by the female head.

The statistics presented here show the diversity of arrangements, roles and strategies employed to finance treatment. To the extent that the customary norm is still valid, the data suggest that heads of households do indeed cover the health costs of their household members, but women and other household members can also actively generate considerable amounts of money to finance treatment, which illustrates how the sick are able to navigate to find money for

Table 9.4a Proportional distribution of assets, savings and relations used during illness in male-headed households (%)

	Patient: Head (N=87)	Patient: Spouse (N=85)	Patient: Other hh member (N=13)
Head	95	58	46
Spouse	2	39	8
Other h'hold member	2	4	46
Total	100	100	100

Source: Household Survey (2005)

Table 9.4b Proportional distribution of assets, savings and relations used during illness in female-headed households (%)

	Patient: Head (N=35)	Patient: Other hh member (N=11)
Head	74	36
Other h'hold member	26	64
Total	100	100

Source: Household Survey (2005)

[11] It should be noted however that the number of children or other household members are small and differences should therefore be taken as being indicative only.

treatment both within their household but also outside it. The next section investigates this diversity by considering five cases in more detail.

Diversity in financing treatment

This section looks at the situation of a widow, a polygamous marriage where one of the wives lives on a separate plot in the village, and three monogamous marriages with different household compositions, wealth status and ethnic background.

Mrs Shuko W. is a 50-year-old Oromo widow who lives in the village with three sons (aged between 10 and 20), three daughters (aged between 8 and 18) and an eight-year-old grandchild. She came to the village about 30 years ago when she got married. When her husband died, she inherited two *timad* of land and some livestock but she does not have many other assets and is in the poorest wealth category. Although she is a member of the Catholic Church and a local *iddir* and *mahber*, she does not actively engage in village labour and credit arrangements, but has good friends and an aunt in the village. In 2004/5 her household was confronted with four illnesses when she and three of her dependents were sick. She suffered headaches for about a month and she had to sell a sheep (for Birr 80) to finance her treatment. After she had recovered, her 18-year-old daughter experienced kidney problems and a cash loan of Birr 175 was needed to pay her medical bill. This was an interest-free loan from one of her friends who had assisted her before. Then her grandchild had TB and needed hospital treatment. Mrs Shuko W. got another interest-free loan, of Birr 200, this time from a labour-sharing partner of her daughter's. And two months later, her son had chest pains and had to go for treatment. Again she was able to secure an interest-free loan, of Birr 185 from a friend who she had never before borrowed from in an informal credit transaction.

In this case, the household was confronted with multiple illnesses and responded with different strategies, using different networks each time to raise cash to pay for treatment.

Mrs Shuko J. is a 42-year-old woman who lives with three of her adult children and her four-year-old son. Her husband lives in a different part of the village with his second wife and four of their children. When he married his second wife, he gave her one *timad* of land so she could take care of herself and her children, as is customary in Oromo culture. With one cow and few other assets, she is in the second-poorest wealth category. She came to the village some 35 years ago when she got married. Although she regularly attends the mosque and is a member of a funeral and a cattle *iddir*, she does not engage in credit or labour-sharing activities in the village. When she was seriously ill with malaria in 2005, she borrowed Birr 100 from her sister, who lives in a rural area some way from Turufe Kecheme, to finance her treatment. She was not assisted by her husband, whose household falls in the middle income category and who owns a considerable amount of land (4 *timad*) and a few head of cattle. He is actively engaged in risk-coping strategies for his second wife. When her uncle died in 2004, he sold a sheep to provide Birr 40 for his bereaved family-in-law. And when the husband and their one-year-old girl got gastritis, he sold part of his harvest in advance to pay for their treatment. And recently when the baby had a fever, the second wife borrowed Birr 30 from one of her friends in the cattle *iddir*.

This case of a polygamous household presents a situation in which the first wife is left to fend for herself, while the husband focuses predominantly on the well-being of his second wife and their children. He is not exclusively responsible for financing treatment as when his daughter fell ill for a second time, her mother (the second wife) secured a loan to cover the treatment costs.

Mrs Werke B. came to live in Turufe Kecheme 10 years ago when she got married. She and her husband live on the plot of her deceased father-in-law with their four children (aged 8 months to 10 years), two brothers (aged 18 and 20), a sister of her husband's (aged 15) and a servant. They are all Oromo and Muslim and are actively engaged in village social life and are members of *iddir*, *mahber* and labour- and credit-sharing arrangements. With 4 *timad* of land, and land that they sharecrop with other village members, they are seen as very successful farmers. And with 2 oxen, other livestock and a wide range of assets, they are among the wealthiest households in the village. When her father-in-law died (in the year before the survey), her husband sold part of the harvest in advance to finance his burial (Birr 2000). The same strategy was used to pay her medical fees when she suffered pain and sought treatment for it (Birr 80). When their six-year-old daughter suffered joint and muscle pain, her husband used some of their savings (Birr 85), and a similar strategy was used when one of their family members needed treatment due to parasites (Birr 80).

In this wealthy family, the male head of household is in control of all expenditures related to health shocks. He covered his father's funeral, his wife's illness and those of their child and a family member. All monetary needs were financed through the family's own savings or harvest; and no one else was approached for assistance, in contrast with the next two cases where the wives financed all the treatment.

Mrs Amerech M. (aged 22) lives with her husband (aged 34) and two sons (aged 1 and 3). She and her husband are Wolayitta and their parents, who are both dead, also lived in Turufe Kecheme. They own one *timad* of land and sharecrop another with someone from the village. With few cattle or other assets, they fall in the second-poorest wealth quintile. Amerech and her husband attend the Kalehiwot Church and are actively engaged in a funeral and cattle *iddir* and in labour-sharing and informal credit networks in the village. When Amerech had stomach ache, she received Birr 50 from a friend in Kuyera to finance medical treatment. Their three-year-old boy had some skin problems that lasted about a month and she spent Birr 30 on treatment, which she financed through the advance sale of part of their harvest. And when their younger son had ear problems, she received a Birr 20 cash loan from relatives in Kuyera to buy ear drops for him.

Mrs Ayene U. was born in Turufe Kecheme and lives with her husband and four children in the village. They are Oromo and Muslim and actively engage in village associations and its social life. They own two *timad* of land and a reasonable number of cattle and other assets and therefore come in the middle wealth category. In 2005 she suffered serious headaches for about a month and was not able to do her domestic activities anymore so had to take one of her sons out of school to help in the house. She also decided to sell some livestock to finance treatment (Birr 100). When, their one-year-old son had diarrhoea two months later, she used some of her savings (Birr 5) for oral rehydration therapy.

The cases here show a diverse picture in terms of whose assets, savings and networks are used to finance treatment. They also shed light on the elements that underlie these arrangements. Some relate to the socio-economic background of the household, such as its composition and wealth status, while others highlight the internal dynamics around responsibilities and the availability of resources to individual household members due to the influence of one's ethnic background. Arrangements are different in polygamous households compared to those in monogamous households or in patriarchal Oromo households compared to more liberal non-Oromo households. In wealthier households, the male head may find it easier to finance treatment simply because more resources are available. If this is not the case, the male head may want to finance treatment but does not have the means to do so and has to ask his wife or other household members to contribute. Alternatively, if other household members have considerable savings or assets, they may finance the treatment and heads or spouses will not have to do so, signalling an intra-household process whereby those with more resources pay the largest share of the medical bill. Yet another option is that the heads have the resources but do not want to spend money on the medical costs of their spouses (in the case of male-headed households) or other household members, who are then left to take care of themselves. In other cases, the wife may chose to fend for herself as she does not want her husband to know about her condition or to interfere in her (choice of) treatment. The cases above do not illustrate the exact intra-household dynamics at play and more in-depth information is needed about the severity of the illness concerned. The cases do show the variations in arrangements and multi-variate analysis is used in the next section to find communalities in the responsibilities and strategies displayed.

A multi-variate analysis: Who finances treatment?

It is customarily the responsibility of the household head to cover the financial costs of illness and the case studies presented in the previous section suggest this practice is indeed common. However, a sizeable minority of spouses who fall ill in male-headed households pay for their own medical expenses. In female-headed households, other household members generally generate their own revenue to finance treatment. This may have to do with the resources available to the head and/or other members of the household but may also reflect the different cultural backgrounds in the village when it comes to the functioning of households and the respective responsibilities for and of different household members.

To explore this issue further, the factors that contribute to the variation in initiatives observed across male-headed households in the village were analyzed.[12] This was done by means of a multi-variate analysis that allows, for example, the effect of the identity of the patient to be isolated from factors such as wealth status, household composition and the type of strategy used. A multinomial logit analysis was performed on the identity of the person whose assets, savings or relations were used to finance the treatment. Multinomial logit regression is used when the dependent variable in question is nominal (a set of categories that cannot be ordered in any meaningful way) and consists of more than two categories. The head, the spouse or other household members were used as categories and the model estimated the influence of a variety of factors related to the probability that a head, a spouse or other household members respectively would use their savings, assets or relationships to finance the treatment of a sick household member.

Factors that may contribute to the observed differences in the dependent variable include those related to both the reported health shock and the strategy used to meet the financial needs for treatment, and the characteristics of the households and individuals involved. Factors related to the health shock and the strategy include dummy variables on the person who experienced the health problem (the head, the spouse or another household member) and dummy variables on the strategies deployed (the sale of assets, the use of savings, informal assistance or another strategy). The omitted dummies in the analysis

---

12 Here the analysis is restricted to male-headed households only as the dynamics in households where both husband and wife are present were of particular interest.

are other household members and other strategies. A number of household characteristics may affect the strategies deployed. When a household is confronted with numerous health shocks, it may be more difficult for the head of the household to protect all members against the consequences. For this reason, the number of shocks reported by the individual over the past year were included in a variable with values ranging from zero to five, with the expectation that the heads would be less likely to undertake a strategy if the household was confronted with more shocks. Other factors that may be relevant at the household level are cultural background, here measured as a dummy variable that equals one when the household head is Oromo. In Turufe Kecheme, this means one belongs to the original population of the area and has a strong patriarchal orientation in the household. Given this tendency, Oromo heads of households were expected to be more involved in the strategies, as this is part of their prescribed responsibility. Heads will also find it easier to cater for all the needs of the individual household members if the household has more resources. For this reason, a wealth indicator was included and the head was expected to be more active in strategies in wealthier households than in poorer households where resources for treatment are less readily available and individual household members may need to cater for their own needs. The wealth indicator used is the factor score on an asset-based wealth index ranging from -2.01 (poor) to 2.43 (rich). The index is based on housing characteristics (toilet facilities and iron roofing sheets) and ownership of assets (a plough, sickle, spade, lamp, spray cart, radio, bicycle, sewing machine, watch, clock, modern bed, blanket, mattress, sofa, table, wardrobe, leather mat and another house outside the village).[13] In the previous sections it was noted that adult household members may share the responsibility of the household head and contribute to risk-coping assets and relations. A variable that counts the number of adults in the household was thus also included and it was expected that other household members would be more actively involved if the number of adults in the household was higher. Differences in the age of the individuals involved were also taken into account.

The results of the multinomial regression analysis are shown in Table 9.5. For simplicity's sake, the table presents positive (+) or negative (-) effects and their statistical significance.[14] The coefficients on the variables in the panel on the spouse and other household members respectively should be interpreted as a

---

[13] For more details on the construction and use of asset-based wealth indices, see Sahn & Stifel (2000) and Dekker (2006) who constructed and reviewed the use of asset-based wealth indices in the Ethiopian context.

[14] The statistical significance of the effect is captured in the p-value, with a lower p-value signalling a higher statistical significance.

change relative to the head of the household. This means, for example, that, all things equal, if a spouse falls ill, it is more likely that she herself will finance her own treatment than that the head of household will use his savings, assets or relations to obtain the finances required for her treatment (positive coefficient with p value of 0.008 on the variable spouse in the spouse panel). Relative to their husbands, a female spouse is less likely to have to use her savings, assets or relationships to finance treatment if she has an Oromo husband and if she is older.

For the likelihood that other household members will use their savings, assets or networks to finance treatment, there is a negative and marginally significant coefficient on wealth (suggesting that the head may have more resources to cater for needs). Relative to household heads, other household members are more likely to finance treatment if there are more adults (including themselves) in their household, suggesting that resident adult children may shoulder responsibility for themselves in the household, or share it with their father. At the same time, other household members are less likely than the household head to use their own resources when the household is confronted with unexpected illness. When taking all these factors into account, age also plays a role. The older the other household members are, the less likely they are to finance treatment costs through their own savings, networks or assets. This may show that heads take care of parents who live with their son or son-in-law.

What emerges strongly in the analysis is that, despite the customary responsibility of the heads of households to provide finance for medical expenditures, spouses in male-headed households often have to use their own networks, savings or assets to generate money to finance healthcare treatment. This is not, however, the case in households with Oromo heads. These differences call for a more detailed analysis of the characteristics of the spouses. The position of a spouse in the household is also likely to be determined by the presence of other wives. The effects of polygamy can be different. Polygamous households may be larger and the head may not be in a position to cater for the needs of all household members (part of this effect is already picked up by the number of adult household members). If this is the case, the effect of polygamy would be similar for spouses and other household members. Alternatively, spouses in polygamous households are more likely to have to cater for themselves, especially women who live on a separate plot and have been allotted a part of their husband's land for themselves, while the husband (sometimes) provides for their children.

To test this, a dummy variable was added to the analysis to equal one if the household head has more than one wife and as an interaction term between this variable and the variable spouse (patient). If the inclusion of these additional variables results in the disappearance of the effect of the patient spouse, the spouse effect is caused by polygamous women. If the 'patient-spouse effect' remains significant after the inclusion of the additional variables, the spouse effect is driven by other unobserved factors. The results of this additional analysis are presented in the third column of Table 9.5. Controlling for polygamous household heads does not change the results for other household members relative to the head of household, but the results in the panel of spouses change considerably. Although the coefficient on the spouse-patient variable is still positive, it is no longer significant. The coefficient on polygamous household is not significantly different from zero but the interaction term between spouse (patient) and polygamous household is. This suggests that the results on spouses in the second column were in fact driven by spouses in polygamous households. If spouses in polygamous households become ill, they are more likely to finance

Table 9.5 Multinomial regression analysis on the identity of the person whose assets, savings or relationships are used to finance healthcare treatment

Category	Variable	Coefficient	p-value	Coefficient	p-value
Spouse	Head (patient)	-		-	
	Spouse (patient)	+	***	+	
	Savings	-		-	
	Sale of assets	-		-	
	Informal networks	+	*	+	*
	Number of shocks	-		-	
	Oromo	-	***	-	***
	Wealth	+		+	
	Adult hh members	+		+	
	Age	-	**	-	
	Polygamous marriage			+	
	Polygamous* spouse			+	**
Other household member	Head (patient)	-		-	
	Spouse (patient)	-		-	
	Savings	-		+	
	Sale of assets	-		-	
	Informal networks	-		-	
	Number of shocks	-	*	-	*
	Oromo	+		+	
	Wealth	-	*	-	*
	Adult hh members	+	***	+	***
	Age	-	***	-	***
	Polygamous marriage			-	
	Polygamous* spouse			-	

Analysis based on 291 observations Pseudo re-squared 0.3594 and 0.3875 respectively.
* significant at 0.10 level, ** significant at 0.05 level, *** significant at 0.01 level.
Source: Household Survey (2005)

their own treatment. This is not the case for spouses in monogamous households: when they are ill, the finances to cover their treatment could come from anybody in the household. Additionally in this second analysis, Oromo women are less likely to finance their treatment themselves, which suggests other cultural influences are at play.[15] The more patriarchal set-up of Oromo households with clear-cut responsibilities for husbands and potentially a limited capacity for women to choose their own strategies and treatment options when confronted with illness was discussed earlier. Either way, this may contribute to the 'protection' of women against health shocks in the context of increasing marketization. This tentatively suggests Oromo households are more likely to operate as a unit from an economic perspective. However attributing this to norms and cultural influences should be done with care, as there is no information about the way the actual practices related to these responsibilities have developed over time in the different ethnic groups in this study, and more particularly in this village. An alternative explanation for the Oromo factor may be related to the settlement history of the village, meaning that many of the Oromo heads are among the original inhabitants and may have preferential access to health facilities, assets and networks that allow them to protect their wives better in times of health problems. The information presented here is inconclusive. It is also important to realize that this analysis was restricted to the simple *use* of risk-coping strategies and the persons within the household who use their savings, assets and relationships to finance the treatment of a household member. This analysis does not include information on the actual quantity and quality of treatment received and the (attained) health status of the household members involved. The detailed information necessary to address these issues is not available at present.

Discussion

In a context of increased monetization and marketization of health and healing and with a limited availability of cash, individuals and households may increasingly depend on risk-coping strategies to finance access to healthcare or healing. Unexpected illness has been seen to contribute to poverty dynamics and it is important to understand the strategies people employ to cope with health shocks. Much of the literature on risk-coping strategies assumes the household is a unit and household members are equally protected against illness. There is now empirical evidence that this is not necessarily the case and that women, in

15 Although many Oromo are also Muslim, the religious factor is not the most important here. In a regression that includes both Oromo and Muslim as an independent variable, the Oromo factor emerges as being significant, and not the Muslim one.

particular, bear the brunt of unequal access to treatment when they are ill. The exact mechanisms that explain these outcomes are, however, not yet fully understood. This chapter contributes to the insights into these mechanisms by questioning whose assets, savings or networks are used when someone in the household needs financing for medical treatment. This question has been empirically investigated here using data from an Ethiopian village where costs related to care and treatment have been rising, and finding treatment is increasingly tied to transactions in the healthcare market. Despite a customary norm that male heads of households are responsible for financing medical expenditures, a wide range of arrangements were found within households. Especially in female-headed households, members are largely responsible for their own treatment as their households only provide limited insurance. Households headed by men are better at meeting the financial needs of medical treatment of members but do not offer full protection either. Spouses and other household members, including adult children, also cater for themselves, either through savings and assets or via networks, although a lack of intra-household insurance is only partly covered by insurance through larger kinship networks. Friends and local organizations play an indispensable role in financing medical expenditures, especially for spouses in male-headed households. When reviewing the different factors at play in these households in a multi-variate analysis, the effect of the identity of the patient remains strong. Controlling for factors such as household composition and wealth, when a spouse is ill she is more likely to use her own resources to finance treatment than her husband's. Further analysis demonstrated that cultural factors do play a role here. It is particularly polygamous spouses who have to fend for themselves, especially when they live in a separate homestead. Spouses with Oromo husbands are much better protected against health shocks. Whether the Oromo factor is culturally embedded (i.e. related to patriarchal structures) or related to the settlement history with potential preferential access to resources is a question for further study, as is the relationship between whose savings, assets and relationships are used and the quality and quantity of the treatment received and the health status attained.

This analysis is a first step to understanding intra-household responsibilities and dynamics and the resulting vulnerabilities. More detailed information is needed to determine whether the observed patterns are driven by choice (with women choosing to finance treatment themselves because they want to choose the treatment and facility without interference from their husbands) or necessity. The latter would be the case if husbands simply refuse to finance treatment when their wives fall ill and the spouses have to fend for themselves. These insights in intra-household risk-sharing arrangements can inform policy makers and practitioners, for example in the field of health insurance of the consequences of the identity of the policy holder, who is typically the household head. The data in this survey suggest that it may be beneficial for women and other household members if all household members are equally included in an insurance policy. The introduction of such a scheme would be beneficial for women if the outcomes observed could indeed be attributed to necessity (i.e. the husband does not provide protection against health shocks). If women themselves choose to act independently, insurance may restrain them from doing so, especially if only one insurance card is provided per household and the household head holds the card.

The data and results presented in this chapter are based on a cross-sectional analysis and add to earlier findings that suggest that households should not be considered a unit where risk is shared. Household members cannot always rely on the resources of the head to finance health expenditures and sometimes members use their own resources or have to use their social networks to pay for medical care. Given the cross-sectional nature of our analysis, it was not possible to address whether the increased costs associated with medical treatment had negatively affected members' chances of finding protection against health shocks within their households. Although the norm suggests the head of the household provide for these expenditures, it is not known if or to what extent this has indeed been the case in the past. The analysis does show, however, that despite a common norm, women experience different realities. These are partly determined by their circumstances, such as age, ethnic background and type of marriage, and also by the way in which they navigate their intra- and extra-household networks.

References

Alwang, J., P.B. Siegel & S.L. Jorgensen (2001), *Vulnerability: A view from different disciplines*. Social Protection Discussion Paper No. 115. Washington, DC: World Bank.

Bevan, P. & A. Pankhurst (1996), *Ethiopian village studies*. Mimeo. Centre for the Study of African Economies, University of Oxford.

Bhattamishra, R. & C.B. Barrett (2010), Community-based risk management arrangements: A review. *World Development* 38(7): 923-932.

Bogale, T., D.H. Mariamand & A. Ali (2005), Cost of illness and coping strategies in a coffee-growing rural district of Ethiopia. *Journal of Health Population and Nutrition* 23(2): 192-199.

Burger, K., J.W. Gunning & B.H. Kinsey (1998), Coping with drought in Zimbabwe. Survey evidence on responses of rural households to risk. *World Development* 26(1): 89-110.

CSA (2004), *Welfare monitoring survey, Analytical report*. Addis Ababa: Federal Democratic Republic of Ethiopia.

CSAE (2010) The Ethiopian Rural Household Survey: http://www.csae.ox.ac.uk/datasets/Ethiopia-ERHS/ERHS-main.html

Dekker, M. (2004), Sustainability and resourcefulness. Support networks in times of stress. *World Development* 32(10): 1735-1752.

Dekker, M. (2006), Estimating wealth effects without expenditure data: An asset-based wealth index for rural Ethiopia. *Ethiopian Journal of Economics* 15(1): 35-54.

Dekker, M. (2008), Intra-household differences in coping with illness in rural Ethiopia. In: M.M.E.M. Rutten, A.H.M. Leliveld & D.W.J. Foeken, eds, *Inside poverty and development in Africa*, pp. 201-224. Leiden: Brill.

Dercon, S. & P. Krishnan (2000), In sickness and in health: Risk sharing within households in rural Ethiopia. *Journal of Political Economy* 108(4): 688-727.

Dercon, S., J. Hoddinnott & T. Woldehanna (2005), Shocks and consumption in 15 Ethiopian villages, 1999-2004. *Journal of African Economies* 14(4): 559-585.

Dercon, S. & J. de Weerdt (2006), Risk-sharing networks and insurance against illness. *Journal of Development Economics* 81(2): 337-356.

Dito, B. (2010), Intra household labour supply, Agricultural shocks and women's bargaining power, Paper presented at the CSAE Conference on Economic Development in Africa. Oxford: Centre for the Study of African Economies. http://www.csae.ox.ac.uk/conferences/2010-EDiA/papers/399-Dito.pdf

Duflo, E. & C. Udry (2004), Intra household resource allocation in Cote d'Ivoire: Social norms, separate accounts and consumption choices. NBER Working Paper No.W10498.

Ellis, F. & T. Woldehanna (2005), Ethiopia participatory poverty assessment 2004-05. Forthcoming.

Federal Ministry of Health (2006), Ethiopian Health Sector Development Program (HSDP) II: Report of the final evaluation of HSDP II, 31 January-March 6, Vol. 1, 2002/03-2004/05. Addis Ababa.

Gezahegn, J., B. Ayele, G. Fulle & M. Tadesse (2006), *Ethiopian village studies II, Turufe Kecheme*. Addis Abeba: Wellbeing and Development Ethiopia. http://www.wed-ethiopia.org/docs/cpii_turufe_no_photos.pdf

Krishna, A.; D. Lumonya, M. Markiewicz, A. Kafuko; J. Wegoye & F. Mugumya (2006), Escaping poverty and becoming poor in 36 villages of central and western Uganda. *Journal of Development Studies* 42(2): 346-370.

Lindelow M. & P. Serneels (2006), The performance of health workers in Ethiopia. *Social Science and Medicine* 62(9): 2225-2235.

Pankhurst, A. & P. Bevan (2007), Unequal structures, unbuffered shocks, and undesirable strategies. Quantitatively informed qualitative investigations into the causes of extreme poverty in rural Ethiopia in 2004. http://www.wedthiopia.org/docs/Extreme_Poverty%20in%20Rural%20Ethiopia.pdf

Rosenzweig, M. & O. Stark (1989), Consumption-smoothing, migration, and marriage: Evidence from rural India, *Journal of Political Economy* 97: 905-926.

Sahn, D.E. & D. Stifel (2000), Poverty comparisons over time and across countries in Africa. *World Development* 28(12): 2123-2155.

Scheil-Adlung, X., G. Carrin, J. Jütting & K. Xu (2006), What is the impact of social health protection on access to health care health expenditure and impoverishment? A comparative analysis of three African countries, extension of social security. ESS Paper No. 24. Geneva: International Labour Organization.

Seebens, H. & J. Sauer (2006), Bargaining power and efficiency: The case of rural Ethiopian households. *Journal of International Development* 19(7): 895-918.

Stierle, F. M. Kaddar, A. Tchicaya & B. Schmidt-Ehry (1999), Indigence and access to health care in Sub-Saharan Africa. *The International Journal of Health Planning and Management* 14(2): 81-105.

Tibandagebage, P. & M. Mackintosh (2005), The market shaping of charges, trust and abuse: Health care transactions in Tanzania. *Social Science and Medicine* 61: 1385-1395.

UNDP (2009), *Human Development Report 2009*. New York: Palgrave Macmillan.

Wagstaff, A. & E. van Doorslaer (2003), Catastrophe and impoverishment in paying for health care: With applications to Vietnam 1993-98. *Health Economics* 12: 921-934.

World Bank & Ministry of Health (Ethiopia) (2005), *Ethiopia: A country status report on health and poverty, Vol. I: Executive Summary*. World Bank Report No. 28963-ET.
http://wwwwds.worldbank.org/external/default/WDSContentServer/WDSP/IB/2005/08/15/000090341_20050815103823/Rendered/PDF/289631ETH0vol1.pdf

Xu, K., D.B. Evans, K/ Kawabata *et al*. (2003), Household catastrophic health expenditure: A multi-country analysis. *The Lancet* 362: 111-117.

10

Can't buy me health: Financial constraints and health-seeking behaviour in rural households in Central Togo

André Leliveld, Corine 't Hart,
Jérémie Gnimadi & Marleen Dekker[1]

By means of a case study in Central Togo, this chapter explores the health-seeking behaviour of rural household members who are faced with a variety of healthcare providers whose services they now have to pay for. The financial costs that come with treatment, as well as vicinity, play an important role in the first illness response, and may prevent people from seeking professional treatment. In the second and third illness responses, financial considerations still play a role but other factors, such as quality of service and the seriousness of the illness, are more important. In academic and policy-making circles, community-based health insurance schemes have been presented as a viable option to overcoming the financial constraints that determine health-seeking behaviour, thus improving the access of household members to professional healthcare. However, the introduction of community-based health insurance schemes should not be seen as an all-inclusive answer to the monetization of healthcare services and the access and financing problems this has created for (poor) rural households in Africa.

1 The authors would like to thank Louvain Développement and Plan Togo for allowing them to use their statistical dataset in the analysis presented in this chapter.

Introduction

This chapter investigates the health-seeking behaviour of rural households in Central Togo facing a diversified and largely monetized healthcare system. As elsewhere in Sub-Saharan Africa, the medical system in Togo is characterized by medical plurality, ranging from local traditional healers to national hospitals, and everything in between. Within this continuum, a wide and bewildering variety of health services are on offer. Health services were first introduced when missionary health facilities were set up and these later became incorporated in colonial and post-colonial government public health services. The last two decades have seen two major shifts in the financing of healthcare services. Firstly, user fees and payment for drugs were introduced to recover at least some of the costs for the health sector, and secondly, when paying for treatment, a shift from kind to cash can be seen. These shifts imply that access to health services has become partly dependent on a household's capacity to raise the cash required to pay for consultations and treatment, medicines and transport costs. For example, the World Bank estimated that Togolese households spent approximately 5% of their total expenditure on health in 1996 (cited in Nubé & Overbosch 2008: 34), and between 1990 and 1998, 50% of total health expenditure in Togo was in the form of privately funded healthcare (figure calculated from Nubé & Overbosch 2008: 31, Table 11). The central questions in this chapter are to what extent the financial costs of using healthcare services determine health-seeking behaviour among rural households in Central Togo, and whether the introduction of community-based health insurance schemes has solved the problems that came with the monetization of healthcare services and the access and financing issues this created for (poor) rural households.

In the literature on health-seeking behaviour in developing countries, financial costs are mentioned as one of the determinants. Others include perceptions of illnesses and how they should be treated, socio-demographic status, the autonomy of women, economic conditions, physical and financial accessibility, and disease patterns and health service issues, such as the availability of staff and drugs, opening hours and waiting times (Shaikh & Hatcher 2005; Tipping & Segall 1995). More specifically for the Central West African region (Burkina Faso, Côte d'Ivoire, Ghana, Mali and Togo), Nubé & Overbosch (2008) mention the geographical location of and distance to the nearest healthcare provider, the poor quality of the staff and services provided, the inadequate supply of care and medicines, trust and mistrust in public health institutions, the gravity of the illness, and financial costs as important factors in explaining the low uptake rates of the modern health system. However, the extent to which the financial costs that come with the use of health services determine the health-seeking behaviour of households in Africa and elsewhere in the developing world is debated. For example, Tipping & Segall (1995), in their annotated bibliography on health-seeking behaviour in developing countries, indicate that the association between a household's socio-economic status and use of healthcare services appears to be undisputed. Richer households make greater use of the higher-quality services, while poorer households make less use of services in general and tend to choose cheaper services. Grobler & Stuart (2007) also found that income significantly affected patterns of healthcare utilization in South Africa although the results from other studies were less robust. Lindelow (2005), for instance, found income to be a relatively unimportant determinant of healthcare choice in Mozambique but the differences could be explained by the costs in combination with the quality of the care provided. And Anyanwu (2007), in a study among Nigerian households, also found that income was less important in deciding on healthcare than other factors such as the distance to a healthcare facility, the severity of the illness and the person's age. When a household member is ill, members attempt to minimize the loss of income rather than the expenditures required to find treatment for the person.

The question about the monetization of health services in Africa determining health-seeking behaviour and health service utilization is interesting from a policy perspective. Recently, a wide variety of public and private organizations (ILO-STEP, national governments, NGOs and private insurance companies) have used the financial costs argument to explain the low utilization rates of health services and to point out the need to improve health-financing systems by introducing insurance schemes. The introduction of health insurance schemes, they argue, would make health services more accessible to a larger group of people (especially the poorer sections of the rural population) and lead to an improvement in the quality of services because providers would be accountable to those who pay insurance premiums. Community-based health insurance schemes have recently been introduced in Central Togo. This chapter uses the findings concerning the determinants of health-seeking behaviour to discuss the intervention logic underlying the introduction of this type of scheme.

The structure of the chapter is as follows. After a brief explanation of the outline of the study and its context, data on health-seeking behaviour among rural households in Central Togo are analyzed. This is followed by a discussion of health costs and financing, and the chapter concludes by relating the findings from the first section to the intervention logic behind the recent introduction of community-based health insurance schemes in Central Togo.

Outline of the study

The data analyzed in this chapter were collected in 2005 by Louvain Développement as part of a context and feasibility study that was commissioned by Plan Togo on the introduction of an alternative health-financing system in Plan Togo's zones of intervention in the Centrale and Plateaux regions (see Map 10.1). The focus of the study was on the health-seeking behaviour of households and not on the utilization of health services.[2] The study explored the factors that influence the response to an illness that may, or may not, involve the use of any particular service and can result in just a single or a succession of healthcare seeking acts. Data on health-seeking behaviour were collected using a complementary mix of quantitative and qualitative methods. A cross-sectional household survey with semi-open questionnaires was conducted among 425 households in 25 villages spread over five districts in the two regions.[3] The questionnaire included questions on the social and economic characteristics of the household and its members, the last time the respondent had been ill, the cause of the illness, the response to the illness, the factors influencing the response to the illness, and the financing of the response. Both the male head and his wife were interviewed in each household. However, fewer women than men answered questions on health-seeking behaviour in the final sample because women were asked whether the last illness in their household was related to them or one of their children. In many cases, it was reported that it was a child who had been ill. In the questionnaire, the questions on illness, illness response and financing were then asked about the child and not the female respondent.

In addition, focus-group discussions were held with male and female adults and children, and semi-structured interviews were conducted with opinion leaders in the villages and districts selected. The focus-group discussions were conducted to gain further insights into the utilization of health services by households and the level of vulnerability of households in relation to their socio-economic profile, and to determine whether basic conditions existed for

---

2 Studies on the process of the utilization of health services focus on the end point of healthcare seeking rather than on the process of healthcare seeking. Studies of health service utilization are often facility based and in the public sector, while studies of healthcare seeking may collect data from health facilities, households or both.

3 Cross-sectional studies rely on recollecting details of illnesses – using accounts of household members – that occurred in the weeks prior to interview. In contrast with longitudinal studies, this may have compromised the accuracy of responses and the recording of specific details, for example of the decision-making process, the sequence of events, and direct and indirect costs of healthcare seeking and its financing. See Tipping & Segall (1996) for a detailed discussion on the pros and cons of cross sectional household surveys in research on healthcare seeking.

Map 10.1 Togo, showing research locations

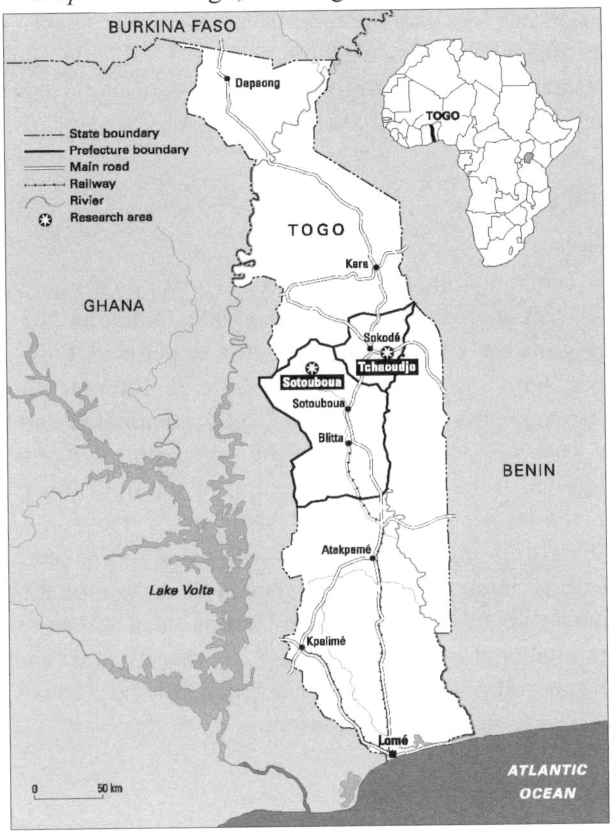

introducing community-based health insurance schemes (*mutuelles de santé*). The interviews with opinion leaders focussed on their perceptions of the feasibility of introducing community-based health insurance schemes in the selected districts. The findings from the sample survey, the focus-group discussions and the interviews have been discussed in a series of reports (Ghesquiere *et al.* 2005; Al Kourdi *et al.* 2005a; Al Kourdi *et al.* 2005b; Aholoukpe *et al.* 2005). A substantial part of this chapter is based on material presented in those reports.[4]

For the quantitative analysis in this chapter, 138 households (with 276 observations at an individual level) out of a total of 425 in the sample survey were used. In 2007, Plan Togo and Louvain Développement introduced community-based health insurance schemes in Sotouboua and Tchaoudjo, two of the districts surveyed in the Central Region. Analysis in this chapter is limited to these

4 See also 't Hart (2010) for further information.

two districts and focuses on members of rural households who are reported to use healthcare services less than the semi-urban and urban households who have been excluded from the analysis. The main reason for this decision was to keep context variables and factors that might influence household members' health-seeking behaviour the same for all the households surveyed.

Context of the study

Regional setting

Sotouboua and Tchaoudjo are two sub-regions (*préfectures*) in Togo's Centrale region, which covers approx. 13,000 km^2 and had a population of about 500,000 in 2005. The region has the lowest population density in Togo. The region's capital is Sokodé, with about 100,000 inhabitants. In 2005 the population of the Soutoboua sub-region was estimated at 135,000 inhabitants and that of Tchaoudjo at about 166,000. The majority of the population is Kotokoli or Kabyè. The former migrated from the southern region of the old Mali kingdom in the late 18th and early 19th century bringing Islam and a tradition of trading. The Kabyè are farmers from the north of Togo who came to the central region over the last few decades looking for fertile land. In general, climatic and soil conditions are favourable to drought-resistant crops such as sorghum, yam and cassava. Rainfall patterns allow for one crop per year, with an annual rainfall of between 1200 mm and 1500 mm, which mainly falls between April and July. The Harmattan is in December and January.

Health conditions and health services

The health status of people in the surveyed areas does not differ much from the national average. Health conditions in Togo reflect the fact that the country is still one of the poorest and least-developed in the world. Life expectancy at birth for men is 52 and 56 for women. The under-five mortality rate per 1,000 live births is 151 for boys and 128 for girls, with the main causes of death being neonatal problems, malaria and diarrhoeal diseases. Under-five mortality rates are higher in the rural areas, and lower among the highest wealth quintile. The maternal mortality ratio per 100,000 live births is 570; immunization coverage in 2004 among one-year-olds was 71% for DTP3 and 70% for measles; and only 2% of children under five were reported to sleep under insecticide-treated nets (World Health Organization 2008).

Regional data on illness patterns are not available but respondents in the household survey were asked to report the last time they were ill. Half of the male respondents had fallen ill in the six months preceding the interview, while in the 12 months before the interview two-thirds of them had been ill. For

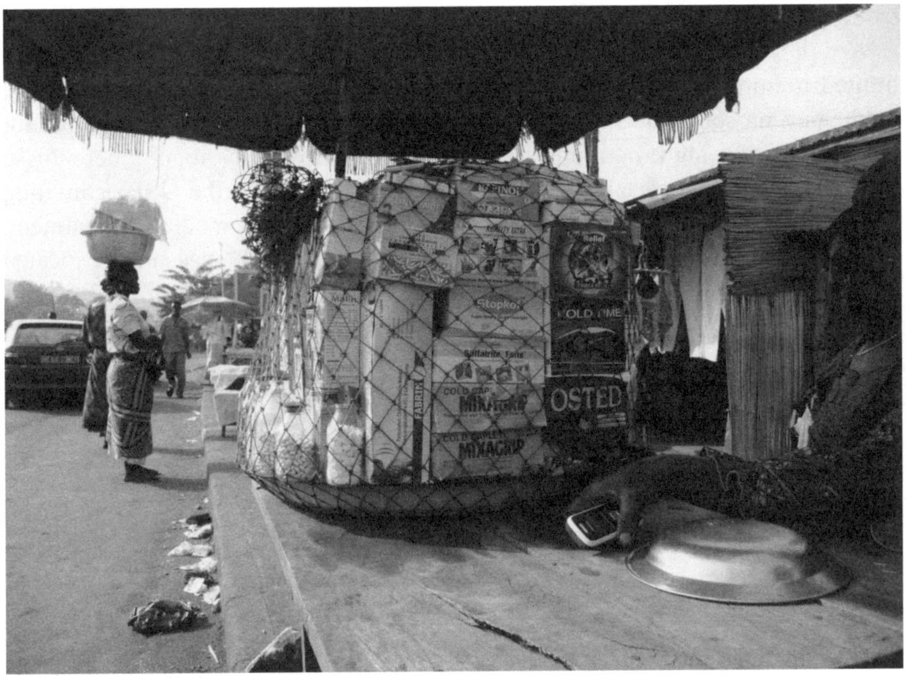

Photo 10.1 Medicine merchant
[Photo: Marleen Dekker]

women and children these figures were 71% and 84% respectively (see Table 10.1). The prevalence of diarrhoeal diseases (one of the main causes of infant mortality) is missing but this may have been reported as 'dysentery'. Respondents only reported physical illnesses and symptoms. To what extent this pattern is related to taboos surrounding mental-health disorders or the way the questions on illnesses were phrased is unclear. The remainder of this chapter focuses on response regarding physical illness.

A range of healthcare services are available in the region. Firstly, there are home remedies that people prepare themselves by collecting herbs. Secondly, medicines can be bought from travelling merchants, herbalists, pharmacies and local dispensaries. Thirdly, private herbalists who specialize in physical injuries and the treatment of aches using plants can be consulted and there are healers who treat diseases (and other problems) that are thought to have an occult or supra-natural background.[5] Public health services at community level include a

[5] In the various languages spoken in the region, these traditional healers are called *Tiw* (Kanye and Kotocoli), *Ouboor* (Bassar), *Ogninkpale* (Tchamba) or *Taada* (Losso).

so-called *Agent de Santé Communautaire* (ASC) and *Unité des Soins Périphériques* (USP). An ASC is a volunteer in the village who has received some limited training in health issues and has a small first-aid box containing basic medicines, mosquito nets and condoms for sale. An ASC is also responsible for childhood screening programmes, informing the community about tuberculosis, HIV/AIDS and other health risks, and referring patients to the USP or inviting these nurses to come to the village to provide preventive or medicinal treatment. USPs are the clinics in rural areas that serve a couple of villages and are located in either one of the villages or along the road between them. USPs offer preventive and curative treatments and hospitalization for a limited number of cases. There are two state-run district hospitals in the town of Sotouboua and Sokodé, a private clinic in Sokodé and *Centres Médico-Social* in the towns.

Table 10.1 Illness prevalence among men, women and children (%)

Type of disease	Men (N=131)	Women (N=42)	Children (N=92)
Malaria	58.8	51.2	44.4
Dysentery	11.5	14.6	29.3
Respiratory diseases	6.1	9.8	8.3
Fracture	4.6	2.4	0.8
Pain in limbs	6.1	2.4	0.8
Anaemia	0.0	0.0	2.3
Cyst	2.3	7.3	2.3
Headache	0.8	4.9	4.5
Other	9.8	7.4	7.3
Total	100.0	100.0	100.0

Source: Household survey 2005

NGOs also provide prevention and awareness programmes.[6] The focus-group report showed that their programmes are more widespread in Tchaoudjo than in Sotouboua (Al Kourdi *et al.* 2005a, Table 3), with programmes to promote hygiene among school pupils, construct school and community latrines, provide boreholes and hand pumps in schools for clean water, de-worm primary-school children, educate local people about health risks related to parasitic infections, and distribute and sell insecticide-treated mosquito nets. The most recent NGO health-related intervention in both sub-regions has been the intro-

6 These NGOs include Plan Togo, ADESCO (*Appui au Développement et la Santé Communautaire*), Radar, GTZ and the Red Cross.

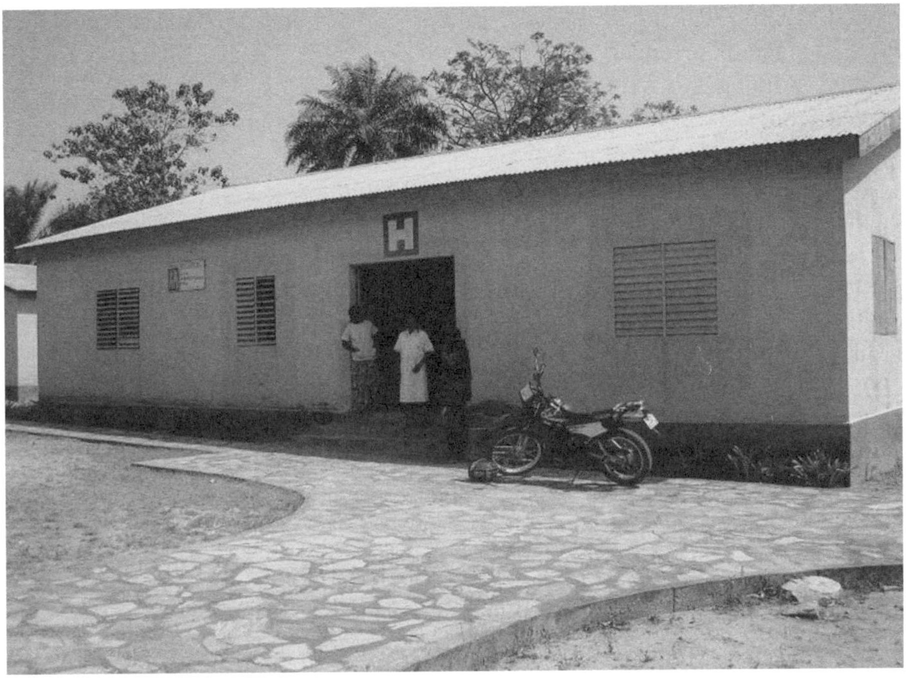

Photo 10.2 *Unité des Soins Périphériques* (USP)
[Photo: Corine 't Hart]

duction of *Mutuelles de Santé,* which are community-based insurance schemes offering coverage for basic health services.[7]

Socio-economic and demographic profile of the households sampled

According to the household survey, the median family size in Sotouboua and Tchaoudjo is 10 persons. Of the families, 26.1% consist of two or more households (*noyau*), with a median household size of 7 persons. In Tchaoudjo, the majority of the households sampled (65.8%) were Kotocoli while in Sotouboua the majority (76.7%) were Kabyè. Of those sampled, 75.4% had at least one child under the age of five, which is important as infants and those over 60 have the highest incidences of illness. 92.8% of the households sampled had one or more children under 18, and 15.9% were made up of people between 0 and 30 years of age. Literacy rates and the level of formal education among heads of households were generally low. 36.2% of the household heads had never at-

7 Implemented by the local NGOs Louvain Développement, ADESCO and Radar, and financed by Plan Togo.

tended school, 30.4% had attended primary school and 25.4% had completed the first stage of secondary school (*secondaire court*). Gender differences were marked. Among the wives of the heads of households, 62.3% had never attended school, 31.2% had attended primary school and only 4.3% had enjoyed some form of secondary or higher education.

The main occupation (82.6%) of the household heads in the survey was self-employment in agriculture, sometimes in combination with keeping animals. 6.5% of the heads of households had a salaried job, and 1.4% were self-employed in trade or in a small business. No consumption or income data were collected in the sample survey so it is not possible to establish different income groups. From the figures presented in the focus-group report (Al Kourdi *et al.* 2005a), it is clear, however, that most rural households live on an average of US$ 1 a day or less, depending on the time of year and incidental windfalls such as the sale of products. In general, the main difference between the less poor and the poorest in both sub-regions is due to the sale of cotton by people in the less-poor group. Polygamous families appear to be richer than monogamous families: the local perception is that one has to be rich to support a polygamous family.

The sample survey provides information on the wealth status of households that allows for a rudimentary calculation of a possessions score (P-score) for each household, drawing on Sender & Smith's (1990) methodology, and more recently applied in Daley (2005) and Leliveld (2008).[8] The higher the P-score, the wealthier a household is (see Table 10.2). Differences in wealth are not very pronounced: the distribution is normal, with the majority of households falling in the middle ranges (3-5), while fewer households are found at the lower and upper ends of the scale. However, significant differences were found between the two districts: in Soutoboua households were generally wealthier than in Tchaoudjo.[9] Significant differences could also be found among villages within the two districts: Aguidagbadé village in Tchaoudjo had relatively more

8 The P-score is a simple index of the level of material well-being of households, providing a rapid indicator of the overall economic status of respondents and households. Households or persons score 0 for the absence or 1 for the presence of several pre-selected visible wealth items. The P-score for each household is calculated by adding up the scores for the selected items. In the survey in Togo, households could score on seven visible wealth items: their roof (metal), floor (cement), walls (cement), the status of ownership of premises, energy used for lighting (other than petroleum), energy used for cooking (other than wood), and the presence of a latrine. No information was collected on cattle ownership, land ownership and land size, or the possession of durable consumption goods.

9 Cross-tabulation between P-scores and region gives a significant relationship at 0.00 (Kendall's tau-b -0.286, t-value -3.769).

Table 10.2 P-scores surveyed households

P-score	No. of households	Percentage
0	0	0.0
1	0	0.0
2	7	6.3
3	26	23.2
4	38	33.9
5	34	30.4
6	7	6.3
7	0	0.0
Total	112	100.0

Source: Household Survey 2005

'wealthier' households, while in Soutoboua, Fazao village clearly has more households with higher p-scores. The latter finding is related to Fazao's location on the Ghanaian border, which offers an easy springboard for men to work as migrants in Ghana. However it should be emphasized that – like income differences – wealth differences among rural households are quite small and rural living conditions can generally be characterized as poor. Calculations using the total sample showed that larger differences in wealth status can be observed between rural and urban households than among rural households *per se*.

Drinking water is mostly obtained from boreholes (89.9%), some of which are equipped with pumps. Of the male respondents, 68.6% reported saving money regularly and in most cases (73.3%), the money was kept at home although 18.9% saved with a micro-finance organization. Only 3.3% reported having a savings account at a bank. Among those interviewed, 80.1% of women reported saving regularly, with 49.5% keeping their savings at home. 19% saved with a micro-finance organization and 31.5% did so with an informal savings group (*tontine*).

Health-seeking behaviour of household members

This section investigates respondents' illness responses for the last time they were ill and the factors behind their choices. In the questionnaire, respondents were asked about the sequencing of health-seeking behaviour. Did they seek treatment in the first place? And, if it was positive, what did they do first? And, if applicable, what did they do second and then even third? Table 10.3 shows the health-seeking behaviour of respondents and reveals three major health-seeking patterns that can be split into various sub-patterns. The main differences are whether respondents started with self-medication or not, and whether they went to a traditional healer or a 'modern' health service provider. A substantial number of respondents (nearly 40%) resorted to a form of self-medication first, either buying medicines from a pharmacy, a travelling merchant or at the market, or gathering free plants and herbs. Cross-tabulation that is not reported here shows that self-medication is only applied in cases of malaria or dysentery (most frequently in cases of diarrhoea).[10] The remaining 60% of respondents sought treatment from a health service provider, either a traditional healer (10%), an ASC (12%) or a USP (25%), or they attended a hospital or clinic (13%). It can be concluded that 50% of respondents went to a modern healthcare provider as a first response to their illness. Illnesses for which they went to a modern healthcare provider included malaria, dysentery and most of the other reported illnesses (see Table 10.1). Traditional healers were visited for cases of malaria and dysentery too, but not for the other diseases reported.

In the survey, 49% of respondents indicated that they had fully recovered after the first treatment, while 16% said they had only partially recovered. Among the latter, almost all sought a second consultation or treatment or both. Columns 4 and 5 in Table 10.3 show the frequency of the various second responses and illustrate how they were a logical next step in the sense that respondents who first relied on self-medication tended to visit a health service provider next, while those who had already consulted a healthcare provider went to see another provider who – according to respondents – could offer better care. In practice, this meant that respondents went to providers who could offer a wider range or different kinds of services than the first provider they saw. People moved from an ASC, with a low range of services, to a USP or hospital with a wider range of services, or from an ASC or USP to a hospital. In some cases, people were seeking a different kind of health service, as is illustrated by the cases in which people after a first or second visit to a modern healthcare provider went to a traditional healer, who are supposed to be better equipped to deal with supra-natural causes of illnesses.

After a second response, 64% of respondents said they were cured, while 17% said they only felt partially recovered. Again, all those who did not feel cured and some of those who felt partially recovered took a further step and sought a third form of treatment. Columns 7 and 8 in Table 10.3 show that these patients either ended up at the hospital or decided to visit a traditional healer. In summary, the health-seeking patterns above show that respondents in a first illness response, unsurprisingly, generally start with self-medication or seek

[10] Approximately 50% of respondents who reported these illnesses used a form of self-medication first.

Table 10.3 Health-seeking behaviour of respondents (N=268)

1	2	3	4	5	6	7	8
1st response	No. (N=268)	Cont'd search	2nd response	No. (N=86)	Cont'd search	3rd response	No. (N=20)
No treatment	4	1	Hospital	1	1	USP	1
Free self-medication	17	12	Bought med.	1	1	Free self-med.	1
			ASC	1			
			USP	10	1	ASC	1
Bought medicines	89	42	Free self-med.	1			
			Bought med.	1			
			ASC	11			
			Trad. healer	3			
			USP	18	4	Trad. healer	1
						Hospital	3
			Hospital	5	2	USP	1
						Hospital	1
ASC	30	7	Trad. healer	1			
			USP	4			
			Hospital	2			
Traditional healer	25	14	ASC	2			
			USP	8	2	Hospital	2
			Hospital	4			
USP	67	18	ASC	1			
			Trad. healer	2			
			USP	3			
			Hospital	9	4	Trad. healer	1
						Hospital	3
Hospital / Clinic	36	10	Bought med.	1	1	Trad. healer	1
			Trad. healer	6	1	Hospital	1
			USP	2	2	Hospital	2
			Hospital	1	1	Bought med	1

Source: Household Survey 2005

treatment from primary healthcare services, and only later as a second and third illness response look for providers offering a wider range or different kinds of services. The next section explores the factors underlying this pattern of behaviour.

Factors affecting health-seeking behaviour

The extensive health-seeking literature identifies a wide range of factors that influence health-seeking behaviour and health service utilization, including people's perceptions of illnesses and how they should be treated, socio-demographic status, the autonomy of women, economic conditions, physical and financial accessibility, and disease patterns and health service issues (Shaikh & Hatcher 2005; Tipping & Segall 1995). This section presents an analysis of the factors that were mentioned by respondents when asked about their choice of illness response. Their answers will be related to some of the factors mentioned in the academic literature. Factors that have not been mentioned by the respondents but may equally explain their health-seeking pattern are also discussed. For the purpose of analysis, the various health-seeking patterns have been grouped into four categories, with the first response making an initial distinction between a group of strategies that start with self-medication, a pattern who starts with the traditional healer, a category combining modern community-based services (ASC and USP), and a category that has a pattern starting with regional health service providers (hospitals and clinics). Table 10.4 presents the results for the factors that were mentioned for the first, second and third illness responses, within each category of health seeking.

The factors mentioned by respondents can be classified into six categories: factors related to financial considerations (expense, flexibility of payment), vicinity (distance to provider), familiarity (known to the respondent; medical history known), the gravity of the illness, the quality of the provider, and the 'other factors' category that includes answers that were given only once or twice. Respondents' answers are thus in line with the factors put forward in other studies on health-seeking behaviour. Table 10.4 shows that financial considerations and the vicinity of the provision or the provider are dominant in deciding about a first illness response. Financial considerations are a major reason for initially choosing for self-medication or for visiting a traditional healer. Respondents refer to the low costs involved in self-medication while also mentioning the favourably viewed flexible terms of payment plus the fact that the traditional healer can be paid in kind, and their reasons for opting for a traditional healer's services. In the focus-group discussions, the role of habits and traditions in self-medication was mentioned but it appeared that in many cases, self-medication is used to allow time to collect the financial means to go for other, in the respondents' perceptions, more effective (and expensive) treatment. In fact, people tend to postpone decisions in order to go for more effective healthcare, and this may harm their health and have a negative effect on the income-generating capacity of the household too. And in the worst-case scenario, people totally forego treatment, which can have a potentially detrimental effect on their long-term health.

The financial considerations expressed by respondents raise questions about whether there is a relationship between the economic status of the household and the respondent and health-seeking behaviour. Recent literature on health-seeking behaviour in developing countries suggests that this relationship is at least ambivalent (Anyanwu 2007; Lindelow 2005), which is in contrast with the older literature that sees the relationship between household income level and health-seeking behaviour as clear-cut (Tipping & Segall 2005). Intuitively, a

Table 10.4 Factors that underlie illness responses by response and health-seeking pattern (% of answers within each health-seeking category)

Basic pattern	Factor	1st response	2nd response	3rd response
Self-medication	financial	50.5	9.3	22.2
	vicinity	20.2	18.5	0.0
	familiarity	17.4	1.9	0.0
	gravity of illness	8.3	27.8	44.4
	quality	1.8	20.4	11.1
	other	2.8	7.4	11.1
Traditional healer	financial	37.5	7.7	33.3
	vicinity	20.8	15.4	0.0
	familiarity	12.5	0.0	0.0
	avity of illness	8.3	61.5	0.0
	quality	4.2	15.4	0.0
	other	16.7	0.0	66.7
Community services	financial	8.4	20.0	12.5
	vicinity	36.8	0.0	0.0
	familiarity	8.4	0.0	12.5
	gravity of illness	10.5	28.0	50.0
	quality	26.3	20,0	12.5
	other	0.0	32.0	12.5
Regional services	financial	11.8	0.0	0.0
	vicinity	38.2	0.0	0.0
	familiarity	17.6	20.0	40.0
	gravity of illness	17.6	50.0	60.0
	quality	14.7	0.0	0.0
	other	0.0	30.0	0.0

Source: Household Survey 2005

relationship between economic status and health-seeking behaviour appears obvious, also given respondents' answers that indicate that financial considerations play a role in the decision-making process. In our findings, no significant relationship could be found between the wealth status of the household (expressed in p-scores) and health-seeking behaviour. But the question is whether this finding allows for robust conclusions. Firstly, some main indicators of wealth – land ownership, precise numbers of cattle and other livestock, the possession of jewellery and other luxury goods – were not measured in the 2005 survey and could thus not be included in the p-score. Secondly, income or consumption data may be a better predictor of health-seeking behaviour than wealth. Thirdly, income and wealth differences between rural households in Central Togo are probably not pronounced enough to generate robust results.

Calculations of the complete sample, including urban households, also show no significant relationship. And fourthly, the outcome may be an indication that households still have limited options in choosing a particular healthcare provider because the provision is not present in or near their village. In other words, in areas with poor health infrastructure, health-seeking behaviour may in fact be supply-driven (and not demand-driven). Given these qualifications, the results presented in this chapter about the relationship between the economic status of households and health-seeking behaviour cannot be taken as conclusive.

In addition to financial considerations, distance to the nearest health service location is an important factor that determines the first response. But distance has a financial aspect too: if the nearest centre is in another village or in town, transport costs will be involved, which could lead people to consider self-medication before any health facility is visited. Indeed a significant relationship between villages with or without a health facility in or nearby the village and the incidence of self-medication was found.[11] This suggests that if a health service is available in or near the village, respondents are more likely to visit the service and resort less to self-medication as a first response.

Table 10.4 shows that for the second and third responses, other factors gain in importance and the financial and distance factors become far less important. The severity of the illness and the quality of the health provider become dominant factors, which indicates that in the second and third response, most people select the most effective treatment, irrespective of the costs involved. Table 10.3 showed that in the second and third response, people visit health services that can provide for a wider range of services, expecting to find more effective treatment from these providers. Leonard *et al.* (2002) found that serious illness made people go for high-quality care in spite of the availability of free treatment. They tended to travel further for cheaper treatment for a minor illness, even if there was other high-quality care closer.

The general perception of the effectiveness of self-medication scored medium (on a scale of bad-medium-good) in the focus-group discussions. Table 10.3 also shows that purchased medicines appear to be more effective than herbal/plant medicines that are collected for free. In the case of purchased medicines, 52% of respondents did not report a second illness response, while in the case of nature-based medicines this percentage was only 30%. The services of the ASC and the USP were ranked as 'good' for their vicinity, the way people were received, the quality of the diagnosis, and the treatment. Some focus-group participants complained about the lack of medical equipment at USPs and the limited possibilities for hospitalization. Compared with other

[11] Significant at the 0.01 level, Lambda 0.141 with T-value 4.36.

modern healthcare providers, USPs were reported to be affordable though more expensive than self-medication and ASCs. In the quality ranking in the focus-group discussions, hospitals were ranked 'medium' to 'good'. The costs involved were mentioned as a negative aspect because they restrict access for those with low purchasing power. Focus-group participants were positive about the quality of care, the availability of medicines, and possibilities for surgery and hospitalization in cases of serious illness.

Opinions about the quality of traditional healers were mixed in the focus-group discussions. Some participants, including adults and older children, refer to their effectiveness in cases of certain injuries such as fractures and snake bites, and the treatment of the spiritual cause of the illness that, according to participants, is not resolved by modern healthcare methods. It is here that perceptions on health and healing meet: to become a healthy person, both are needed. Alternatively, praying and the church or the mosque are also mentioned as necessary resources in the healing process: 'believing in God cures all diseases, there is a complementarity between the medicine that takes care of the body and the Church that takes care of the spirit' (translation of a quote in Al Kourdi *et al.* 2005a: 41). Other participants, however, rejected any perceived positive attributes of the traditional healer, mentioning the false hopes they create, their ineffectiveness and the unrest they create in social relationships.

Many of the factors affecting health-seeking behaviour that are mentioned in the wider literature were also mentioned one way or another by our survey respondents or in focus-group discussions. One factor, namely female autonomy, that is explicitly mentioned in the literature was not mentioned by respondents because it is considered a hidden factor. In many societies men play a paramount role in determining the health needs of women and since men are the decision-makers and in control of all the household resources, they decide when and where women should seek treatment. This may have severe repercussions on the health of women and their children (Shaikh & Hatcher 2005), and the Togolese context is no exception in this respect. On the question of who decides on the first response in the case of the illness of a woman or a child, 49% of women claimed that their husband or another male family member (brother, husband's brother) did so. The majority of women (60%) who reported having decided themselves chose self-medication as a first response. The majority of women (87%) who reported that others made the decision about their treatment visited a health facility or traditional healer as a first response. As these services are on average more expensive than buying cheap medicines at the market or collecting herbs and plants, this finding could suggest that women lack the financial resources to visit more expensive health services and have to ask their husband or other male persons for money to pay for such services. Strictly speaking, they do not ask for approval to visit a more expensive health service but for the money that will facilitate access to this service. In this way, men have a large say both in the amount that is spent and the health service that is visited. Financial constraints may prevent women from choosing the health service provider she wants because her husband or another male family member influences her choice of health facility. This can prevent her from recognizing and voicing her concerns about health needs, resorting first to a health-seeking pattern she is in control of and thus seeking self-medication. This may well have a negative effect on her health or that of her children.

A main conclusion from the analysis above is that the financial costs that come with treatment play an important role in determining health-seeking behaviour. Together with vicinity, financial considerations are the most important in the first illness response, and determine whether someone chooses self-medication or visits a traditional or modern healthcare provider. In the second and third illness response, financial considerations still play a role but other factors such as quality, vicinity and the seriousness of the illness are more important. If the first illness response is based more on financial considerations than on issues of quality, the severity of the illness or effectiveness, this may stand in the way of recovery. As mentioned earlier, self-medication may lack a satisfactory diagnosis, which can lead to a deterioration in a person's condition and make further treatment more complicated and expensive. People postpone seeking effective healthcare, which may negatively affect their health and lead to adverse effects in the income-generating capacity of the household as well. And in the worst-case scenario, people even forego treatment, with potentially detrimental effects on their long-term health. The following sections discuss how people in the surveyed areas deal with health costs and how alternative health-financing systems can reduce the role of financial considerations in decisions in health-seeking behaviour.

Health costs and sources of financing

It is well known that illness is a significant risk for people in developing countries (Dekker 2004; Dekker & Wilms 2010; Dercon *et al.* 2005; Leliveld 2006) and can have considerable financial effects on the household affected. This has also been observed for rural households in Central Togo. First of all, there are the financial costs, such as charges for consultations, medication, transport and, in some cases, hospitalization. Table 10.5 shows that at least 75% of respondents had to pay the full costs of their treatment.

On average, 10% said they had to pay some of the costs incurred, while the remainder claimed that their treatment was free. However, these free treatments were closely related to self-medication through the collection and use of plants

Table 10.5 Incidences of full or partial payment of treatment for adults and children (by consult and % of N)

Source	Payment of full cost of treatment? Yes	Partial	Free
Men			
1st consult (N=122)	77.9	9.8	12.3
2nd consult (N=58)	88.9	11.1	0.0
3rd consult (N=13)	76.9	7.7	15.4
Women			
1st consult (N=34)	85.3	8.8	5.9
2nd consult (N=12)	75.0	16.7	8.3
Children			
1st consult (N=88)	89.8	2.3	8.0
2nd consult (N=26)	92.3	3.8	3.8

Source: Household Survey 2005

and herbal medicines. This means that households had to pay for any treatment from traditional or modern healthcare providers. The household survey did not indicate levels of costs but the focus-group discussions gave some indications. About 4% of the total annual budget of households in Sotouboua was spent on health and the figure was about 1% in Tchaoudjo (Al Kourdi *et al.* 2005a: 31, 33). However, it was noted that there is a wide discrepancy in the reporting of health-related costs. For example in the focus-group discussions, a large number of 'other expenses' were mentioned, including unforeseen costs due to illness and access to clean water. These can also be seen as being health-related. In three other districts where focus-group discussions were held, health costs were reported to be much higher at between 20% and 38% as a result of a different system of classification. Out-of-pocket expenditures on healthcare that exceed 10% of a household's total budget are referred to as 'catastrophic payments' (Pradhan & Prescott 2002; Wagstaff & van Doorslaer 2003). The 10% threshold is seen to approximate the burden at which a household is forced to sacrifice other basic needs, deplete its productive assets, incur debt or become impoverished (Russell 2004).

The focus-group reports also indicate that traditional healthcare is not necessarily cheaper than modern healthcare. Not only do traditional healers demand fees comparable to those demanded by modern healthcare providers but respondents also mentioned that in many cases they have to visit a traditional healer more often than a modern provider before they are cured. The difference between traditional healers and modern healthcare providers though is the flexibility and kind of payment demanded as some traditional healers allow clients to pay in instalments and in kind. This is an important reason for choosing a traditional healer over modern healthcare providers.

Table 10.6 gives an overview of how respondents paid their healthcare costs when a household member became ill. Households use costly risk-coping strategies to pay for medical care and reduce spending on basic needs, use their savings or sell household or productive assets. There are major differences between men and women, and men are usually responsible for deciding how health costs are to be covered. Men mentioned the depletion of savings and the selling of stock and family assets as the main ways of financing healthcare costs whereas women mentioned their husband's savings as their major source of finance. Women appear to have some degree of freedom in decision-making given the fact that they talked about family solidarity and selling their commercial stock, which are sources the men did not mention. Putting a child *en gage*, a practice whereby a child is sent to work at a relative's place in return for a loan, is another way in which health costs can be financed. As soon as the parents have paid off the loan, the child returns home as the child's labour at the relative's home is in fact the payment of interest.[12] One would expect this could be found between the wealth status of households and this practise. One explanation is that the regions surveyed have a strong history of migration and a

Table 10.6 Sources of financing for healthcare costs, by men and women and by consultation (% of N)

Source	Men			Women & Children	
	1st (N=109)	2nd (N=53)	3rd (N=11)	1st (N=110)	2nd (N=28)
Savings of head of household	38.0	34.0	27.3	22.7	10.7
Money from wife/husband	4.6	1.9	0.0	35.5	35.7
Own money	0.0	0.0	0.0	1.8	7.2
Loan from family member	10.2	11.3	18.2	6.4	3.6
Family solidarity	0.0	0.0	0.0	6.4	10.7
Loan from money lender	0.0	0.0	0,0	0.9	0.0
Sale of stock for subsistence	23.1	26.4	18.2	3.6	7.1
Sale of commercial stock	0.9	0.0	0.0	9.1	7.1
Sale of family assets	2.8	5.7	0.0	0.0	0.0
Child '*mise en gage*'	6.5	13.2	9.1	0.0	0.0
Combination	13.9	7.6	27.3	15.4	17.9

Source: Household Survey 2005

12 This practice should be distinguished from a form of child trafficking in which older children are sent by middlemen to earn money for their family in towns or neighbouring countries.

tradition of sending children to stay with aunts or uncles (Human Rights Watch 2003). This may explain why the term *enfant en gage* only exists in the Kotocoli language (*tolma*) and why the practice was mostly mentioned by Kotocoli households.

Other studies have shown that the above-mentioned strategies are expensive and can endanger a household's future economic status by depleting its finances through indebtedness and its future income-generating capacity by selling off productive assets (Dekker & Wilms 2010; Scheil-Adlung *et al.* 2006). This, in return, increases the risk of ending up or being trapped in poverty. Illness is likely to reduce a household's income if people cannot work and may result in additional expenditures to cover the costs of treatment. Bogale *et al.* (2005) and Krishna *et al.* (2006) have demonstrated how the cost of illness contributes significantly to the impoverishment of households in rural Ethiopia and Uganda respectively. Respondents were asked about the effects of illness on the family. Men mentioned, in descending order of importance, declining income and poverty (26%), the disruption of work rhythms (14%), indebtedness (8%) and the depletion of assets (2%), or a combination of these. Women mentioned similar points in more or less the same order, although they added children's labour, which was second in importance for them (15%). Respondents were asked what measures they had taken to deal with these adverse effects of illness on the family. Men mentioned raising additional income (20%), preventing illnesses (16%), and saving more (14%), or a combination of these, while women talked about generating more income (20%), restricting the number of births in the family (13%), saving more (7%) and preventing illness (6%), or a combination of these factors.

Overcoming financial constraints: Community-based health insurance

Health risks leave rural households in Togo vulnerable to serious losses as a result of negative health shocks, and force them to undertake costly strategies to manage their income and assets in the face of health risks. This lowers the mean income earned. Other studies have shown that welfare costs due to shocks and having to forego profitable opportunities have been found to contribute to persistent poverty (Dercon 2005; Elbers *et al.* 2007). In this context, reducing the financial burden of healthcare by having health insurance and seeking earlier medical treatment to shorten the duration of an illness will reduce the number of workdays lost, improve productivity and enhance a household's long-term welfare (Dekker & Wilms 2010; Jütting 2004; Young *et al.* 2006). More indirectly, when households are better protected against high medical costs, they are less likely to have to rely on other risk-coping strategies and may be able to accumulate savings and assets, and thus improve their general welfare.

In line with these arguments, policy debates have placed a great deal of emphasis on developing health insurance products for the poor. Health-financing systems through general taxation or the development of social health insurance are generally recognized as being powerful methods of achieving universal coverage with adequate financial protection for all. But many low-income countries are experiencing difficulties in achieving universal financial protection (van Ginneken 1999). Most recognize the impediments to universal financial protection and so other methods are therefore being explored including the direct involvement of communities in health financing. In the past, cost recovery for healthcare via user fees was established in many developing countries as a response to severe constraints on government finance. User-fee policies were also seen as a possible expression of community financing. However, studies have alerted decision-makers to the negative effects of user fees on the demand for care, especially among the poorest households (McPake 1993).

The involvement of the community in health financing was partly spurred by the Declaration of Alma Ata in 1978, which urged maximum community participation in the organization of primary healthcare (Carrin *et al.* 2005). Community financing for health is seen as a mechanism whereby households in a community (the population of a village, district or other geographical area, or a socio-economic or ethnic population group) finance or co-finance the current and/or capital costs associated with a given set of health services. At the same time, they are expected to participate in the management of the community financing scheme and the organization of the health services. Various forms of community financing exist, with the most common being the payment of user fees for healthcare at the point and time of use. An innovative form of community financing that emerged in the second half of the 1980s and has received increasing attention from policy makers in the last decade is community-based health insurance (CBHI). CBHI is a common denominator for voluntary health insurance schemes organized at community level that are labelled alternatively as mutual health organizations, medical aid societies, medical aid schemes or micro-insurance schemes (Carrin *et al.* 2005). The common characteristics are that they are run on a non-profit basis and apply the basic principle of risk sharing.[13]

Togo has adopted and implemented the Bamako Initiative (1987) with a view to promoting primary healthcare through community participation in the

---

13 Churchill (2006) defines micro-insurance as insurance that operates by risk pooling, is financed through regular premiums and is tailored to the poor who would otherwise not be able to take out insurance. For a review of studies on micro-insurance, see Dercon & Kirchberger (2008).

management and funding of the health sector. In 1991, the Ministry of Health decentralized the healthcare system and the national health policy advocated the participation of the people in defining their healthcare needs in 1996. Togo's national health policy aims to provide access to quality healthcare for all. At the same time, the government's objective is to improve social protection for vulnerable sectors of the population. Its social protection policy is geared principally to developing new strategies for caring for the most vulnerable as a way of mitigating the demise of family solidarity by putting in place new mechanisms and structures. CBHI is viewed as a promising channel for giving the poor a voice, extending social protection and increasing (modern) health service utilization. Togo has also set up a national framework for consultation on mutual health insurance schemes to learn from experiences in the field and define a national strategy to support these initiatives.

In 2006, the NGO Louvain Développement, in collaboration with Plan Togo, ADESCO and Radar, started preparing to establish two CBHIs in Tchaoudjo and Sotouboua to improve the affordability and quality of healthcare and make it more accessible to the population. CBHIs take the form of mutual associations (in French *mutuelles de santé*) with the aim of ensuring financial access without delay to basic health services throughout the year. Two CBHIs in Sotouboua and Tchaoudjo began in May 2008. Members have to pay a FCFA 500 (€ 0.76) registration fee and an annual premium of FCFA 2,040 (€ 3.11).This payment insures a nuclear family for a year and covers treatment costs at a USP or CHR/CHP, 50% to 70% of costs for consultations, medicines, minor surgery, pre- and post-natal care, childbirth at a USP, and 50% to 100% of the costs of paediatric (including hospitalization) and gynaecologic care at a CHR/CHP. In 2008, CBHIs had 2478 and 2023 patients in Tchaoudjo and Sotouboua respectively and these figures doubled in 2009 to 4,254 and 4,363 respectively, which represents about 5% of the target population and is in line with experiences elsewhere in the developing world.

There is no indication yet whether CBHI has made a difference in health-seeking behaviour among member households. Data on these issues have recently been collected to be included in the analysis presented here. However, some preliminary observations can be made. A positive contribution can be seen in a CBHI scheme in its potential to reduce the importance of the financial costs argument, which plays a significant role in the first illness response. Belonging to a CBHI may allow a larger group of households to refrain from self-medication as a first response, which often involves postponing vital treatment, and to seek adequate healthcare immediately. CBHI may encourage household members to obtain adequate treatment in an earlier stage of their illness and thus contributes to better levels of health among men, women and children. In this sense, the introduction of a CBHI scheme can be seen as an answer to the increasing monetization of healthcare in Togo, and Africa in general, and the way this shapes health-seeking behaviour and health service utilization.

At the same time, the introduction of CBHI reinforces the process already set in motion. To become a member of a CBHI scheme, a contribution has to be paid and a new financial consideration is thus added to a household's decision-making concerning health. A comparison of CBHI membership lists for 2009 with those in the 2005 survey reveals that about 6% of the households sampled have became members of a CBHI scheme. Cross-tabulation between the household poverty score and CBHI membership does not indicate a significant relationship but no members can be found in the lowest wealth category.[14] Paying the premium may still form the biggest obstacle to participation and the focus-group discussions showed that the poorest may have a reduced capacity to contribute because the monthly balance between their income and expenditure is regularly negative or zero (Al Kourdi *et al.* 2005a). Although CBHI may improve women's access to healthcare services as it reduces the financial costs argument that forces women to choose self-medication first, a CBHI scheme does not resolve women's unequal access to their households' financial resources and the pronounced gender differences in decision-making on health issues. In particular, when there is only one insurance-policy card for each household and the card is given to the household head (usually a man), as is the case in Togo, this may further complicate women's access to healthcare services. In addition, CBHIs do not cover all forms of treatment and all the costs involved. The focus is on biomedical healthcare provided by modern health service providers and CBHI only provides for the immediate expenses that come with the health shock, for example the costs of treatment, transport, medicine and possible hospitalization. However, other long-term costs, like those resulting from chronic disease and the loss of income-generating capacity, may need complementary social insurance schemes.

Concluding remarks

This chapter has explored the health-seeking behaviour of rural household members who are facing a variety of healthcare service providers in a context where most health services have to be privately paid for in cash. The financial costs of using these services, together with the vicinity, play an important role

---

[14] A significant relationship can be found between the level of education of the household head and CBHI membership. The higher the level of education, the more likely CBHI membership is. The data also show that relatively more households in Fazao were members than in one of the other villages. Anecdotal evidence suggests that Fazao's village leaders played an important role in promoting CBHI membership.

in the first illness response and may initially prevent people from seeking professional treatment. In later responses, financial considerations still play a role but other factors, such as the quality of the services and the gravity of the illness, are more important. Community-based health insurance schemes have been presented by policy makers and scholars as a viable option to overcome the financial constraints that determine health-seeking behaviour, and thus improve household members' access to professional healthcare. However, the introduction of community-based health insurance schemes only partly solves the problems that have emerged with the monetization of healthcare services and the access and financing problems this has created for (poor) rural households in Togo. Further research is needed on how far the introduction of (community-based) health insurance – being a manifestation of the monetization of the healthcare sector itself – improves access for the poorer strata of the population to healthcare services. For these poorest households, the cash payment of insurance premiums may form another barrier to professional healthcare, and force people to continue with costly, poverty-enhancing, risk-coping strategies when confronted with illness. To increase equitable access to healthcare for special groups, such as children or the very poor, exemption from payment or a lower premium could be considered through public subsidies. But the feasibility of such options needs further investigation.

References

Agbéré, A. & K. Kouassi (2004), *Dix-sept pratiques familiales et communautaires-clés en matière 'Prise en charge Intégrée des maladies de l'enfant': Analyse de la situation dans les cinq districts d'appui de Plan Togo*. Lomé: Plan Togo.

Aholoukpe, A.A., Y. Al Kourdi, G. Ghesquière & J. Gnimadi (2005), *Etude de contexte en de faisabilité pour la mise en place d'un système alternatif de financement de la santé dans 5 districts de la Région Centrale et des Plateaux; Rapport de l'enquête leaders d'opinion*. Cotonou: Louvain Développement, Coordination Afrique de l'Ouest & Plan Togo.

Al Kourdi, Y., G. Ghesquière, J. Gnimadi & I. Valcke (2005a), *Etude de contexte en de faisabilité pour la mise en place d'un système alternatif de financement de la santé dans 5 districts de la Région Centrale et des Plateaux; Rapport de l'enquête qualitative Focus Group adulte.,* Cotonou: Louvain Développement, Coordination Afrique de l'Ouest & Plan Togo.

Al Kourdi, G., J. Gnimadi, & G. Guesquière (2005b), *Etude de contexte en de faisabilité pour la mise en place d'un système alternatif de financement des soins de santé dans les districts sanitaires de Blitta, Sotouboua, Tchamba, Tchaoudjo et l'Est Mono, enquête quantitative*. Lomé: Louvain Développement, Coordination Afrique de l'Ouest & Plan Togo.

Anyanwu, J.C. (2007), Demand for health care institutions services: Evidence from malaria fever treatment in Nigeria. *African Development Review* 19(2): 304-344.

Bogale, T., D.H. Mariamand & A. Ali (2005), Cost of illness and coping strategies in a coffee-growing rural district of Ethiopia. *Journal of Health Population and Nutrition* 23(2): 192-199.

Carrin, G., M.P. Waelkens & B. Criel (2005), Community-based health insurance in developing countries: A study of its contribution to the performance of health financing systems. *Tropical Medicine and International Health* 10(8): 799-811.

Churchill, C. (2006), What is insurance for the poor?. In: C. Churchill, ed., *Protecting the poor, A microinsurance compendium*. Geneva: International Labour Organization.

Daley, E. (2005), Land and social change in a Tanzanian village, part 2: Kinyanambo, 1920s-1990. *Journal of Agrarian Change* 5(4): 526-572.

Dekker, M. (2004), Sustainability and resourcefulness. Support networks in times of stress. *World Development* 32(10): 1735-1752.

Dekker, M. & A. Wilms (2010), Health insurance and other risk-coping strategies in Uganda: The case of Microcare Insurance Ltd. *World Development* 38(3): 369-378.

Dercon, S. (2005), Risk, insurance and poverty: A review. In: S. Dercon, ed., *Insurance against poverty*. Oxford: Oxford University Press.

Dercon, S., J. Hoddinott & T. Woldehanna (2005), Vulnerability and shocks in 15 Ethiopian villages, 1999-2004. *Journal of African Economies* 14(4): 559-585.

Dercon, S. & M. Kirchberger with J.W. Gunning & J.P. Platteau (2008), *Literature review on microinsurance*. Geneva: International Labour Office.

Elbers, C., J.W. Gunning & B. Kinsey (2007), Growth and risk: Methodology and micro-evidence. *World Bank Economic Review* 21(1): 1-20.

Ghesquière, G., Y. Al Kourdi, J. Gnimadi & I. Valcke (2005), *Etude de contexte en de faisabilité pour la mise en place d'un système alternatif de financement de la santé dans 5 districts de la Région Centrale et des Plateaux; Rapport de l'enquête qualitative Focus Group enfants*, Cotonou: Louvain Développement, Coordination Afrique de l'Ouest & Plan Togo.

Grobler, C. & I.C. Stuart (2007), Health care provider choice. *The South African Journal of Economics* 75(2): 327-250.

Human Rights Watch (2003), *Borderline slavery: Child trafficking in Togo*. New York: Human Rights Watch.

Jütting, J. (2004), Do community-based health insurance schemes improve poor people's access to health care? Evidence from rural Senegal. *World Development* 32(2): 273-288.

Kouassi, B., ed. (2008), *Pauvreté des ménages et accès aux soins de santé en Afrique de l'Ouest*. Paris: Karthala.

Krishna, A., D. Lumonya, M. Markiewicz, A. Kafuko, J. Wegoye & F. Mugumya (2006), Escaping poverty and becoming poor in 36 villages of central and western Uganda. *Journal of Development Studies* 42(2): 346-370.

Leliveld, A. (2006), Poverty trap or safety net? Dynamics in social security arrangements in Ugandan rural economies. Paper presented at 'The end of poverty in Africa?' conference, African Studies Centre, Leiden, 16-17 March.

Leliveld, A. (2008), The social security function of land in Mbarara District, Uganda. In: M. Rutten, A. Leliveld & D. Foeken, eds, *Inside poverty and development in Africa: Critical reflections on pro-poor policies*, pp. 169-201. Leiden: Brill.

Lindelow, M. (2005), The utilization of curative health care in Mozambique: Does income matter? *Journal of African Economies* 14(3): 435-482.

McPake, B. (1993), User charges for health services in developing countries. *Social Science and Medicine* 36: 1397-1405.

Nubé, M. & G.B. Overbosch (2008), Health in Central West African countries: Commodities and disparities. In: B. Kouassi (ed.), *Pauvreté des ménages et accès aux soins de santé en Afrique de l'Ouest*, pp. 13-49. Paris: Karthala.

Pradhan, M. & N. Prescott (2002), Social risk management options for medical care in Indonesia. *Health Economics* 11: 431-446.

Russell, S. (2004), The economic burden of illness for households in developing countries: A review of studies focusing on malaria, tuberculosis, and human immunodeficiency virus/acquired immunodeficiency syndrome. *American Journal of Tropical Medicine and Hygiene* 71(2): 147-155.

Scheil-Adlung, X., G. Carrin, J. Jütting & K. Xu (2006), What is the impact of social health protection on access to health care health expenditure and impoverishment? A comparative analysis of three African countries. Geneva: International Labour Organization.

Sender, J. & S. Smith (1990), *Poverty, class and gender in rural Africa: A Tanzanian case study*. London: Routledge.

Shaikh, B.T. & J. Hatcher (2005), Health seeking behaviour and health service utilization in Pakistan: Challenging the policy makers. *Journal of Public Health* 27(1): 49-54.

't Hart, C. (2010), *Mutuelles de santé in Central Togo*. Leiden: African Studies Centre, mimeo.

Tipping, G. & M. Segall (1996), How to do (or not to do)…; Using a longitudinal illness record to study household health care decision-making in rural communes in Vietnam. *Health Policy and Planning* 11(2): 206-211.

Tipping, G. & M. Segall (1995), *Health care seeking behaviour in developing countries: An annotated bibliography and literature review*. Brighton: Institute of Development Studies.

van Ginneken, W. (1999), Social security for the informal sector: A new challenge for the developing countries. *International Social Security Review* 52: 49-69.

Wagstaff, A. & E. van Doorslaer (2003), Catastrophe and impoverishment in paying for health care, with applications to Vietnam 1993-98. *Health Economics* 12: 921-934.

World Health Organization (2008), *World Health Statistics 2008*. Geneva: World Health Organization

Young, P., P. Mukwana & E. Kiyaga (2006), *Microinsurance: Exploring ways to assess its impact*. Washington, DC: Microfinance Opportunities/IRIS.

11

Marriage, commodification and the romantic ethic in Botswana

Rijk van Dijk

Many groups in Botswana perceive marriage as a social panacea in the fight against HIV/AIDS. Christian, Pentecostal groups attach great value to the institution and feel that it promotes healthy relationships and thus a healthy society. In pursuing a moral agenda on relationships, they appeal to middle-class life-styles and encourage consumptive patterns and glamorous weddings. This adds enormously to the cost of a wedding. While marriage is perceived as a road towards healing the social order and rescuing society from the further spread of AIDS, the pursuit of social health has become part of a highly commoditized market involving the splendour that a middle-class 'white wedding' requires. This chapter explores how patterns of commodification and the marketization of marriage are affecting social institutions and concerns, making the fight against AIDS part of the overall rise in consumptive patterns that mark social life in today's Botswana. These patterns are impacting on ideas and practices that are considered part of establishing a healthy society and contribute to a process of middle-class social differentiation. While the contradictions in the concerns about AIDS that this process gives rise to are noted by the people and (Christian) groups involved, they remain unresolved.

Introduction

There is a literature that applauds Christianity's changing public role in Africa and the way it is engaging with the problem of HIV/AIDS in many African societies (Prince *et al.* 2009). Christian groups have become involved in care, prevention and treatment and are particularly active in promoting behavioural change (Dilger *et al.* 2010; Becker & Geissler 2009; Dilger 2007, 2009; Burchardt 2009). In awareness-raising and counselling programmes, Christian groups are emphasizing a theology and morality of sexual relations in an attempt to make societies healthier. One way of doing so, they believe, is to propagate conjugal marital relations and promote marriage as the exclusive site of sexuality and the social panacea in the fight against HIV/AIDS (Amanze 2007; Christiansen 2009a; Togarasei *et al.* 2008; Smith 2007).

Two schools of thought are emerging as to whether counselling and/or awareness-raising practices have significance with regard to AIDS and marital practices. One school of thought that is emerging on the basis of experiences in Uganda acknowledges the huge impact of behavioural change on reducing AIDS infection rates. Public programmes have emphasized the need to reduce the numbers of sexual partners, and the importance of using of condoms and remaining faithful to one partner in marriage. This, in Museveni's terms, is propagated as a 'zero-grazing' public philosophy (Gusman 2009; Christiansen 2009b). In the literature, this is seen as one of the most important factors in creating real behavioural change and one that has had a measurable impact on infection rates (Epstein 2007; Green *et al.* 2006; Allen & Heald 2004).

There is however another body of literature emerging that sees policies that promote marital relationships, which are supported by Christian faith-based organizations (FBOs), as producing another set of dangers (Parikh 2007; Smith 2007, 2008, 2009; Mokomane 2005; Togarasei e*t al.* 2008). This literature argues that marriage is becoming the most important source of AIDS infection in Africa as women are left with increasingly little space to negotiate safe sex with their partners. Demanding the use of condoms when married signals the woman's deep distrust of her partner's level of faithfulness, and this may jeopardize the marriage. The literature shows how this usually backfires on the wife who is seen as being the 'troublemaker' who should be reprimanded by her in-laws and subsequently even by her own family for being so distrusting (divorce is generally understood as either 'being sent back', i.e. to the home of the wife's father, or 'going home' if there is agency on the part of the woman).

In the world of Christian AIDS-intervention programmes, these insights are considered disturbing as they disrupt and disqualify the nature, aims and intentions of much of the faithfulness programme and (pre-)marital counselling. If marriage is turning out to be a major source for HIV infection, as this literature demonstrates, the Christian doctrines that have been so forcefully promoted may have in fact produced an unforeseen but devastating dark side. Most of the safe-sex practices that have been promoted in countries such as Uganda and Botswana have focused on the use of condoms (the C of 'condomize' in the ABC strategy), yet this promotion did not receive much support. In fact, there has been staunch opposition to it from Christian circles and specifically from

Pentecostals (Bornstein 2005). The conundrum is that the promotion of faithfulness and marriage as a social vaccine against AIDS without opening a space for women to negotiate safe-sex practices has turned marriage into its opposite. Faithfulness, marriage and counselling practices are co-producers of the problem.

The promotion of marriage in Botswana as the social panacea against AIDS has run into a new difficulty: the increased commodification of weddings. This chapter demonstrates that although Christians, and in particular Pentecostal groups, are promoting marriage, they are also promoting a middle-class style of weddings. They are encouraging consumptive patterns and a glamorous style. Pauli (forthcoming) describes the way Namibian weddings have become status markers for the middle classes too. Whereas marriage is seen as a road to healing the social order and rescuing society, the trajectory of social health has become a highly commoditized market with all the splendour a 'white wedding' involves. This is leading to a rise in conspicuous consumptive patterns in Botswana today. The point is that while marriage is being promoted as a social remedy in the fight against HIV/AIDS, becoming married has become an enormously costly affair which only a few can afford.[1] This contribution explores how patterns of commodification and marketization of marriage may affect social institutions and can impact on ideas and practices that are considered part of the process of social healing. While these contradictions are noted by people and Christian groups in everyday situations, they remain unresolved.

Breaking chains, breaking culture and the counselling of contestation

Botswana's latest nationwide AIDS awareness-raising programme is the 'Who is in your sexual network?' campaign. This government and international-donor-sponsored campaign addresses 'multiple concurrent partnerships' and aims to increase awareness of the dangers of entering and maintaining networks of sexual relations. It highlights how the HIV virus is capable of spreading through relationships of multiple partners and social chains. The slogan of the campaign is 'Break the Chain!' (*O Icheke!*). Campaign leaflets and brochures demonstrate how curtailing sexual networking breaks the chain and stops the spread of the virus.

---

1 A literature is showing the steady decline in marriage rates in Botswana as evidenced by data from censuses held in 1981, 1991 and 2001 (Mookodi 2004: 123). See also Gaisie (2000).

Map 11.1 Botswana

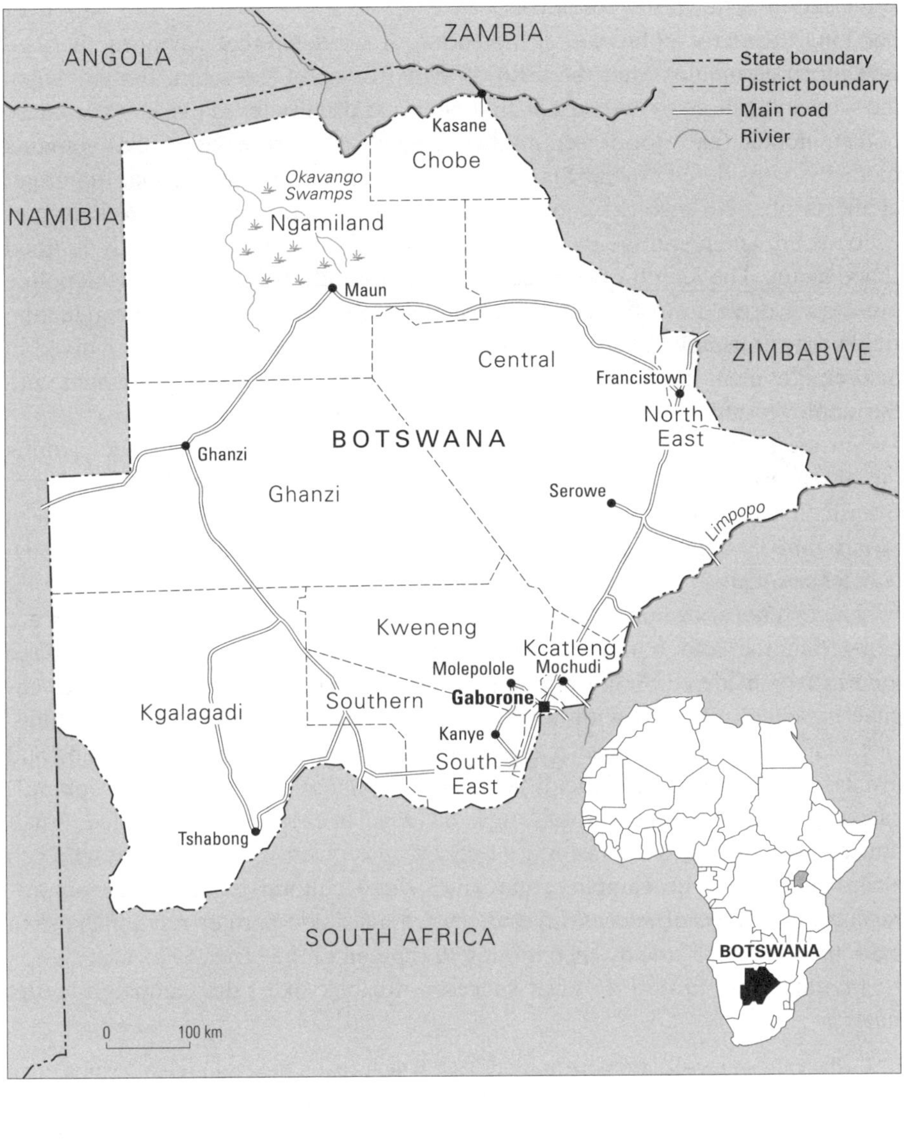

The campaign material and its mediatized messages do not limit themselves to a discussion of breaking networks. However there is the a priori assumption of their existence. The message covers a widely expanding domain in which a range of relationships and social circumstances that may be conducive to the emergence of these networks are brought into orbit. In a way, the campaign message displays a level of cultural sensitivity that is intriguing: the interventionism that is propagated in the campaign espouses a notion of cultural contestation at a variety of levels. Take for example the way the notion of breaking the chain is directed at the period of seclusion that young mothers go into for three months after the birth of their first child (botsetsi). It starts when the woman is about to deliver her first born and usually takes place at the house of her mother (and not at her in-laws' home). The presence of the woman's mother is considered crucial for training her daughter in motherhood. Important elements of socio-medical knowledge are transmitted, moral and spiritual precautions are taken and the daughter will be taught how to get her body in good shape again. The length of time can vary considerably, although in Molepolole (an hour's drive from the country's capital Gaborone where I am conducting fieldwork), it usually lasts about three months. As more women are involved in paid employment however, this length of seclusion needs to be negotiated with the employer and an additional connotation of being on vacation can emerge.

For the *O Icheke!* campaign, the crucial aspect of this period of seclusion is the absence of the husband or male partner. Men are supposed to stay away from their partners during this period and their mothers-in-law are expected to ensure this. Couples take the idea of absence, separation and paucity in sexual contact seriously.

The *O Icheke*! campaign sees this practice as one of the reasons why men are being tempted into multiple partnerships. Abstinence for a period of three months is considered highly problematic for men and encourages people to engage in sexual relations with others. The campaign addresses this issue alongside other culturally induced reasons for multiple concurrent relationships and discusses why these are difficult to break. *Botsetsi* is put in the same 'cultural' category as the phenomenon of 'sugar daddies' or *inyatsi*; the so-called 'small houses', which means the keeping of concubines or mistresses by men who can afford to do so. The campaign perceives these cultural practices as compromising the chance of successful and rewarding single-partner relationships, in particular marriage, and as encouraging the spread of the virus.

In attempting to define 'what success will look like', the campaign-leaflet states:

> ... the campaign will promote a mindset in which sex is linked to relationships, love and emotional commitment. This will be complementary to promotion of primary partnerships because men currently find it easy to mentally de-link looking for sexual satisfaction elsewhere and their emotional commitment to their partner. (MCP-Campaign leaflet, March 2009, p. 14)

For young women tempted into relationships with sugar daddies (the so-called 'Ma14' relationships), the campaign says it wants to establish that:

> … the main motivation for or function of young women's relationships with men will shift from being about material gain to being about finding love and commitment. (*Ibid.* p. 10)

While the campaign is heavily supported and staffed by Christian circles alongside governmental organizations, international donors and other civil-society organizations, there are a number of features about the promotion of single relationships that this 'break the chain' stands for.

The first is the promotion of marriage in Botswana where there is a 'reluctance to marry'. Indicating that marriage is in crisis in the country, the campaign highlights the fact that less than 20% of the adult population is married (see also Mookodi 2004; Heald 2006), and suggests that many relationships are unstable and cohabitation is common. The campaign stresses that while marriage itself is in dire straits, stable relationships in the form of marriage should be regarded the most important social panacea against AIDS.[2] Alternative relations, such as cohabitation, polygamy or multiple concurrent relationships, are considered immoral because they impede the social responsibility that everyone should feel in the fight against HIV/AIDS. The programme's national coordinator views cohabitation as 'one of the greatest sins this country is facing' (Interview, November 2009) and thinks marriage should be promoted because cohabitation cannot ensure stable and single-partner relationships.

The national coordinator of the 'Break the Chain' campaign explained that the influence and involvement of Christian representatives is important. Christian voices are to be found at the various levels of the campaign's organization, and activities are required to tie in with local-level activities in Christian organizations regarding the provision of counselling and advice. The Christian message is regarded as relevant in circles where counselling is offered, such as those related to the functioning of the state-sponsored voluntary HIV testing and counselling centres known as *Tebelopele* (literally: vision).

The second point about the 'Break the Chain' campaign is its call for an emotionalization of relationships. Words such as 'love' and 'commitment' are brought into play as ways of introducing a changing understanding of the nature and quality of a relationship. Single-partner relationships, and preferably marriage, need to be emotionalized to create better, more stable and longer-lasting relationships. This emotionalization is being pursued by breaking the culture of

---

2 Also the long-term government vision for Botswana 's future, known as 'Vision 2016' talks about the need for a strengthening of the marital institution in the fight against the disease, when it says: 'The emphasis on a strong family unit will encourage responsible parenting and the institution of marriage. It will provide the social foundation for the eradication of problems such as the high incidence of teenage pregnancies, adultery, prostitution, street children and the spread of HIV.'

silence about intimate sexual matters. There is a rationality of emotions at play here that indicates that as soon as these matters can be put into words and communicated between a couple, the relationship will deepen and become more stable.

The promotion of marriage as a social panacea and the emotionalization of single-partner relationships fall within a wider spectrum of the 'behavioural change' policy that the Botswana government and Christian groups are promoting (Heald 2006; Nkomazana 2007). Since the mid-1990s there has been a new social contract between the state and religion in Botswana in the fight against AIDS (Amanze 2007; Nkomazana 2007; Togarasei *et al.* 2008). Important players are the Pentecostal churches, not because the mainline churches are not playing a substantial role in providing care, treatment and prevention but because of the relative significance of their voice on moral issues. In an organization such as BOCAIP,[3] which emerged in the mid-1990s too, many Pentecostal churches joined forces to provide support and staff, seeing this as an important vehicle for spreading ideological messages. In the ABC campaign, Pentecostals have become known for emphasizing the 'B', which stands for 'being faithful' (as against the 'C' for using the condom). Pentecostal groups, such as well-known churches like Bible Life, Winners Chapel, Christ Ambassadors and the Apostolic Faith Mission, have organized a multitude of (pre-) marital counselling and marriage-enrichment seminars, meetings and workshops (Togarasei 2010).

Following the initiative taken by the Seventh Day Adventists, they have invested in training and the professionalization of staff involved in counselling, writing manuals for fellow counsellors and organizing marital counselling practices within their own congregations. Often these Pentecostal churches have well-trained marriage officers who are ordained to solemnize a marriage but who also act as trusted advisors within their communities. A young, recently married couple explained to me in Molepolole in 2009 how they had gone to one of these counsellors when they were preparing their wedding for legal, emotional and sexual advice, instead of going to their parents or relatives within their respective families. 'Yes' the young man said in the interview, while his young wife was sitting next to him, 'the counsellor explained to my wife that my sexual appetite was going to be enormous during the first weeks of our marriage and asked her to be patient with me! But he also said that I should take care of her orgasm as well because we both should enjoy it.'

---

[3] This is the Botswana Christian AIDS Intervention Program, a faith-based umbrella organization established in the mid-1990s in response to the Botswana leadership's call on the churches to join hands in fighting the disease.

This is a new kind of openness about sexuality and intimacy that Pentecostalism does not refrain from voicing. On the contrary, it has been made part of its emotionalizing of marriage, of creating a particular language of love and commitment that runs counter to customary and cultural conventions.[4] The Pentecostal notion of breaking with the past (Meyer 1998; van Dijk 1998), which has become a dictum in Pentecostalism throughout Africa, is also made relevant in counselling on marital life, sexuality and intimacy. At times when reflecting on sermons from the pulpit, audiences may sometimes wonder whether 'this is still the church', as one of the pastors at the Bible Life Church explained to me. Yet the idea that cultural models of informing young people about marriage and sexuality running short of commitment and contradicting Christian principles of the exclusionary nature of sexuality with the marital bond is highly conducive to this Pentecostal stand. Marital counselling within these circles is contesting culture and customs in particular ways. The emotionalization in terms of love, commitment and intimacy of the marital bond is part of a rationalized strategy (including training, the professionalization of staff and services, and the writing of manuals) in how, when and where local culture should be critiqued and contested.

Educating emotions, affective institutions and the romantic turn

A new social contract is emerging that has been forged between Christianity and public/government policy-making regarding behavioural change, in this case related to the institution of marriage. The situation in Botswana is in no way unique. In countries like Uganda and Nigeria, marriage has been publicly promoted as the social panacea for the disease, though this dictum is criticized in the social-sciences literature that indicates that marriage in these countries is also turning out to be a major source of HIV infection (Ojo 1997; Smith 2007, 2008, 2009 for Nigeria; Parikh 2007 for Uganda; Allen & Heal 2004 for a comparison of Uganda and Botswana).

The Christian campaign of tying sexuality exclusively to marriage, and thus increasing the social profile of marriage as belonging to a proper social order, runs counter not only to infidelity or multiple, concurrent partnerships but also to culturally held notions of adulthood. A great deal of marital counselling and awareness-raising takes place in the lives of couples when the time of abstinence from pre-marital sex is long past. Marriage counselling has little impact on what socio-cultural patterns and demographic statistics in Botswana show

4 An extensive literature is emerging on African situations in which notions of cultural conventions, discretion and intimacy, and on the other hand new forms of openness about these matters, are being studied. See Bochow (2008, 2010); Geissler & Prince (2007a, 2007b); Hirsch & Wardlow (2006) and Hirsch *et al.* (forthcoming).

for the preferred age of first birth (before the age of 25) and the preferred age of marriage (in one's early thirties). The timing of the birth of one's first child and marriage are unrelated demographically and indicate different processes of identity formation, namely that of adulthood through motherhood and adulthood through marriage. The two should not be confused and should be understood in view of their gendered nature as well as their specific functions. While the first form of adulthood is obviously related to reproduction, the second, which is produced through marriage, is related to authority, to the licence to speak, to having an opinion and to taking decisions in family affairs, inheritance and the ownership of property. Many couples have one or more children before they marry and have therefore achieved adulthood in just one sense, while marriage as another form of adulthood protects the inheritance rights of spouses and children. The Christian emphasis on pre-marital abstinence and tying sexuality to marriage exclusively in this sense seems to have a counter-cultural objective.

Another important factor in attaining adulthood is spending and having spending power. The social status of being an adult is enhanced if the person can be seen to be spending money on cars, clothes, the home, food and alcohol. This link between adulthood and spending power is not new and has always been part of the migration experience to South African mining complexes for men in the past. However it has increasingly become linked to adulthood through marriage. Weddings in Botswana have become hugely costly affairs with weddings now ranging from a spectacular BP 100,000 to even BP 200,000.[5] This forces many couples to take out a bank loan to cover the costs of their wedding and leaves them with debts that usually take years to repay. The national newspaper *Mmegi* reported this development in an article entitled 'Couples tied in knots of debt' (*Mmegi*, 17 October 2008) stating that:

> Weddings have become big business and everything about them is expensive. Many have been known to take loans to finance their weddings, sometimes perceived as being a waste, since you pump in so much money into a one-day event.

Marriage is not only becoming an impoverishing institution but also one that increasingly fewer people can afford. Cynically, the call for marriage can be seen as a social panacea that makes this 'social medicine' a luxury for the lucky few.[6] How has this commodification of the institution emerged and what shape is it taking?

Studying the development of marriage at a time of AIDS in Molepolole, an agricultural town of more than 60,000 inhabitants on the edge of the Kalahari

---

5 The exchange rate in July 2010 was: Botswana Pula (BP) 1,000 = US$ 144.

6 I am not suggesting here that there is a causal relationship between social class and fidelity but marriage has become a social status marker (Pauli forthcoming) which also highlights the idea of marriage as a social medicine.

and sometimes called the 'largest village of Africa', shows the many sides of this commodification, which has been taking place nationwide in rural and urban situations alike. In this town, the three different systems that Botswana's laws recognize as a valid marital relationship are to be found. The first concerns marriage under customary law, as performed at the court of the Kwena paramount chieftaincy (*Kgosi Sechelle*). The *Kgosi* holds court at a place known as the *Kgotla*. The second system is the one provided by the District Commissioner (DC) who registers and ordains marriages under Dutch Roman law. The third concerns religious marriages that can be ordained by recognized marriage officers appointed by religious bodies such as churches and mosques. A religious marriage ceremony is the only way a legal polygamous marriage can be registered, a provision that caters for Botswana's Islamic minority. These systems are not mutually exclusive, so a Christian wedding can (and in most cases is) registered by the District Commissioner because this provides for marital security under Dutch Roman law. This is significant for the arrangement of property relations and inheritance purposes.

Lastly, in addition to the *Kgotla*, the churches, BOCAIP and the DC, the other institutional actor that is important in relation to marriage in Molepolole is the traditional doctor (sing: *ngaka*; plural: *dingaka*) who can be invited on behalf of the groom's side of the family to perform important functions in arranging a wedding. All *dingaka* are supposed to be supervised by the Kwena *kgosi* but involving these traditional healers depends on the family's interest in doing so as the authority concerning the actual arrangement of a marriage lies in the hands of elderly family representatives, and their approval is more important than the authority behind any of the three systems mentioned above.

There is a long established literature on marriage in Botswana as provided by anthropological studies such of that of Schapera (1940, 1950) and later that of Kuper (1982) and the Comaroffs (1991) who all took an extensive interest in studying Tswana "Laws and Customs". This involved also the Kwena of Molepolole as being one of the eight "principal Tswana-speaking tribes" with a seat in the national House of Chiefs. The work of Griffiths (1997) in the 1980s contributed to a legal-anthropological understanding of marriage systems in this area. Yet this literature is now in need of revision for two important reasons; first of all, the unprecedented growth of Botswana's wealth and prosperity as a result of becoming one of the world's leading producers of high-quality diamonds. This is combined with the country's exceptional access to the European beef market, which has made livestock farming in Botswana a highly profitable business for many. The Tswana bovine culture received a boost as cattle rearing, which any self-respecting Tswana man is involved in, is a guaranteed source of wealth.

The second important change in Botswana society in recent years has been the arrival of AIDS, although this has not been studied in terms of its impact on marital practices. While Botswana's relative affluence and its small population meant that preventive systems as well as education and training programmes were put in place and reached large sections of the population, the spread of the disease has been unparalleled. High levels of sexual networking by men and women alike as well as unstable family lives due to patterns of labour migration were identified as important reasons for the rapid spread of the virus (Hope 2000; Upton 2003). Perhaps remarkably, the real pressure in terms of marital arrangements stems less from the impact of AIDS and the need for AIDS testing and safe-sex practices but from the expense of getting married and the debts and conflicts that arise as a result of conspicuous consumption.

The following three cases provide a glimpse of how couples arrange their weddings (*linyalo*) and what specific issues need to be addressed in terms of its commodification.

The first case is that of the wedding of Couple R. The groom was 31 and had a job in IT, and the bride was 30 and was working in the banking sector. The couple met in 2005 and had a baby in the same year. To open the way for marriage, the groom's parents were required to meet those of his partner because they needed to deal with the accusation on the part of the bride's parents that 'your child has messed up our yard'. This is an expression that indicates the illicit nature of the sexual relationship the young man initiated. Negotiations can only start if and when a 'repair payment' (*Thlaga legora*, literally: a fine for 'jumping the fence') for the parents of the bride has been agreed upon. Commonly, the man responsible for getting a woman pregnant is not obliged to take care of the mother and the child. Parents sometimes try to enforce such arrangements with the help of the law, but in practice the success of such demands is limited.

In the process of getting married, a payment of one head of cattle had to be made to open the way. At the so-called *patlo* that followed the negotiations for the bride price, which is paid by the man and his family to the bride and her family, this was set at the usual *lobola* of eight head of cattle. Of these, the groom had to provide two, while the others were provided by uncles, his siblings and even one by the *kgotla* to which he belonged. But this was only the start of what the couple explained was a wedding that they estimated would cost BP 200,000 in total (about five times an annual average salary in Molepolole). This was partly to cover the *patlo* (the engagement) and the rest to pay for the actual wedding days (in the plural as it was to be celebrated at the parental homes of both the bride and the groom).

Before the *patlo* takes place, the woman must ensure that she has new clothes, so the groom has to provide her with new clothes, shoes, underwear, sheets, blankets, pillows, lamps, an umbrella, soap and so on. Her mother is also to be provided with the customary short blankets, the so-called 'German print' that they put on their shoulders as a sign of their maturity and authority.

A big decorated tent has to be erected for the wedding, and food and drinks for the hundreds of guests has to be bought and prepared, including the slaughtering of one or two head of cattle. New outfits and shoes are bought for the bride and groom as they will change clothes several times during the wedding, and clothes for all their best man and the matrons of honour also need to be bought. A wedding cake, usually costing around BP 6,000, and wedding rings have to be purchased. Firewood and transport must be arranged. Cards are printed and sent out well in advance, and pastors are invited to lead the prayers and the white wedding in church, which is an entirely separate event. A traditional doctor has to be arranged to cleanse the places where the wedding will be held, prepare the food and guard the fires. He will charge about one head of cattle or the equivalent in monetary terms (BP 1,500). Music and a video man have to be arranged and a photographer will be hired to make a photo shoot on the wedding days. Careful planning is required to ensure that every stage in the entire wedding process is recorded on video and in photos.

The couple was largely responsible for covering the expense themselves. Relatives may contribute towards the cost of the cattle and support parts of the programme, but in this case it became clear from the start that the couple would assume most of the costs. They decided to take out a large bank loan as they were both in paid employment and could ensure a monthly servicing of the loan. They were thus able to borrow a considerable sum (the man BP 80,000 and the woman BP 40,000). The remaining BP 80,000 needed came from their savings and small donations from relatives and friends, particularly on the groom's side. They are aware that paying off the loan will take them between five and ten years because of the interest charged on it (about 20% annually).

By comparison, the cost of the wedding of Couple M in February 2008 was half that of what Couple R paid. However this couple was also forced to take out a bank loan because they are from a poor family and could not count on substantial financial support from their families. They both had modest salaries in the period prior to their wedding so needed longer to save up for the event. When they got married, the groom was 41 and the woman was 39. As she had a better-paid job than her husband, her loan was twice as big as his (BP 30,000) but this was not considered a source of shame. The groom had to take charge of the *lobola* and could not count on much support in getting the eight head of cattle together, a factor that influenced the time it took for them to get married. On the wedding days, however, they managed to have the expensive tents, all the decorations, the food, the drinks and the transport required to give the wed-

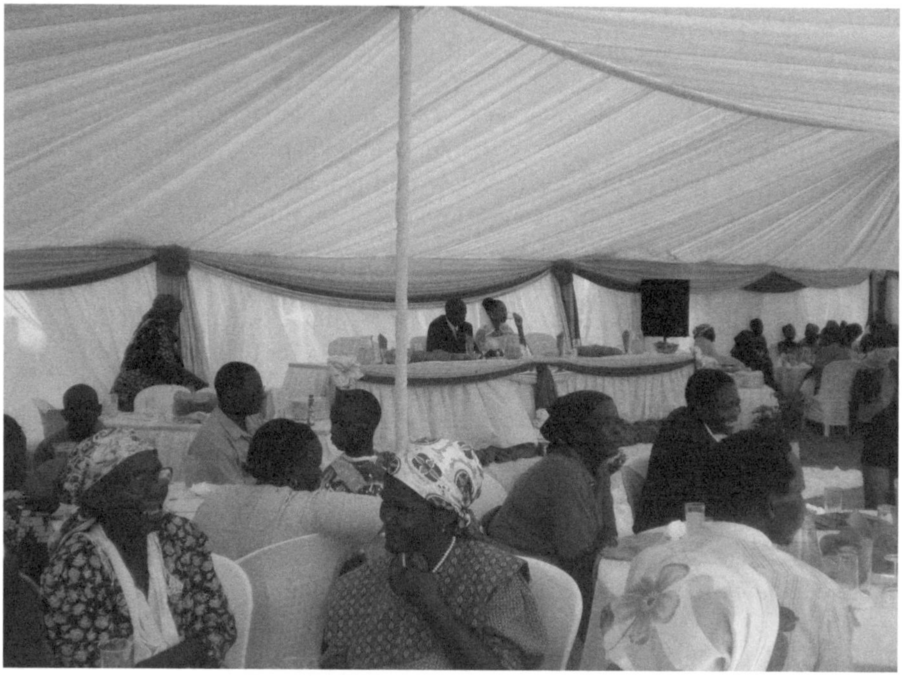

Photo 11.1 A sumptuous wedding in Molepolole
[Photo: Rijk van Dijk]

ding the status it should have. While the wedding was thus a huge success and brought prestige to them and their families, they are now faced with the reality of paying off their bank loans.

The third case is the wedding of Couple K in 2009. Neither the bride nor the groom had a job; both are from poor families and neither could expect their relatives to contribute in financial terms. Still the notion of having an impressive wedding loomed large and every effort was made to generate the money required to make it a prestigious event. However BP 100,000 or BP 200,000 was far beyond their means and the only way the groom could generate the minimum amount needed was to sell some of his precious cattle to raise an estimated BP 30,000. In addition, he had to provide the cattle for the *lobola* as none of his uncles were able to help him, and he had to pay the one of head of cattle for the child that was born prior to their wedding to make amends for 'jumping the fence'. As neither of them had jobs they could not apply for a bank loan. Postponing the marriage allowed them to raise money by selling cattle at a time when they could get a better price for them at market. The whole process of preparing for the wedding, selling the cattle and saving money took more than five years.

These cases show the enormous costs involved in marriage and how the poorer and less well educated are even prepared to sell their sole source of social security, namely their cattle. This would normally be the last or most desperate thing one would do for a consumerist purpose and indicates how strong the social pressure to marry in style is. Important sacrifices need to be made.

For the older generation, this is entirely new. In the 1950s, couples would not have spent more than one to two months of their earnings on getting married. The wages of most Batswana then came from working in the South African mines and provided a monthly income of around BP 600. A *lobola* of eight head of cattle would have been the most significant element in the wedding: this would amount to many months of hard work and would only have been achievable with the support of relatives.

What the above examples demonstrate is not only the competitive consumerist pattern in which the institution of marriage has become captured but also the dwindling *relative* significance of the value of the *lobola* payment. Particularly in the first example, the value of the bride price was marginal compared to the value of all the other items. The value of an average cow for the *lobola* is estimated at BP 1,500, which means that the *lobala* represents a total value of BP 12,000, whereas the expense of hiring a tent plus the trappings already exceeds that amount by far (about BP 16,000),and that is before all the other items are included.

While the *lobola* is considered traditionally as the most important 'test' of a man's readiness to start the marriage process, the significance of this entry ticket into adulthood is increasingly becoming more symbolic and the real demonstration of the capacity to spend money is now located elsewhere. In a strange sense, the *lobola* has become the easiest part of the entire process as many of the other elements are not only more expensive but require much more organization, such as arranging a loan.

Another point of interest is the age at which marriage is now taking place. Looking at marriage registrations recorded at the DC's office in Molepolole in 2008 and 2009 shows the age at which men and women are marrying nowadays (Figures 11.1 and 11.2).

The mean age of marriage is in the 30 to 39 years bracket, an age at which many will already have one or more children from this or another relationship, and which further complicates marriage negotiations between the parents. The couples indicated that one obvious reason for marrying relatively late was the parental demand to be 'prepared', meaning that the couple and the groom in

Figure 11.1 Number and age of men and women registering their marriages in Molepolole, 2008 (N = 383)

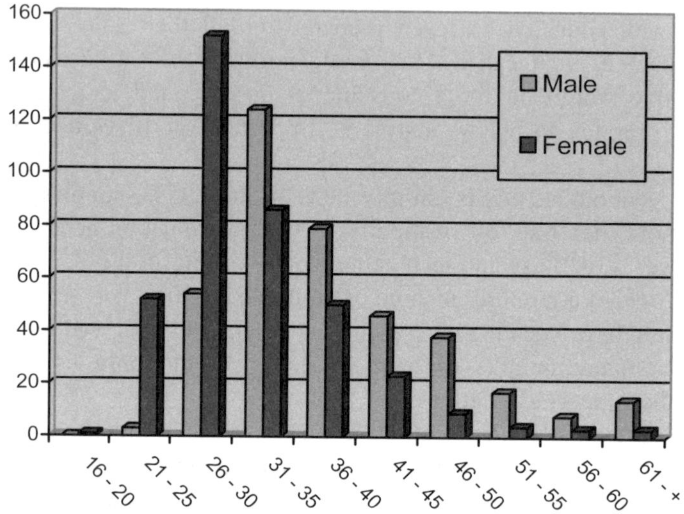

Figure 11.2 Number and age of men and women registering their marriages in Molepolole, 2009 (N = 295)

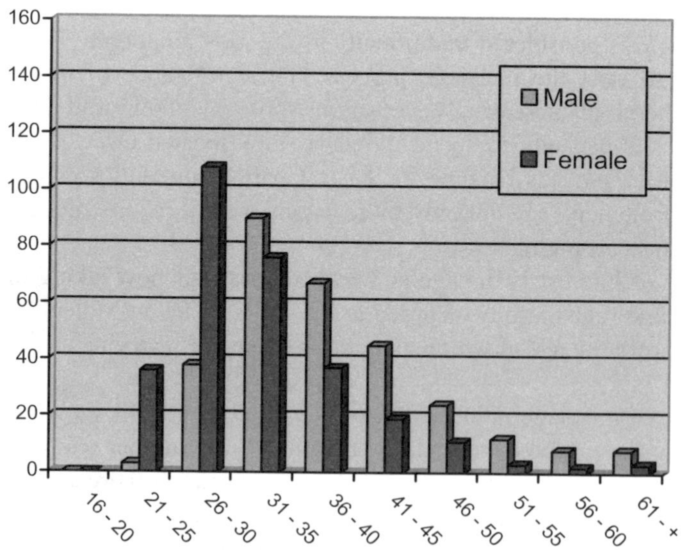

particular had to have the necessary financial resources to pay for the wedding. There is a sense of diminishing support from relatives and an expectation of greater independence on the part of the couple to accumulate the resources necessary. The way the couples in some of the above cases talk of being from poor families also indicates that there is increasingly less expectation that parents or other relatives will help out.

Mobility and ideology

While the previous examples demonstrate the rising costs for marriage and how this is becoming unaffordable for the lower social economic classes, there are a number of other factors that must be taken into account in understanding the significance and the power of the dynamic at play. One is that while the middle classes appear able to spend enormous amounts of money on a wedding, poorer people can no longer keep up with the expense yet feel pressure to try to do so. Marriage is turning into an impoverishing institution. The large bank loans and the high interest rates connected to them are indicative of the real danger that the people getting married will ultimately end up slipping down the social ladder. Marriage may leave them impoverished or deplete their securities.

It is becoming clear that the customary, traditional marriage, in which the *kgotla* plays a crucial part, is no longer considered viable or attractive. The sober and modest form of customary marriage revolves around the payment of a *lobola* and the celebration of the movement of the woman to the groom's parental home, at which point vast quantities of food will be prepared for all the guests. As one of the couples in the above examples put it: 'a wedding without tents and decorations is no wedding. You might as well forget all about it if you can't do that. You will be so embarrassed and your parents will come and talk to you. No, they won't like it at all.'

While customary marriage is at the lower end of the scale of stratification, the Christian, white wedding, and specifically those in the Pentecostal churches, are at the upper end of the scale. Pentecostalism is in a sense the proverbial 'greedy ideology' (Thoden van Velzen & van Beek 1988); i.e. an ideology that seems to place higher and higher demands on its people. Pentecostals promote the commodification of marriage. The white wedding with its expensive dresses and surroundings is the ideal and a sign of the progress and prosperity by which so much of Pentecostalism in Africa is marked (Gifford 2004, 2007; Marshall 1993; Maxwell 1998; Meyer 1999, 2004; van Dijk 2002, 2004). In general, (financial) success is a sign of the benevolence of God and every Pentecostal will do his/her utmost to signal this divine presence. Success and prosperity relate to the notion of progress in the way these marriages are moving away from what is considered 'traditional', and therefore morally and spiritually inferior and backward. Pentecostals in Molepolole do not criticize the *lobola*; on the contrary, some would even say it is Biblical. Yet they still challenge the authority of the elders in the way they demand the presence of traditional healers, the insistence on alcoholic drinks and the customary advice given to the young couple.

An important link between commodification and progress is the Pentecostal promotion of the nuclear household. Couples have to establish nuclear households (where the man is perceived to be the head of the household) as this strengthens the notion that a couple is able to fend for itself; i.e. without the influential presence of the extended family, and defend their interests against traditional obligations *vis-à-vis* the wider family. The ways in which couples therefore stand on their own regarding marriage expenses and bank loans is, from the Pentecostal perspective, a significant element in being or becoming fully independent.

Expenses are not the only issue in becoming a modern, married person: behaviour and moral conduct are of equal importance. An ideal, fully fledged Pentecostal white wedding requires a specific kind of moral conduct before the wedding, which is marked by abstinence and Christian courtship. The ideal in the Pentecostal sense is when the couple has lived according to the principles of Christian courtship in the pre-marital period (other forms of Christianity in Molepolole are more relaxed about this). This means that there will have been complete abstinence of sexual activity and the couples' movements will have been closely monitored. They should only meet when other people are around, should never enter each other's bedrooms, should hardly touch one another to prevent 'temptation' and should display a keen interest in attending abstinence clubs and pre-marital counselling. While the white Christian wedding is centred around church celebrations much more than the festivities at the couple's parental homes, there is no noticeable reduction in cost so one cannot economize by marrying in a Pentecostal fashion. The demands placed on the couple relate to discipline and the pursuit of middle-class bourgeois values. The Pentecostal pastors put forward clear demands about how the marriage and the wedding are to be conducted, and intervene in some of the traditional elements that otherwise would be part of the ritual order of things. They do not reject the payment of *lobola* but condemn the presence of traditional healers for cleansing purposes. Pastors will do the praying (i.e. the spiritual cleansing) and the sanctifying of the places where the wedding is to be conducted.

The most important objection the Pentecostals have is against the preparation and consummation of the *nama ya thsiamo* (the meat of righteousness), which is meat specifically prepared for the couple to eat on the Friday evening before the wedding celebrations. Customarily, the *nama ya thsiamo* is prepared by the *dingaka* and is meant to strengthen and protect the marriage. The couple have to 'take a bite' (*molomo*) of this meat, which is taken from the right side of a slaughtered cow and this will signal consummation of the marriage, which can only broken ritually (following divorce or death). Pentecostal churches are vehemently against such practices as they 'play with the devil'. The only way in which a marriage can be spiritually strengthened and protected is through elaborate prayer and invoking the 'pouring of the blood of Christ'. Another element that will be objected to is the presence of alcoholic beverages: alcohol must not be present at any point during the wedding process.

In general terms, the tying of sexuality to marriage (cf. Bochow 2008), which the Pentecostals forcefully proclaim, makes the attainment of the ideal of this form of white wedding practically impossible for most couples. Children will usually have been born during this or previous relationships, and the age at which marriage takes place means that virginity is unlikely. The effect of Pentecostal demands is however something that one could call a 'middle-classization' of a marriage ideology that goes hand in hand with a process of commodification. In Molepolole, as in the whole of Botswana, upper-middle-class families are becoming members of Pentecostal churches. These are groups in society that can live up to the ideals of progress and prosperity, that can afford the costly styles that Pentecostalism demands, and that can afford some independent distance from the often poorer and more traditional family members. While white weddings are certainly not limited to Pentecostal circles, Pentecostal churches are known to place great emphasis on the public morality of the event. These groups tend to have strict rules of conduct for their teenage children or children in their early twenties and who still live with their parents. In this pursuit of such bourgeois ideals of a virgin wedding and some control over pre-marital relations, they find support in precisely the kind of activities that are promoted by BOCAIP in its fight against AIDS. In a sense, the AIDS pandemic has contributed to the strengthening of these marriage ideals as there are important reasons for controlling sexuality, for abstinence and for promoting faithfulness in marriage. Youth from middle-class families that attend school are part of abstinence clubs, are subjected to the abstinence activities that BOCAIP youth counsellors organize in Molepolole and are members of the youth ministries of the Pentecostal churches. Having a boyfriend or girlfriend is reformulated as a 'problem', likewise the use of condoms. They should only be used 'if one is no longer capable of restraining oneself', as one counsellor explained to me.

Although the Pentecostal churches in Molepolole are well aware of the fact that people are tending to marry later and that their message of pre-marital abstinence is falling on deaf ears, they are holding onto a notion of setting a public agenda of strict behavioural codes that will 'uplift marriage'. In this sense, pre-marital counselling and abstinence are not enough. Marital counselling is, in their view, equally important and the reason why these churches are employing counsellors who have been trained to perform their duties. Specific organizations have been established that concern themselves with the training of marriage counsellors and the writing and publishing of counselling materials and manuals. Some organizations even operate commercially, such as the former Seventh Day Adventist pastor Mpofu's FALIMAC Inc. Having its headquarters in Gaborone's business-park is evidence of the ease with which Pentecostalism relates to processes of commodification. Most of these manuals are written from a Christian perspective, through proclaiming to be neutral, and often have questions for couples to answer such as: 'Are you born-again?'.

There are contradictions in this ideology of tailoring marriage to the demands of the middle classes. One is obviously that whereas the Pentecostal marriage ideology subscribes to and underscores the position of the husband as the head of the household, the faith has been doing little to address the issue of men and fidelity within marriage. While men are generally perceived to be the greater liability when it comes to ensuring faithfulness in marriage, the Pentecostal ideology is doing little to create a more equal power balance between couples to reduce this problem. In traditional counselling practices, brides are usually told never to ask where their husbands have been. In other words, the authority and license of men to deal with there own affairs and their own relations in the way they want are held to be of great importance. While Pentecostal churches feel they should replace this traditional counselling with counselling they feel best fits a Christian relationship, the idea that marital relations can be improved if there is room for greater equality between the sexes is not part of this intervention. Pentecostal Christianity prohibits part of the marriage proceedings and the structures of authority, but other elements are not contested such as the undisputed power relations that favour men.

All in all, the Pentecostal marriage, its practices of premarital/marital counselling and the faith's messages about abstinence and faithfulness create a perspective in which Pentecostalism appears to harbour and signal moral superiority. It looks down on customary and *kgotla* marriages and on marriages that take place in missionary mainline churches because of their lukewarm attitudes to elements of tradition and the use of alcohol. Pentecostalism has presented an agenda for 'uplifting' marriages that are registered under Dutch Roman law with the District Commissioner by adding a neutral form of Christian counselling to this administrative system.

Conclusion: Commodification and romance

The effect of this intertwining of commodification and religion is that a social stratification of different positions of the institution of marriage has occurred, not only in terms of economy but also in ideology. In its consumerist patterns of expense and competition regarding the style of conducting a wedding as well as in the rise of Pentecostal-assumed moral superiority over marriage, Pentecostalism has produced a particular social stratification for the institution of marriage. For the poor, less educated, less affluent, less Pentecostal-inspired, it is harder to conduct a viable and respected marriage. The costs are too high, the burdens too great, the time for preparation too long and the moral constraints too stringent. The result is that not only are couples remaining unmarried but also that the system of authority in society is coming under more pressure than ever before. As long as the older generation maintains the principle that somebody's voice can only be heard in matters relating to the family, its resources or inheritance patterns when one is married and has thus 'become an adult', the new generation will lose out and not be able to stand up for their own interests in the context of the wider family. The contradictory situation is that precisely in a society where it is important that the voice of the younger generation is being heard on matters relating to family life in a context of AIDS, attaining a marital status that allows them to speak is becoming increasingly difficult. While young couples are pursuing expensive, white weddings because of middle-class and romantic ideals, the commodification of marriage that they are involved in, in fact runs counter to their own interests.

The institution of marriage in Botswana, its engulfment in commodification and its increasing embrace by Christianity, and Pentecostalism in particular, can be linked to what Campbell (1987, 2006) has called the 'Romantic Ethic'. Contesting Weber's 'Protestant Ethic', Campbell argues that much of the success of the rise of capitalism was not related to Christianity instilling a Protestant work ethic of labour and production, combined with a moral lifestyle in which saving and family values were deemed important, but that there was a crucial change in patterns of affect, emotions and appetites. In this perspective, life has been increasingly realized by pursuing consumption, which was geared to fulfilling desires and emotions related to aspiring levels of a middle-class lifestyle. In other words, the question is whether in the pursuit of marriage and the ways in which certain (new) emotions and consumptive patterns have become important for a society such as Botswana's, something akin to Campbell's Romantic Ethic can be seen. This involves a language of emotions that informs economic behaviour, such as commodification.

Botswana society has experienced unprecedented economic growth and has become a middle-income-earning society based on its successful, diamond-driven economy. Middle-class aspirations have taken hold, although wealth is still unevenly divided (Good 2006). Enormous expense is put into attempting to meet middle-class styles and aspirations and Pentecostalism appeals to the middle classes due to its high standards of education and income. The neoliberal economy has brought wealth to Botswana and this specific type of Christianity is well-versed in entrepreneurialism and operating in a neo-liberal market, with its leaders being perceived as religious entrepreneurs (van Dijk 2010; Gifford 2004; Werbner 2004).

The interesting point about establishing a link between emotions and a romantic ethic is that it provides a framework of understanding for the significance of commodification at a different level. Commodification becomes a tool, an instrument for the expression of romantic emotions such as love, commitment, fidelity and affection. In other words, commodification is required to emotionalize marriage, or, in Pentecostal jargon; to 'make it deeper'. All the expenses needed to show these emotions of love to one another and the social environment demonstrate this depth. The result of this is that commodification is considered a tool that produces healthy marriages. And a healthy institution of marriage is considered synonymous with a healthy social order.

References

Allen, T. & S. Heald (2004), HIV/AIDS policy in Africa: What has worked in Uganda and what has failed in Botswana?. *Journal of International Development* (16): 1141-1154.

Amanze, J., ed. (2007), *Christian ethics and HIV/AIDS in Africa*. Gaborone: Bay Publishing.

Becker, F. & P.W. Geissler, eds, (2009), *AIDS and Religious Practice in Africa*. Leiden: Brill.

Bochow, A. (2008), Syncretism and antisyncretism in marriage patterns in Kumasi: The role of Pentecostal charismatic churches. In: A. Adogame, M. Echtler & U. Viercke, eds, *Unpacking the new: Critical perspectives on cultural syncretization in Africa and beyond*, pp. 239-266. Hamburg: LIT Verlag.

Bochow, A. (2010), *Intimität und Sexualität vor der Ehe. Gespräche über Ungesagtes in Kumasi und Endwa, Ghana.* Hamburg: LIT Verlag.

Bornstein, E. (2005), *The spirit of development: Protestant NGOs, morality, and economics in Zimbabwe*. Stanford: Stanford University Press.

Burchardt, M. (2009), Subjects of counselling: Religion, HIV/AIDS and the management of everyday life in South Africa. In: F. Becker & W. Geissler, eds, *Aids and religious practice in Africa*, pp. 333-358. Leiden: Brill.

Campbell, C. (1987), *The romantic ethic and the spirit of modern consumerism*. Oxford: Basil Blackwell.

Campbell, C. (2006), 'All you need is love': From romance to romanticism: The Beatles, romantic love and cultural change. *Etnofoor* 19(1): 111-127.

Christiansen, C. (2009a). When AIDS becomes part of the Christian family. Dynamics between kinship and religious networks in Uganda. In: C. Leutloff-Grandits, A. Peliekis & T. Thelen, eds, *Social security in religious networks. Anthropological perspectives on new risks and ambivalences*, pp. 23-42. Oxford: Berghahn.

Christiansen, C. (2009b),The new wives of Christ: Paradoxes and potentials in the remaking of widows' lives in Uganda. In: F. Becker & P.W. Geissler, eds, *AIDS and religious practice in Africa*, pp. 85-116. Leiden: Brill.

Cole, J. & L.M. Thomas, eds (2009), *Love in Africa*. Chicago: University of Chicago Press.

Comaroff, J. & J. Comaroff (1991), *Of revelation and revolution, Vol. 1: Christianity, colonialism and consciousness in South Africa*. Chicago: University of Chicago Press.

Dilger, H. (2007), Healing the wounds of modernity: Salvation, community and care in a Neo-Pentecostal church in Dar es Salaam, Tanzania. *Journal of Religion in Africa* (37): 59-83.

Dilger, H. (2009), African sexualities revisited: The morality of sexuality and gender in the era of globalization and AIDS. In: C. Pope, R.T. White & R. Malow, eds, *HIV/AIDS: Global frontiers in prevention/intervention*, pp. 124-136. London: Routledge.

Dilger, H., M. Burchardt & R. van Dijk, eds, (2010), The redemptive moment: Antiretroviral treatment (ARTs) and the production of new religious spaces in Africa. Special Issue of the *African Journal of AIDS Research* (*AJAR*).

Epstein, H. (2007), *The invisible cure: Africa, the West, and the fight against AIDS*. New York: Farrar, Straus & Giroux.

Gaisie, S.K. (2000), Family structure, gender and fertility in Botswana. *Pula: Botswana Journal of African Studies* 14(2): 130-147.

Geissler, W. & R. Prince (2007a), Christianity, tradition, AIDS and pornography. In: R. Littlewood, ed., *On knowing and not knowing in anthropology*. London: UCL Press.

Geissler, W. & R. Prince (2007b), Life seen: Touch and vision in the making of sex in western Kenya. *Journal of Eastern African Studies* 1(1): 123-149.

Gifford, P. (2004), *Ghana's new Christianity. Pentecostalism in a globalising African economy*. London: Hurst & Co.

Gifford, P. (2007), Expecting miracles: The Prosperity Gospel in Africa. *Christian Century*, July 10.

Green, E.C., D.T. Halperin, V. Nantulya & J.A. Hog (2006), Uganda's HIV prevention success: The role of sexual behavior change and the national response. *AIDS and Behavior* 10(4): 335-346.

Griffits, A. (1997), *In the shadow of marriage. Gender and justice in an African community*. Chicago: Chicago University Press.

Gusman, A. (2009), HIV/AIDS, Pentecostal churches, and the 'Joseph Generation' in Uganda. In: P. Prince, Ph. Denis & R. van Dijk, eds, Christianity and HIV/AIDS in East and Southern Africa. Special Issue of *Africa Today* 56(1): 67-86.

Heald, S. (2006), Abstain or die. The development of HIV/AIDS policy in Botswana. *Journal of Biosocial Science* 38: 29-41.

Hirsch, J.S. *et al.*, eds (forthcoming), *The secret: Love, marriage, and HIV*. Nashville: Vanderbilt University Press.

Hirsch, J.S. & H. Wardlow (2006), *Modern loves. The anthropology of romantic courtship and companionate marriage*. Ann Arbor: University of Michigan Press.

Hope, K.R. (2000), Mobile workers and HIV/AIDS in Botswana. *AIDS Analysis Africa* 10(4): 6-7.

Kuper, A. (1982), *Wives for cattle: Bridewealth and marriage in Southern Africa*. London: Routledge.
Livingston, J. (2009). Suicide, risk and investment in the heart of the African miracle. *Cultural Anthropology* 24(4): 652-680.
Marshall, R. (1993), Power in the name of Jesus, social transformation and Pentecostalism in western Nigeria revisited. In: T. Ranger & O. Vaughan, eds, *Legitimacy and the state in twentieth-century Africa*, pp. 213-246. London: Macmillan.
Maxwell, D. (1998), 'Delivered from the spirit of poverty?': Pentecostalism, prosperity and modernity in Zimbabwe. *Journal of Religion in Africa* 28(3): 350-373.
Meyer, B. (1998), 'Make a complete break with the past'. Time and modernity in Ghanaian Pentecostalist discourse. In: R.P. Werbner, ed., *Memory and the postcolony*, pp. 182-208. London: Zed Books.
Meyer, B. (1999), Commodities and the power of prayer. Pentecostalist attitudes towards consumption in contemporary Ghana. In: B. Meyer & P. Geschiere, eds, *Globalization and identity: Dialectics of flow and closure*, pp. 151-176. Oxford: Blackwell.
Meyer, B. (2004), Christianity in Africa: From African independent to Pentecostal-charismatic churches. *Annual Review of Anthropology* (33): 447-474.
Mokomane, Z. (2005), Cohabitation in Botswana: An alternative or a prelude to marriage? *African Population Studies* 20(1): 19-37.
Mookodi, G. (2004), Male violence against women in Botswana. A discussion of gendered uncertainties in a rapidly changing environment. *African Sociological Review* 8(1): 118-138.
Nkomazana, F. (2007), Christian Ethics and HIV/AIDS in Botswana. In: J. Amanze, ed., *Christian ethics and HIV/AIDS in Africa*, pp. 48-69. Gaborone: Bay Publishing.
Ojo, M.A. (1997), Sexuality, marriage and piety among Charismatics in Nigeria'. *Religion* 27: 65-79.
Parikh, Sh.A. (2007), The political economy of marriage and HIV: The ABC approach, 'safe' infidelity, and managing moral risk in Uganda. *American Journal of Public Health* 97(7): 1198-1208.
Pauli, J. (forthcoming), *Celebrating distinctions. Marriage, elites and reproduction in rural Namibia*. Cologne: Cologne University.
Prince, R., P. Dennis & R. van Dijk (2009), Engaging christianities: Negotiating HIV/AIDS, health, and social relations in East and Southern Africa. Introduction to Special Issue: R. Prince, P. Dennis & R. van Dijk, eds, Christianity and HIV/AIDS in East and Southern Africa. *Africa Today* 56(1): v-xviii.
Schapera, I. (1940), *Married life in an African tribe*. London: Faber & Faber.
Schapera, I. (1950), Kinship and marriage among the Tswana. In: A.R. Radcliff-Brown & D. Forde, eds, *African systems of kinship and marriage*, pp. 140-165. London: Oxford University Press.
Smith, D.J. (2007), 'Modern marriage, men's extramarital sex, and HIV risk in Nigeria. *American Journal of Public Health* 97(6): 997-1005.
Smith, D.J. (2008), Intimacy, infidelity, and masculinity in southeastern Nigeria. In: W. Jankowiak, ed., *Intimacies: Love and sex across cultures*, pp. 224-244. New York: Columbia University Press.

Smith, D.J. (2009), Managing men, marriage and modern loves: Women's perspectives on intimacy and male infidelity in southeastern Nigeria. In: J. Cole & L.M. Thomas, eds, *Love in Africa*, pp. 157-180. Chicago: University of Chicago Press.

Thoden van Velzen, H.U.E. & W. van Beek (1988), Purity, a greedy ideology. In: W. van Beek, ed., *The quest for purity. Dynamics of puritan movements*. Berlin: Mouton de Gruyter.

Togarasei, L. (2010), Life, death and healing in the age of HIV Anti-retroviral therapy: Christian reflections. In: H. Dilger, M. Burchardt & R. van Dijk, eds, *The redemptive moment: Antiretroviral treatment (ARTs) and the production of new religious spaces in Africa*. Special Issue of the *African Journal of AIDS Research* (*AJAR*).

Togarasei, L., M. Haron, K.E. Jensen, S. Mmolai, F. Nkomazana & L. Sebina (2008), *An assessment of the capacity of faith-based organizations for HIV prevention in Botswana*. Gaborone: Associated Printers.

Upton, R.L. (2003), 'Women have no tribe'. Connecting carework, gender, and migration in an era of HIV/AIDS in Botswana. *Gender & Society* 17: 314-322.

van Dijk, R. (1998), Pentecostalism, cultural memory and the State: Contested representations of time in postcolonial Malawi. In: R. Werbner, ed., *Memory and the postcolony: African anthropology and the critique of power*, pp. 155-181. London: Zed Books:

van Dijk, R. (2002), Religion, reciprocity and reconstructing family responsibility in Ghanaian Pentecostal diaspora. In: D.F. Bryceson & U. Vuorela, eds, *The transnational family. New European frontiers and global networks*, pp. 173-196. Oxford: Berg.

van Dijk, R. (2004), Negotiating marriage: Questions of morality and legitimacy in the Ghanaian Pentecostal diaspora. *Journal of Religion in Africa* 34(4): 438-468.

van Dijk, R. (2010), Social catapulting and the spirit of entrepreneurialism. Migrants, private initiative, and the Pentecostal ethic in Botswana. In: G. Huwelmeier & K. Krause, eds, *Travelling spirits. Migrants, markets and mobilities*, pp. 101-117. New York: Routledge.

Werbner, R. (2004), *Reasonable radicals and citizenship in Botswana. The public anthropology of Kalanga elites*. Bloomington: Indiana University Press.

List of authors

Akinyinka Akinyoade is currently the country coordinator for Nigeria for the Tracking Development project at the African Studies Centre in Leiden. He has also done research on the dynamics of reproductive behaviour in rural coastal communities in southern Ghana, and regional comparisons between the socio-economic correlates of fertility references and contraceptive use in Nigeria. His other research interest is higher education and he has investigated access to higher education in Nigeria and the effects of SAPs on tertiary education in Ghana.
aakinyoade@ascleiden.nl

Nadine Beckmann is a researcher and deputy director of the Fertility and Reproduction Studies Group at the University of Oxford. After being awarded her PhD in anthropology at the University of Oxford, she conducted research on the politicization of AIDS activism, biological citizenship and medical governance in Tanzania at the Department of Peace Studies in Bradford, and lectured in international development at the University of Leeds. Her work focuses on the intersections of sexuality, illness and well-being, and the interplay between bio-medicine and alternative forms of addressing illness, particularly in Muslim communities. Her research interests also include notions of morality and uncertainty, and living with HIV/AIDS.
nadine.beckmann@anthro.ox.ac.uk

Christine Böhmig is a nurse and medical anthropologist. She has been working as a tutor at University College Utrecht, the Netherlands since 1999 and also teaches courses in cultural anthropology, medical anthropology and qualitative research methods. In March 2010 she was awarded her PhD at the University of Amsterdam for her research on the work and perceptions of nurses in a Ghanaian academic hospital. Her research interests are hospital ethnography, trans-cultural care, religion and health, African belief systems and qualitative methodologies.
c.bohmig@uu.nl

Marleen Dekker is a development economist and human geographer. Her research is interdisciplinary in nature, combining methods and insights from economics, human geography and sociology. She studies the role of social networks in accessing (informal) insurance, markets and local socio-economic

development. Risk and coping strategies were the focus of her PhD work in Zimbabwe and her post-doc project in Ethiopia, and remain central in her current work on community-based health insurance in Togo and ways of dealing with the economic crisis in Zimbabwe.
mdekker@ascleiden.nl

Dick Foeken is a senior researcher at the African Studies Centre in Leiden where his main research interests are urban poverty, urban agriculture and urban water supply in Africa. He has published extensively in *Geoforum*, *Habitat International*, *Journal of Peasant Studies* and *Political Geography* and his latest books include *"To subsidise my income": Urban farming in an East-African town* (2006) and *Inside poverty and development in Africa: Critical reflections on pro-poor policies* (co-edited, 2008).
dfoeken@ascleiden.nl

Corine 't Hart is a graduate of Leiden University's Research Masters in African Studies (2009), for which she did research on peace education in a Congolese refugee camp in Tanzania. She then conducted a qualitative study on healthcare and solidarity for the ASC/PLAN project on community-based health insurance in Togo. She is currently working for the Society of African Missions in a centre for street girls in Arusha, Tanzania.
corienthart@hotmail.com

Jérémie Gnimadi is a development economist who is managing the programme on health insurance for the NGO Louvain Developpement in Benin and Togo in West Africa. In his previous position, he was responsible for the feasibility and evaluation studies of different mutual health-insurance and food-security programmes for Louvain Developpement in these countries.
jgnimadi@louvaindev.org

Wijnand Klaver is a nutritionist working on food and nutrition security at the African Studies Centre in Leiden and the Centre for Development Innovation at Wageningen University and Research Centre. His specific areas of expertise are the methodology of research, and the planning, monitoring and evaluating of food and nutrition security in rural and urban areas. He carries out household surveys on health, nutrition and urban agriculture in relation to poverty alleviation.
klaver@ascleiden.nl

André Leliveld is an economist at the African Studies Centre in Leiden. Since the late 1980s he has been conducting research on (informal) social-security arrangements in Africa. His ongoing research is on community-based health insurance in Togo and social-security arrangements in rural Uganda. He is also involved in a comparative study of the development trajectories of four African and four Asian countries. Wth Marcel Rutten and Dick Foeken, he co-edited *Inside poverty and development in Africa; Critical reflections on pro-poor policies* (2008).
leliveld@ascleiden.nl

Alice Mboganie Mwangi is a lecutreer in the Department of Food Science, Nutrition and Technology at the University of Nairobi, Kenya where she teaches human nutrition and heads the Unit of Applied Human Nutrition. She has a PhD in human nutrition and biotechnology from Wageningen University, the Netherlands and has published in *Ecology of Food and Nutrition*, *Food and Nutrition Bulletin* and *European Journal of Clinical Nutrition.* She has participated in various national steering committees on food and nutrition issues and is currently a member of the Interim Council implementing the Kenya Nutritionists and Dieticians Bill 2007.
amwangi@uonbi.ac.ke

Kenneth Ombongi was awarded his PhD in African history at the University of Cambridge, UK and is now a lecturer in the Department of History at the University of Nairobi. His research interests and publications focus on how the state has shaped the understanding and utility of bioscience, medicine and public health policy in Africa. He is also interested in the dynamics of development and electoral politics in Africa. He is currently a partner in the MOSQGUIDE project sponsored by the World Health Orgnization on the 'Best practice guidance on the deployment of genetically modified mosquitoes as a disease control measure in the developing countries'.
kombongi@hotmail.com.

Samuel Owuor is a senior lecturer in the Department of Geography and Environmental Studies at the University of Nairobi, Kenya, where he has been teaching urban geography since 1995. He was awarded his PhD in urban geography at the University of Amsterdam and has published in *Geoforum*, *Development Southern Africa*, *Flux* and *Hekima*. He has written a number of chapters in books and *Bridging the urban-rural divide: Multi-spatial livelihoods in Nakuru town, Kenya* (2006).
samowuor@yahoo.com

Bukola Adeyemi Oyeniyi used to be the Acting Head of the Department of History and International Relations at Redeemer's University, Nigeria and is currently working on his PhD at the Institute for History at Leiden University, the Netherlands. His works have appeared in *African Affairs*, *Journal of AIDS Research in Africa* and many other publications, and he is the author of *Mobility and social conflicts in Yorubaland, 1893 to 1983* and *The Ife-Modakeke conflicts*.
b.oyeniyi@hum.leidenuniv.nl

Marcel Rutten is a geographer at the African Studies Centre and Radboud University, Nijmegen. He has been doing longitudinal research on land, water and food security in Africa since the early 1980s and his current research projects are on sustainable water management, combining indigenous and modern technical and institutional knowledge; resource conflicts and (eco)tourism. His main publications include *Selling wealth to buy poverty* (1992), *Out for the count: The 1997 general elections and prospects for democracy in Kenya* (with A. Mazrui & F. Grignon, 2001) and *Inside poverty and development in Africa* (co-edited, 2008).
rutten@ascleiden.nl

Robert Thornton has been Professor of Anthropology at Witwatersrand University, in Johannesburg ince 1992. Prior to this, he lectured in anthropology at the University of Chicago (1977-78), the University of Cape Town (1979-1989) and Rutgers University, US (1990-1992). He specializes in Southern and Eastern Africa, HIV/AIDS, sexuality, ethnography, community development, and medical and political anthropology. He has published over fifty articles in major journals and is the author of three books, the latest being *Unimagined community: Sex, networks and AIDS in Uganda and South Africa* (2008).
Robert.thornton@wits.ac.za;

Wouter van Beek is an anthropologist at the African Studies Centre in Leiden and Professor of Religious Anthropology at the University of Tilburg. He has done extensive research on two West African groups, the Kapsiki/Higi of northern Cameroon and northeastern Nigeria, and the Dogon of central Mali. His main research themes are religion, ecology and tourism (as both his study areas are on the tourist circuit in West Africa). His current research links local religions, such as those of the Kapsiki/Higi and the Dogon, to the wider dynamics of religion in the world.
vanbeek@ascleiden.nl

Rijk van Dijk is an anthropologist at the African Studies Centre in Leiden. He has done extensive research on the rise of Pentecostal movements in urban areas of Malawi and Ghana and his current work focuses on the transnational dimensions of Ghanaian Pentecostalism, particularly in relation to the migration of Ghanaians to the Netherlands and Botswana, and religious engagement with HIV/AIDS in Botswana. He has co-edited *The quest for fruition through Ngoma (*with Ria Reis & Marja Spierenberg, 2000), *Situating globality: African agency in the appropriation of global culture* (with Wim van Binsbergen, 2004) and a thematic issue of *Africa Today (*with Ruth Prince& Philippe Denis) on 'Christianity and HIV/AIDS in East and Southern Africa' (2009).
DijkR@ascleiden.nl

AFRICAN DYNAMICS

ISSN 1568-1777

1. Bruijn, M. de, R. van Dijk and D. Foeken (eds.). *Mobile Africa.* Changing Patterns of Movement in Africa and Beyond. 2001. ISBN 978 90 04 12072 6
2. Abbink, J., M. de Bruijn and K. van Walraven (eds.). *Rethinking Resistance.* Revolt and Violence in African History. 2003. ISBN 978 90 04 12624 4
3. Van Binsbergen, W. and R. van Dijk (eds.). *Situating Globality.* African Agency in the Appropriation of Global Culture. 2004. ISBN 978 90 04 13133 7
4. Abbink, J. and I. van Kessel (eds.). *Vanguard or Vandals.* Youth, Politics and Conflict in Africa. 2005. ISBN 978 90 04 14275 4
5. Konings, P. and D. Foeken (eds.). *Crisis and Creativity.* Exploring the Wealth of the African neighbourhood. 2006. ISBN 978 90 04 15004 8
6. Bruijn, M. de, R. van Dijk, and J-B. Gewald (eds.). *Strength beyond Structure.* Social and Historical Trajectories of Agency in Africa. 2007. ISBN 978 90 04 15696 8
7. Rutten, M., A. Leliveld and D. Foeken (eds.). *Inside Poverty and Development in Africa.* Critical Reflections on Pro-poor Policies. 2008. ISBN 978 90 04 15840 5
8. Ellis, S. and I. van Kessel (eds.). *Movers and Shakers.* Social Movements in Africa. 2009. ISBN 978 90 04 18013 0
9. Dekker, M. and R. van Dijk (eds.). *Markets of Well-being.* Navigating Health and Healing in Africa. 2010. ISBN 978 90 04 20110 1